NYFCH

THE
HANDBOOK
OF
FRACTURES

Neuro Levels ✓

C5 - Deltoid
C6 - Wrist extensors
(ECRL and ECRB)

C7 - Elbow extensors (triceps)
C8 - Finger flexors to middle finger
(FDP)

T1 - Small finger abductor
(Abductor digiti minimi)

L2 - Hip flexors (iliopsoas)
L3 - Knee extensors (quadriceps)
L4 - Ankle dorsiflexors (tibialis anterior)
L5 - Long toe extensors (EHL)
S1 - Ankle plantar flexors
(Gastrocnemius, soleus)

THE HANDBOOK OF FRACTURES

EDITORS

Clayton R. Perry, M.D.
Associate Professor
Department of Orthopaedic Surgery
Washington University School of Medicine
St. Louis, Missouri
Director of the Fracture Service
Barnes Hospital
St. Louis, Missouri

John A. Elstrom, M.D.
Clinical Assistant Professor
University of Illinois
Chicago, Illinois
Chairman, Department of Surgery
Northern Illinois Medical Center
McHenry, Illinois

Arsen M. Pankovich, M.D.
Clinical Professor
Department of Orthopaedic Surgery
New York University Medical Center
New York, New York
Director of Orthopaedic Surgery
New York Hospital Medical Center of Queens
Flushing, New York

McGRAW-HILL, INC.
Health Professions Division

New York St. Louis San Francisco Auckland Bogotá
Caracas Lisbon London Madrid Mexico City Milan
Montreal New Delhi San Juan Singapore
Sydney Tokyo Toronto

34567890   DocDoc   9876

ISBN   0-07-048590-9

This book was set in Times Roman by TCSystems, Inc.
The editors were Jane E. Pennington and Mariapaz Ramos Englis;
the production supervisor was Richard Ruzycka;
the project was managed by Spectrum Publisher Services, Inc.;
the cover designer was José R. Fonfrias;
R. R. Donnelley and Sons was printer and binder.
This book is printed on acid-free paper.

Library of Congress Cataloging-in-Publication Data

The handbook of fractures / editors, Clayton R. Perry, John A. Elstrom, Arsen
   M. Pankovich.
      p.   cm.
   Includes bibliographical references and index.
   ISBN 0-07-048590-9 (alk. paper)
   1. Fractures—Handbooks, manuals, etc.   I. Perry, Clayton.
II. Elstrom, John A.   III. Pankovich, Arsen.
   [DNLM: 1. Fractures—surgery—handbooks.   2. Orthopedics—
methods—handbooks.   WE 39 H238 1994]
RD101.H24   1994
817.1'5—dc20
DNLM/DLC
for Library of Congress   94-29661

This book is dedicated to Monica,
without whose help it would not have been possible,

and to my sons, Clay and Kevin

Contents

Contributors

KEITH H. BRIDWELL, M.D.
Associate Professor
Division of Orthopaedic
  Surgery
Washington University School
  of Medicine
St. Louis, Missouri [14]

C.M. COURT-BROWN, M.D., FRCS Ed. (Orth)
Orthopaedic Trauma Unit
Royal Infirmary of Edinburgh
United Kingdom [20]

KENNETH A. DAVENPORT, M.D.
Attending Surgeon
Marquette General Hospital
Marquette, Michigan [18]

JOHN A. ELSTROM, M.D.
Clinical Assistant Professor
University of Illinois

Chairman
Department of Surgery
Northern Illinois Medical
  Center
McHenry, Illinois [3, 6, 7,
  and 8]

MARK GONZALEZ, M.D.
Associate Professor
Department of Orthopaedic
  Surgery
University of Illinois
Chicago, Illinois

Chief, Section of Hand
  Surgery
Cook County Hospital
Chicago, Illinois [13]

MICHAEL E. JOYCE, M.D.
Assistant in Surgery
Division of Orthopaedic
  Surgery
Washington University School
  of Medicine
St. Louis, Missouri [5]

ENES KANLIC, M.D., M.S., Ph.D.
Instructor
Division of Orthopaedic
  Surgery
Washington University School
  of Medicine
St. Louis, Missouri [17 and
  22]

LAWRENCE G. LENKE, M.D.
Assistant Professor
Division of Orthopaedic
  Surgery
Washington University School
  of Medicine
St. Louis, Missouri [14]

The numbers in brackets show the chapter numbers of each contributor.

CARL H. NIELSEN, M.D.
Assistant Professor
Department of Anesthesia
Washington University School
   of Medicine
St. Louis, Missouri [4]

MICHAEL F. O'BRIEN, M.D.
Fellow
Division of Orthopaedic
   Surgery
Washington University School
   of Medicine
St. Louis, Missouri [14]

**ARSEN M. PANKOVICH,
   M.D.**
Clinical Professor
Department of Orthopaedic
   Surgery
New York University Medical
   Center
New York, New York

Director of Orthopaedic
   Surgery
New York Hospital Medical
   Center of Queens
Flushing, New York [21]

CLAYTON R. PERRY, M.D.
Associate Professor
Department of Orthopaedic
   Surgery
Washington University School
   of Medicine
St. Louis, Missouri [1, 2, 5, 6,
   9, 10, 16, 17, 19, and 22]

DONALD L. PRUITT, M.D.
Assistant Professor
Division of Orthopaedic
   Surgery
Washington University School
   of Medicine
St. Louis, Missouri [11
   and 12]

D. KEVIN SCHEID, M.D.
Associate Professor
Department of Orthopaedic
   Surgery
Indiana University
Indianapolis, Indiana

Orthopaedic Education
   Director
Methodist Hospital Trauma
   Center
Indianapolis, Indiana [15]

**ROBERT C. SCHENCK,
   Jr., M.D.**
Assistant Professor
Department of Orthopaedic
   Surgery
The University of Texas
Health Science Center at San
   Antonio
San Antonio, Texas [19]

Preface

Fracture management is fundamental to orthopaedic practice. In developing this book, we wanted a portable handy reference written for the practicing orthopaedic surgeon. It is not always convenient to refer to the large published tomes for quick management decisions. Our aim has been to create a concise, organized, and readily accessible reference for fracture management. In order to fulfill our objectives, it has been necessary to publish a pocket-size book that can be readily carried.

We have attempted to bring together the basic elements that the reader must know in order to diagnose, classify, and manage specific fractures. Despite the small trim size of the book, we have maximized the use of illustrations to avoid excess use of words in the text and to better present fracture classification and management procedures. We present a balanced overview of fracture management; it is not our intention to discuss some of the more controversial issues that can be read elsewhere. Despite this, the author's philosophy of management may be evident, and we encourage the reader to also review other literature for specific technical procedures. In keeping with this scope, we decided to omit references within the text, but to include a more practical list of reading material entitled ''Selected Readings.''

The organization of this book is simple. Initially, there are general chapters that cover clinical evaluation, methods of fixation, nonoperative techniques, anesthetic techniques, and fracture healing and bone grafting. Thereafter, each chapter specifically examines fractures organized by anatomy, starting with the glenohumeral joint and working down to the foot. For ease of accessibility, we have divided each chapter into identical sections: anatomy, fracture classification, diagnosis and initial management, radiographic examination, and associated injuries. Bolding of key words within the text is designed to help the reader quickly identify relevant material. The glossary at the end of the book defines terms that are not defined within the text itself, thus, it can be used as a quick reference.

This book is a collaborative effort, representing the method of fracture management from a small group of active orthopaedic trauma surgeons. The editors would like to acknowledge the expertise provided by a select group of contributing authors. We hope that we have fulfilled our goal in providing a practical, accessible guide for all persons involved in the care of fracture management.

1 | Clinical Evaluation

Clayton R. Perry

A history and physical examination are obtained from all patients who have sustained a fracture or dislocation. Unlike patients with complex medical problems, the diagnosis of a fracture or dislocation is relatively obvious. The key is not to miss an associated injury.

The elements of a **history** are where, when, and how the injury occurred. A **past medical history** is obtained to determine if there are preexisting conditions that alter the choice of management (e.g., a recent myocardial infarction mitigates for closed management of a fracture, or a prior injury may have compromised function of the extremity). Hand dominance and occupation are documented. A **social history** regarding the use of alcohol, tobacco and drugs is obtained.

A complete **physical examination** of cardiovascular, respiratory, gastrointestinal, genitourinary, and neurologic systems is performed. The examination then focuses on the area of the injury, distal to the injury, and one joint proximal to the injury. The patient is asked to localize his or her pain. The area is inspected for open wounds and deformity, then it is gently palpated to elicit pain and to determine the position of underlying bones and joints. Active and passive range of motion of surrounding joints is determined. The circulatory status is determined by palpating pulses, looking for capillary refill in the nail beds, and assessing the color of the skin (blue, pink, or white). The neurologic system is evaluated by determining whether sensation is intact, and whether voluntary movement and deep tendon reflexes are present.

A specific, detailed pattern of examination of the musculoskeletal, vascular, and neurologic systems of the upper and lower extremities follows.

Upper Extremity, Musculoskeletal System: Flexion of distal interphalangeal joints of the fingers and thumb indicates intact flexor profundus and flexor pollicis longus. Flexion of the proximal interphalangeal joints of an individual finger, while the remaining digits are held in extension, indicates an intact flexor superficialis. Interphalangeal extension indicates intact interossei and extensor hood; metacarpal phalangeal extension—extensor digitorum; wrist dorsiflexion and palmar flexion—flexor carpi radialis, ulnaris and extensor carpi radialis longus, radialis brevis, and ulnaris. Radial or ulnar deviation indicates that the contralateral flexor or extensor is not functioning. Forearm pronation with elbow extended indicates an intact pronator teres; with a flexed elbow, an intact pronator quadratus. Forearm supination indicates an intact supinator or biceps; forearm pronation with elbow flexed—brachialis and biceps;

1

elbow extension— triceps; initiation of glenohumeral abduction and ability to maintain the humerus abducted 60°—rotator cuff; the deltoid, pectoralis major, and trapezius are palpated as they contract. The phalanges, metacarpals, radius, ulna, and humerus are palpated along their lengths. Range of motion of joints is measured by degrees with full extension expressed as 0°. Wrist motion is expressed as degrees of dorsiflexion and palmar flexion with neutral being 0°. Forearm rotation is expressed as degrees of supination and pronation with neutral being 0°. Glenohumeral motion is measured while stabilizing the scapula with one hand to estimate the contribution of scapulathoracic motion. Bringing the elbow forward is glenohumeral flexion; posteriorly is extension.

Upper Extremity Vascular System: Pulses are palpable in the axilla (axillary artery), the antecubital fossae medial to the biceps tendon (brachial artery), and radial to the flexor carpi radialis tendon at the wrist (radial artery). A palpable radial pulse indicates a systolic pressure of at least 80 mmHg. The Allen test indicates an intact ulnar artery. It is performed by compressing the radial and ulnar arteries at the wrist after the patient has made a fist. When pressure is taken off the ulnar artery the hand becomes pink. Capillary refill is assessed by compressing the nail beds and observing the return of oxygenated blood.

Upper Extremity Neurologic System: Sensory function is assessed by determining the ability to differentiate sharp from dull. Intact sensation on the sides of a digit indicates an intact digital nerve. Sensation on the dorsum of the first web space indicates an intact radial nerve. The median nerve is assessed by stimulation of the palmar aspect of the distal index finger; the ulnar nerve at the ulnar aspect of the fifth finger; the musculocutaneous nerve at the dorsum of the forearm; and the axillary nerve in the "policeman's badge" distribution over the deltoid. The **motor component of the neurologic system** is assessed by determining the ability to actively contract a given muscle. Abduction of the fingers indicates an intact ulnar nerve; palmar abduction of the thumb, an intact median nerve; thumb and wrist extension, the radial nerve; deltoid contraction, the axillary nerve. An intact deep tendon reflex indicates that the arc consisting of an efferent nerve from the tendon, the spinal cord at the level of the motor neurons supplying the muscle, and the afferent nerves to the muscle is intact. When peripheral nerves are intact, deep tendon reflexes are the best way to assess nerve root function. Presence of the biceps reflex indicates an intact musculocutaneous nerve and C5 root; brachioradialis and triceps reflexes are indications of radial nerve function and C6 and C7 roots, respectively.

Lower Extremity Musculoskeletal System: Foot eversion indicates intact peroneal longus and brevis. The anterior tibialis dorsiflexes the ankle and is palpable at its insertion on the navicular; ankle plantar flexion indicates an intact triceps surae; knee extension—quadriceps femoris; knee flexion—intact hamstrings; hip extension—gluteus maximus; hip abduction—gluteus medius. The bones of the foot, the tibia, the patella, and the femoral condyles are palpated. Range of motion of the joints is measured. Ankle motion is documented as degrees of dorsiflexion and plantar flexion with neutral being $0°$. Hip motion is measured while stabilizing the pelvis with one hand to minimize lumbosacro and sacroiliac motion. Evaluation of the ankle ligaments is described in Chapter 21. Evaluation of the knee ligaments is described in Chapter 19.

Lower Extremity Vascular System: Pulses are palpable lateral to the base of the first metatarsal (dorsalis pedis), behind the medial malleolus (posterior tibial), and in the popliteal fossae (popliteal artery). Capillary refill is observed in the nail beds.

Lower Extremity Neurologic System: Intact sensation on either side of a digit indicates an intact digital nerve; in the first web space—deep peroneal nerve; lateral side of the foot—sural and superficial peroneal nerves; medial dorsum of the foot—saphenous nerve. **Motor system:** Contraction of the anterior tibial, peronus longus and brevis indicates an intact common peroneal nerve; triceps surae—tibial nerve; quadriceps femoris—femoral nerve; hamstrings—sciatic nerve. Intact deep tendon reflexes of the triceps surae indicate an intact S1 nerve root; patellar tendon—L4 nerve root.

Two extremity injuries bear special mention: open fractures and compartment syndromes. **Open fractures** are graded I to III, with III being the most severe and having the highest incidence of complications (i.e., osteomyelitis and nonunion). **Grade I** open fractures have wounds less than 1 cm in length; **grade II** wounds are more than 1 cm in length, but clean without devitalization of tissue; **grade III** wounds are contaminated, with devitalized tissue, or associated with comminuted fractures and vascular injury. Grade III fractures are further divided into three groups. **IIIA** are without periosteal stripping, or a vascular injury; **IIIB** have periosteal stripping; **IIIC** have an associated vascular or significant nerve injury.

Compartment syndromes are caused by elevated hydrostatic pressure in a closed fascial space or compartment. There are many causes of elevated pressure, including contusion of muscle, a bleed into the compartment, and occlusion of venous outflow from the compartment. As hydrostatic pressure increases, the capillary beds and arterioles collapse, shunting blood through the compartment via larger arteries without supplying the structures within the compartment. This results in more ischemia, increased swelling, and higher pressures. The physical signs of compartment syndrome are increased **pain,** and the extremity involved has normal sensation; **pain with passive stretch** in which very slight, gentle motion elicits severe pain; **paresthesia of nerves** traversing the compartment is most valuable in assessing the anterior compartment of the leg as indicated by decreased sensation in the first web space (deep peroneal nerve); **hard tense compartments,** the most equivocal sign; **elevated pressures** when measured with a manometer, the most objective sign and used to confirm compartment syndrome when the clinical signs are equivocal. Note that the lack of pulse and pallor, signs of arterial occlusion, are not necessarily present. The management of compartment syndrome is surgical release of the involved compartments and delayed primary closure or skin grafting after swelling has subsided. The sequelae of an untreated compartment syndrome can be acute, involving muscle necrosis and myoglobinuria resulting in renal shutdown or chronic, resulting in muscle scarring, contractures, and nerve compression.

INITIAL MANAGEMENT OF PATIENTS WITH MULTIPLE INJURIES

The emergency management of the multiply injured patient is divided into two phases: the initial assessment and management, and the secondary survey and management. When the multiply injured patient presents, the focus is on identifying and managing life-threatening injuries. The first priority is to ensure an **adequate airway.** This is done while an assistant stabilizes the head to prevent flexion or extension of the neck. All multiply injured patients are considered to have a cervical spine injury until proven otherwise. The mouth is opened, inspected, and cleared of loose bodies. The chin is lifted and a nasal airway is inserted. **Inability to secure the upper airway** is indication for an immediate cricothyroidotomy. Uncontrollable hemorrhage in the upper airway, fracture of the larynx, or displaced fractures of the facial bones, particularly the mandible, are the most frequent obstacles to securing the upper airway.

After the airway has been established, the next priority is to ensure that the patient is **breathing.** If not, respiration is assisted with a bag and mask or the patient is intubated. Arterial blood gases are drawn. Dark blood indicates decreased oxygenation. Assuming that the blood is arterial, that the upper airway is secured, and that the patient is ventilating, the cause of decreased oxygenation is usually a pneumothorax, a hemothorax, or a flail chest. The chest is inspected for open wounds and paradoxical motion. An open sucking wound suggests the diagnosis of pneumothorax. Paradoxical motion indicates a flail chest. The neck is inspected to determine if the trachea is deviated; deviation of the trachea indicates a pneumothorax on the side toward which the trachea is deviated. The chest is auscultated, percussed, and gently palpated. Absence of breath sounds and tympany indicate a pneumothorax. Absence of sensation suggests a hemothorax. Crepitus on palpation indicates fractured ribs and a flail chest. Pneumothorax is managed by covering the chest wound to prevent the ingress of air and by inserting a large bore needle in the midclavicular line at the second intercostal space. Flail chest is managed by positive pressure ventilation.

After the upper airway and breathing are secured, the next priority is assessment of **circulation.** Capillary refill and peripheral pulses are an approximate measure of adequacy of circulation. Inadequate circulation indicates shock that is assumed to be due to blood loss. External blood loss is controlled with application of sterile dressings and direct pressure. Fluids and blood products are administered via large bore lines. Initially 2 L of Ringer's lactate is administered while blood is being typed and crossed. In absolute emergencies type O rh negative blood is administered. MAST suits (military antishock trousers) are used to increase peripheral resistance. MAST suits have the added advantage of immobilizing lower extremity fractures and decreasing intrapelvic volume if there is a displaced pelvic fracture.

After the airway has been secured, ventilation is adequate, and fluid resuscitation has started, the **secondary survey and management** begin. The secondary survey is a more detailed physical and radiographic examination of the patient. Procedures performed concurrently at this time may include insertion of chest tubes (in place of an intercostal needle); intubation (oral if there is no cervical spine injury, nasotracheal if there is a cervical spine injury); catheterization of the bladder; and insertion of arterial and central lines. In addition, a detailed history of the injury is obtained from the patient or witnesses to the injury.

The physical examination is performed in an orderly fashion starting at the head and including the neck, eyes, ears, face, nose, mouth, chest, abdomen, rectum, bony pelvis, external genitalia, extremities, and neurologic system. The basic elements of the examination are inspection, auscultation, and palpation. The response to stimuli (e.g., reaction of the pupils to light) is noted, and open wounds are examined.

Open wounds are managed acutely by removal of gross contaminants, obtaining material for anaerobic and aerobic cultures, and administration of broad spectrum antibiotics. Wounds are irrigated and covered with sterile dressings. **Fractures and dislocations** are reduced or aligned and splinted or placed in traction to facilitate transport. MAST suits temporarily immobilize the fractured pelvis.

Fractures and dislocations in the multiply injured patient are not immediately life-threatening. They are definitively managed as soon as life-threatening injuries have been treated and stabilized. **Early stabilization** (within 24 h of injury) of long bone fractures decreases the incidence of adult respiratory distress syndrome (ARDS) and fat embolus. The management of isolated fractures is straightforward. Multiple fractures are stabilized according to the following parameters: **debridement of open wounds** is a primary goal; **early mobilization** of the patient is a primary goal; therefore, stabilization of a tibial fracture is useless unless an associated fracture of the femur is also stabilized. The **surgeon's facility with available techniques** is the primary determinant of the duration and adequacy of the procedure (e.g., external fixation vs. intramedullary nailing vs. plating of a grade III open tibia).

2 | Methods of Fixation

Clayton R. Perry

There are four basic methods used to stabilize fractures: rigidly, with screws and plates; dynamically, with wires or lag screws; with intramedullary nails; and with external fixaters. The distinction among these methods is not always clear. Intramedullary nails and external fixaters allow controlled motion through the fracture and thus could also be considered dynamic fixation. In this chapter each of these basic methods of fracture fixation is further described.

RIGID FIXATION

The Association for the Study of the Problems of Internal Fixation (AO/ASIF group) revolutionized fracture surgery by introducing techniques and implants which rigidly stabilized anatomically reduced fractures. Fixation is so stable that postoperative immobilization is not required, thus speeding rehabilitation and eliminating cast disease. The mobilization aspect of the ASIF methods cannot be overemphasized: immobilizing an extremity in which a fracture has been reduced and stabilized is counterproductive. The primary disadvantages of rigid fixation are that an extended surgical exposure is necessary and consolidation of the fracture by primary bone healing is prolonged. Stable fixation is achieved using interfragmentary screws and plates.

Interfragmentary fixation with screws is performed in such a way that a compression force is exerted across the fracture site. This is done by "lagging" the fragments together. This technique involves traversing the reduced fracture with a screw. One fragment is fixed with the screw threads; the second fragment lies under the head of the screw. Screw threads are functionally absent in the second fragment, either because the diameter of the hole equals the diameter of the screw threads, or because the portion of the screw in this fragment is smooth. As the screw is rotated, it advances, and the head of the screw moves the second fragment toward the first, applying compression across the fracture (Fig. 2–1).

Plates function in one of four ways: to neutralize forces across the fracture, to apply compression across the fracture, to act as a buttress, or to act as a tension band.

A **neutralization** plate isolates the fracture from extrinsic forces. It is applied after the fracture fragments have been lagged together. The plate is fastened to the bone without applying compression across the fracture site. An example of a neutralization plate is a one-third tubular plate used to stabilize a lateral malleolar fracture that has been lagged together with an interfragmental screw.

7

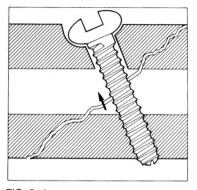

FIG. 2–1   Lag-screw technique.

A **compression** plate applies a compressive force across the fracture. It can be used to stabilize only simple fractures because compression across a comminuted fracture results in shortening. The most frequently used method of applying compression is to fasten the plate to one fracture fragment and then insert screws that are eccentrically located in the holes of the plate. Tightening the screws moves the plate, thus compressing the fracture. An example of a compression plate is a dynamic compression plate used to stabilize a transverse diaphyseal fracture of the ulna.

A **buttress** plate functions as a buttress. That is, it prevents a fragment of bone from moving centrifugally. It also prevents shortening. The plate does not necessarily have to be fixed to the fragment to function as a buttress. One example of a buttress plate is a T plate stabilizing a split-depressed fracture of the lateral tibial plateau.

A **tension band** plate is always applied to the tension side of the bone. It cannot be used on comminuted fractures. As the bone is axially loaded, the tension band plate prevents angulation at the fracture site. Directly under the plate there are distraction forces across the fracture and the plate is loaded in tension. The side of the fracture opposite the plate is loaded in compression. An example of a tension band plate is a dynamic compression plate applied to the lateral cortex of the femur to stabilize a transverse diaphyseal fracture.

DYNAMIC FIXATION

Dynamic fixation allows controlled motion between fragments after they have been stabilized. The disadvantage of dynamic fixation is that we occasionally underestimate or overestimate the amount of controlled motion that will occur. Underestimation leads to a fracture which is stabilized with its fragments distracted. Overestimation leads to uncontrolled collapse of a fracture and loss of reduction. The three techniques by which dynamic fixation is achieved are: tension band wires, the sliding compression screw, and cerclage wires.

Tension band wires function similarly to tension band plates. They are always applied to the tension side of the bone. As the bone is loaded, distraction forces occur across the fracture directly under the wire and compression forces occur across the fracture through the opposite cortex. This method of stabilization can be used only for simple transverse fractures. If interfragmentary fixation is used to align the fracture prior to insertion of the tension band wire, it must allow for axial motion. If screws are used, the threads do not cross the fracture site; and if Kirschner wires are employed, they are inserted parallel to each other. Tension band wires are used most frequently to stabilize fractures of the olecranon and patella.

Sliding compression screws are used to stabilize fractures around the hip. They allow controlled shortening of the fracture to a more stable position. Sliding compression screws are inserted parallel to the long axis of the femoral neck. They are either inserted directly through the lateral cortex (i.e., for a femoral neck fracture), or are attached to a side plate on the lateral cortex of the femur (i.e., for an intertrochanteric fracture). Postoperatively, when the patient bears weight, the screws slide through the lateral cortex of the femur or through the side plate and the fracture impacts until bone-to-bone contact across the fracture site prevents further shortening. For these devices to function effectively, it is important to remember that when multiple screws are used they must be parallel; when adjunctive fixation is used, it must allow shortening (e.g., cerclage wires); and the potential length that the fracture can shorten must not exceed the length that the device can shorten.

Cerclage wires are always used with other methods of fixation because they will not adequately stabilize a fracture when used alone. It is essential that as the fracture shortens or displaces, the cerclage wire tightens. These wires are an effective method of adjunctive fixation for intertrochanteric, subtrochanteric, and diaphyseal fractures of the femur, but not for supracondylar fractures of the distal femur in which the fragments ''telescope'' together (Figs. 2–2 and 2–3).

INTRAMEDULLARY NAILS

The advent of intramedullary nails revolutionized the management of diaphyseal fractures of the femur and tibia. Today there are intramedullary nails designed to stabilize fractures of all long bones. They are usually inserted closed (i.e., without opening the fracture site, using fluoroscopic guidance). The advantages of intramedullary nailing are a low incidence of implant failure due to the fact that they are load

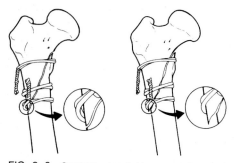

FIG. 2-2 Cerclage wires tighten, preventing shortening of a subtro-chanteric fracture.

sharing versus load bearing, minimal soft tissue irritation due to their intramedullary location; a low incidence of infection because they are inserted without opening the fracture, and rapid healing by external callus. The disadvantages of intramedullary nailing are the difficulty of the technique, frequent insertion site symptoms, and the limitation of intramedullary nailing to diaphyseal fractures.

There are three parameters used to describe intramedullary nails: rigid or flexible, reamed or nonreamed, and dynamic or static. The majority of intramedullary nails are **rigid.** One rigid nail is used to stabilize a fracture. On cross section, most rigid nails are hollow. Some are slotted along their length, whereas others are "closed sectioned." Rigid nails are designed to approximate the shape of the bone that they are used to stabilize (e.g., femoral nails have an anterolateral bow which approximates that of the intact femur). They are inserted through a single insertion portal. For the femur, the portal is in the piriformis

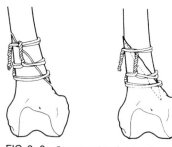

FIG. 2-3 Supracondylar fracture fragments "telescope"; therefore, cerclage wires do not prevent shortening.

fossa, between the base of the femoral neck and the greater trochanter. For the tibia, the portal is posterior to the patellar tendon. The Grosse-Kempf femoral nail is an example of a rigid nail.

Flexible intramedullary nails are distinct from rigid intramedullary nails in that more than one is used to stabilize a fracture; usually more than one insertion portal is used; they are smaller in cross section; and all flexible nails are solid. Flexible intramedullary nails control rotation through the fracture when more than one insertion portal is used and the tips are flared in the metaphysis. The major disadvantage of flexible intramedullary nails is that they cannot be statically locked, thus they are indicated only for axially stable fractures. Examples of flexible intramedullary nails are Rush rods and Ender nails.

Reaming denotes sequential enlargement of the medullary canal with flexible drills. Enlarging the medullary canal allows a larger intramedullary nail to be used. Because the strength of the nail increases in proportion to the cube of its radius larger nails minimize implant failure. In the management of nonunions, reaming reinjures the bone, theoretically stimulating the healing process to begin again. The primary disadvantage of reaming is that it is a tedious process. Reaming destroys the endosteal circulation. This may be important in open fractures in which there has been periosteal stripping, and in fractures which have been previously managed with plates and screws. In both instances reaming may destroy the only remaining blood supply to the bone and result in segmental devascularization. Most rigid nails are reamed.

Dynamic nails are not fastened to the bone. They act as intramedullary splints, aligning the fracture. A **static nail** is "locked," or attached to the bone proximal and distal to the fracture, usually with screws that perforate the cortex and then go through the nail. Placement of locking screws can be difficult and is either done freehand with fluoroscopic guidance, or with the aid of guides that are fastened to the driving end of the nail. Locked nails are either statically locked or dynamically locked. Static locking prevents shortening and rotation through the fracture site. However, it also prevents impaction at the fracture site and converts the nail into a load-bearing device. Therefore, there is a high incidence of implant failure. Static locking extends the indications for intramedullary nails to fractures that are rotationally or axially unstable.

Dynamically locked nails are attached to the bone on only one side of the fracture. This increases the stability of fixation of the locked fragment. At the same time, the disadvantages of preventing impaction and of converting the nail into a load-bearing device are avoided.

The **reconstruction nail** is a specific type of locked nail used for proximal femur fractures. It is characterized by the proximal locking screw or screws being inserted up the femoral neck into the femoral head. Reconstruction nails can be locked distally, making them statically locked.

EXTERNAL FIXATION

External fixation is accomplished by driving pins through the bone proximal and distal to the fracture site. The pins are then fastened rigidly together with clamps and rods. These clamps and rods are known as the "external frame." The ideal external frame is simple, rigid, and allows access to open wounds. The theoretic advantages of external fixation are that the construct is relatively stable, therefore loss of reduction will not occur and the risk of infection is minimized because minimal surgical exposure is necessary and an implant is not left in the wound. The practical advantage of external fixation is that it can be applied quickly. This is particularly important in unstable multiple trauma patients and in the management of hemodynamically unstable patients with Malgaigne or "open book" pelvic fractures. The practical disadvantages of external fixation are that the pin sites become infected and there is a high incidence of nonunion following its use for certain types of fractures (e.g., fractures of the tibial diaphysis). There are three basic types of external fixaters: uniplanar frames, multiplanar frames, and small wire circular frames. **Uniplanar frames** are simple frames used to manage diaphyseal fractures. They are applied quickly and do not obstruct access to the underlying extremity.

Multiplanar frames are more rigid, more difficult to apply, and obstruct access to the extremity. However, they can be used for a greater variety of fractures than the simple unilateral frame (e.g., metaphyseal fractures).

Small wire circular frames use wires which are tensioned instead of larger diameter pins to hold the bone to the external frame. The wires are driven through the bone, fastened to one side of the ring, then tensioned and fastened to the other side of the ring. The advantage of small wire circular fixaters is that they can be used to stabilize intraarticular fractures. The disadvantages are that they are less stable than conventional fixaters, they obstruct access to the extremity, and they are technically difficult to apply.

External fixaters are increasingly important in the management of the posttraumatic complications of malunion and nonunion. The external frame is made in such a way that it can be manipulated to gradually lengthen or shorten the bone through the nonunion and to correct angular deformity. In the most specialized example of this technique, an "internal lengthening" can be performed to fill in segmental defects of long bones.

SELECTED READINGS

Browner BD, Edwards CC: The Science and Practice of Intramedullary Nailing. Philadelphia, Lee & Febiger, 1987.

Maiocchi A, Bianchi M, Aronson J: Operative Principles of Ilizarov. Baltimore, Williams & Wilkins, 1991.

Muller ME: AO Manual of Internal Fixation, 3d ed. New York, Springer-Verlag, 1991.

3 | Nonoperative Techniques

John A. Elstrom

The nonoperative techniques covered in this chapter are splints and casts, traction, and arthrocentesis.

SPLINTS AND CASTS

Splints and casts immobilize and support the injured extremity and thereby reduce pain, prevent injury of structures in the proximity of a fracture, and maintain alignment after reduction. Splinting and casting are also used postoperatively to provide additional stabilization when fixation is tenuous, or to maintain surrounding joints in a position of function (e.g., following open reduction of an ankle fracture to prevent equinus deformity). Splinting and casting are accomplished with plaster or synthetic materials such as Fiberglas. Splints differ from casts in that splints are not circumferential and, therefore, allow swelling of the extremity without a significant increase in pressure within the splint. Casts are circumferential and swelling within the cast increases pressure, potentially resulting in a compartment syndrome. Casts tend to immobilize an extremity more completely than a splint.

Many of the **fundamental rules of splinting and casting** are identical. Ideally, at least one joint proximal and one joint distal to the injury are immobilized. Prior to immobilization, fractures are reduced and, if possible, the extremity is placed in a position of function (e.g., the hand is immobilized with the metacarpophalangeal joints at 90° and the interphalangeal joints at 0°). The extremity is padded to prevent pressure sores and neurovascular compression. Incisions or wounds are covered with a sterile dressing. A layer of stockinette is followed with cast padding appropriate to the type of material being used. Bony prominences (e.g., the posterior aspect of the heel and malleoli) and areas where nerves pass over bone (e.g., the medial elbow and the fibular neck) are protected with extra padding, foam, or felt. The splint or cast material is moistened with cold or room temperature water to give a prolonged setting time and decrease the heat of reaction which could burn the skin as the material sets. This is especially important if the patient is anesthetized and cannot complain of pain. Fingertip indentation is avoided as it will result in pressure necrosis of the skin. Splints and casts covering damaged skin or surgical wounds should not be allowed to get wet.

The following **techniques of cast application** are used with plaster or synthetic materials. Fatigue prevents the patient from holding the **upper extremity** in the desired position during cast application. If an assistant is not available, a short or long arm cast is applied by using fingertrap traction to the index and long fingers with counter traction over the flexed elbow. The material is rolled on and carefully molded to prevent the cast from slipping or the fracture from displacing. **Short arm casts** are applied far enough proximally and with appropriate three-point molding to create an oval cross section to prevent them from sliding down the forearm like a glove. To prevent forearm rotation, the cast is extended above the elbow. To prevent elbow flexion and extension, the cast is extended to the proximal arm.

Casts are applied to the **lower extremity** with the patient sitting and the foot supported by a bolster or an assistant. The ankle is positioned in neutral to prevent equinus contracture. Because the limb varies in diameter, the padding is torn on the side of the larger diameter (i.e., proximal part of the padding) to conform the padding material to the limb. The padding is overlapped 50 percent. The cast material is then applied from the metatarsal heads to the upper limit of the cast. Short leg casts extend to the tibial tubercle. Patellar tendon-bearing casts are molded over the patellar tendon and patella, but allow knee flexion. Long casts extend to the groin. Tucks in the cast material are taken on the side of the smaller limb diameter again to conform the material to the limb. Longitudinal splints (i.e., a posterior splint at the ankle and medial and lateral splints at the knee) provide additional support. Molding of the cast material along the medial aspect of the tibia and over the lateral malleolus increases stability. The cast is trimmed by removing excess material with scissors or a cast saw, pulling the stockinette over the edge of the cast and wrapping it with additional cast material. Trimming of the cast should allow toe flexion and avoid pressure against the fifth toe. To prevent the cast from slipping on wood and linoleum floors, a cast shoe or rubber walking heel is applied. The rubber walking heel is advantageous when a limited axis of loading of the lower extremity is desired (e.g., to avoid force transmission through fractured metatarsals). The rubber heel is placed proximal to the fracture.

The **technique of splinting** usually involves the use of a casting material which hardens after it is applied. However, there are other types of splints which are preformed. These preformed splints are used at the accident site (e.g., aluminum universal arm and leg splints, ladder splints, and inflatable splints) and seldom are left in place after the initial evaluation is completed. Preformed splints used for definitive management are the cervical collar, figure of eight splint, and knee immobilizer.

The **upper extremity** is splinted while the arm is in fingertrap traction or held by an assistant. Plaster or synthetic material 4 to 5 in. wide and 5 to 10 thicknesses is used. When plaster is used, the splint is conformed to the extremity with a gauze wrap and an Ace bandage. The material is applied from the metacarpal heads to the proximal extent of the splint. A short arm splint is applied to the volar surface of the forearm and extends to the olecranon. The sugar tongs splint starts on the volar surface of the hand and forearm and wraps around the elbow ending on the dorsal surface of the hand. The thumb spica splint extends from the tip of the thumb along the radial aspect of the forearm to just below the flexion crease of the elbow. The radial styloid is padded to prevent injury to the superficial branch of the radial nerve.

The **lower extremity** is splinted with the patient sitting and the ankle in neutral. The ankle is splinted with a sugar tongs splint. The splint extends down the medial aspect of the leg under the foot and then back up the lateral aspect of the leg. When a posterior splint is applied it must be thicker than the sugar tongs splint, and additional splints are used medially or laterally to provide additional support. To prevent thermal injury, cold water is used and excessively thick splints and heavy wrapping are avoided.

Complications of splinting and casting include pressure sores, burns, and skin irritation. **Pressure sores** occur when sensation is reduced (e.g., diabetic peripheral neuropathy); decreased sensation is a major concern when splinting and casting. To minimize the incidence of skin breakdown, bony prominences are padded and the splint or cast is changed frequently. Pain underneath a splint or cast is a complaint that is taken seriously and managed by windowing of the cast over the involved area, or cast removal and inspection of the skin.

Burns following the application of a splint or cast occur most commonly when plaster is used and the material is excessively thick. To minimize the incidence of burns, cold water and adequate padding are essential.

Skin irritation beneath the splint or cast can often be controlled with the use of mild analgesics, such as aspirin, and the use of a hair dryer set on room temperature to blow cool air underneath the cast. Powders and ointments should not be applied to the skin under the cast in hopes of drying or lubricating the skin.

TRACTION

Traction is used temporarily to splint or definitively manage fractures. Traction is applied through the skin (skin traction), or via a pin inserted into a long bone (skeletal traction).

The disadvantage of **skin traction** is that it can result in skin breakdown. The danger of skin breakdown limits the length of time it can be utilized (48 h) and the amount of weight applied (10 lb). The advantage of skin traction is that it does not require insertion of a pin. Skin traction is applied via adhesive strips applied to the skin, or more frequently, via "Buck's" boot. Buck's traction is used to temporarily splint hip fractures prior to surgery. It employs a prefabricated soft synthetic boot held in place with Velcro straps through which 5 to 7 lb of weight is applied. A pillow is placed beneath the knee slightly flexing it. The most common error is that the patient slides down in bed and the weights rest on the ground or the boot lies against the end of the bed. A push box between the end of the bed and the opposite foot prevents the patient from sliding down in bed.

Skeletal traction is used most frequently to temporarily manage acetabular and femoral fractures, and occasionally fractures of the distal humerus and distal tibia. More weight can be applied for a longer period of time via skeletal traction than via skin traction.

Basic **rules of skeletal traction** are as follows: skeletal traction is contraindicated when there is damage to the ligaments of the joint proximal to the pin site; radiographs in traction are obtained immediately after application, then, as required for adjustments, and weekly; and the neurologic and vascular status of the extremity is examined daily.

The **technique of pin insertion** is described as follows: the area is shaved and scrubbed prior to pin insertion; local infiltration anesthesia (taking care to infiltrate the periosteum and skin on both sides) and parenteral sedation are used; pins are inserted from the side most vulnerable to neurovascular damage so that the point is accurately applied to the bone (e.g., medial to lateral in the distal femur and the calcaneus and ulnar to radial in the proximal ulna); the skin is incised with a No. 11 blade; the pin is drilled by hand through the bone; the skin on the opposite side is incised as it is tented by the point of the pin; and stability of the pin is evaluated by pushing proximally and distally on one end of the pin to see if the bone moves with the pin—the "toggle test."

Pin selection is based on the following considerations: threads prevent the pin from loosening and sliding in the bone; threaded pins must be larger caliber than smooth pins because the threads weaken the pin; smooth pins that are threaded in their midportions are especially useful; and threaded pins are not used when the pin will pass near a neurovascular bundle (e.g., through-and-through olecranon pin), for fear of the soft tissues being wrapped around the pin and causing a neurovascular injury. **Traction maintenance** is: support of the part distal to the pin; twice-daily cleaning of the pin sites with sterile saline or peroxide, sterile dressings, and release of skin under tension to prevent necrosis.

For **acetabular and femoral fractures,** the pin is inserted through the distal femur at the flare of the condyles, or through the proximal tibia 2 cm posterior and 1 cm inferior to the tibial tubercle. As longitudinal traction is applied via the pin, the leg is supported with slings (Fig. 3–1) or in a frame. The frame used most frequently is the Thomas ring with a Pierson attachment. The Pierson attachment is an outrigger which slides up and down the Thomas frame to compensate for the length of the femur and allows knee flexion (Fig. 3–2). Depending on the size of the patient, between 15 and 30 lb of longitudinal traction is appropriate initially.

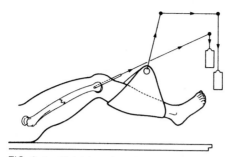

FIG. 3-1 Skeletal traction using a sling to support the calf.

The safest type of **olecranon** pin is a screw with an eyelet, inserted at 90° to the long axis of the ulna. A through-and-through pin can be used, but the ulnar nerve must be protected. Olecranon traction is supplemented with skin traction to support the hand and forearm. Five to 10 lb of longitudinal traction is applied initially. The **calcaneal** pin is inserted 2 cm distal and 2 cm posterior to the medial malleolus. The leg is supported on a frame and weight of 5 to 10 lb is applied initially.

ARTHROCENTESIS

Arthrocentesis, or aspiration, of a swollen painful joint is both therapeutic and diagnostic. Strict adherence to aseptic techniques is essential:

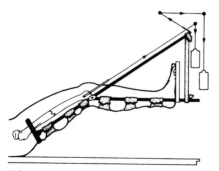

FIG. 3-2 Skeletal traction using a Thomas splint and Pierson attachment.

the area through which the joint is aspirated is shaved and scrubbed, and sterile gloves are used. Local infiltration anesthesia is optional. Large joints are aspirated with a 19-gauge needle. Smaller joints of the fingers and toes are aspirated with a 22-gauge needle, but the smaller diameter makes obtaining fluid difficult. The larger the syringe, the more negative pressure is generated which tends to draw obstructive particles into the needle opening.

The **contraindications** to arthrocentesis are periarticular sepsis and uncorrected coagulopathy. Tubes for synovial fluid cell count, microscopic examination, and culture should be available in the event that an effusion suggestive of an acute inflammatory arthritis is found.

The **knee** is aspirated with the patient supine and the joint extended. The needle is directed posterior to the quadriceps tendon at the superior pole of the patella.

The **ankle** is aspirated via the interval between the extensor hallucis longus tendon and the medial malleolus, or just proximal and medial to the tip of the lateral malleolus and below the level of the joint line.

Aspiration of the **hip** is done with the aid of fluoroscopy. The patient is supine and the hip is extended. A spinal needle is inserted lateral to the femoral artery and 2 cm distal to the inguinal ligament. It is directed toward the inferior aspect of the femoral head and neck. The resistance of the hip capsule is apparent as the needle enters the joint.

Shoulder aspiration is performed with the patient sitting and the humerus in neutral or slight external rotation. Unless the patient is unusually large, a 1.5-in. needle is used. The needle is inserted lateral to the coracoid process and below the acromioclavicular joint. It is directed posteriorly into the interval just medial to the biceps tendon and near the junction of the supraspinatous and subscapularis tendons.

The **elbow** is aspirated with the patient sitting and the elbow in 80° of flexion. A tense hemarthrosis can often be palpated in the interval between the lateral epicondyle, radial head, and olecranon. The needle is passed medially through the center of this triangular area.

4 | Anesthetic Techniques

Carl H. Nielsen

Physicians without specialty training in anesthesiology can safely employ the following techniques of sedation and regional anesthesia for short surgical procedures, provided that a few basic rules are followed. Drugs are never administered to a patient without a plan for establishing an airway, administration of oxygen, and immediate management of an overdose or unwanted side effect of the administered drug. Also, the following techniques are to be used only on healthy, nonpregnant patients without allergy to the drugs.

SEDATION

Midazolam (Versed) has a wide margin of safety, but may cause respiratory depression and/or overdose with rapid injection. Dosage is reduced for geriatric patients. Midazolam is administered intravenously as a single 0.03 mg/kg dose. The dose may be repeated after 5 min if the patient needs additional sedation. Midazolam has no analgesic properties, but mental function may be impaired for hours after administration.

ANALGESIA

Opioids rarely provide complete analgesia for even minor procedures, but used as adjuncts to sedation and/or regional anesthesia, they add to patient comfort. All opioids are potent dose-dependent respiratory depressants. Avoid intramuscular (IM) injection because duration of onset is slow and variable. Use morphine, 2.5 mg; meperidine, 25 mg; or fentanyl, 50 μg. One of these is administered through an IV. The dose may be repeated for a total of 10 mg of morphine, 100 mg of meperidine, or 100 μg of fentanyl.

REGIONAL ANESTHESIA

Infiltration techniques inhibit excitation of sensory nerve endings and provide sensory anesthesia. Intravenous regional anesthesia (IVR) is usually classified as an infiltration block, although the exact mechanism of action is unclear. Peripheral nerve blocks involve reversible blockade of nerve action potentials along all types of nerve fibers and are called conduction anesthesia.

Bier Block

Bier block, or IVR, is a suitable technique for operative procedures on the hand and forearm with a duration of less than 1 h. The technique may also be used for foot and lower leg anesthesia, but the quality of anesthesia is not as good as for the upper extremity. The following diseases of the limb are contraindications for the use of IVR: infection, malignant tumor, and vascular insufficiency.

A 20- or 22-gauge canula is placed and secured in a vein distal to the limb to be anesthetized. A tourniquet is placed as proximal to the limb as possible. For longer-lasting procedures, two tourniquets or a double tourniquet must be used. The limb below the tourniquet(s) is exsanguinated by compression. The tourniquet(s) is inflated to a pressure 100 mmHg above the systolic blood pressure. The source of the pressure must be calibrated and must maintain the desired preset pressure. A regular cuff, sphygmomanometer, and bulb with release valve are inadequate as a tourniquet for IVR. Immediately after exsanguination, a single dose of 50 ml of 0.5% (250 mg) lidocaine (Xylocaine) is injected in the indwelling canula. Complete IVR of the leg requires about

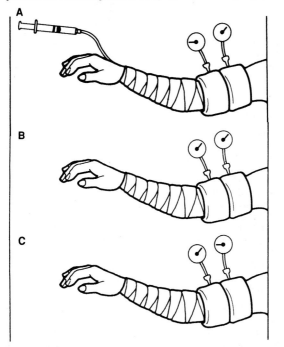

FIG. 4–1   Bier block. (*a*) The distal tourniquet is deflated and anesthetic is injected. If there is tourniquet pain, the distal tourniquet is inflated (*b*), and the proximal tourniquet is deflated (*c*).

75 ml of local anesthetic. Use lidocaine only from a sealed single dose vial without epinephrine. The canula may be removed after the injection. Satisfactory anesthesia is obtained in 10 min. When two tourniquets are used, the distal is now deflated. If the patient complains about the tourniquet pain before completion of the operation, the distal cuff is inflated, and about 20 s later the proximal cuff is deflated (Fig. 4–1). At completion of the operation, the tourniquet is deflated. This is not to be done until at least 15 min have elapsed postinjection. Early release of the tourniquet may bring about a systemic reaction to the lidocaine.

Nerve Block

The following nerve blocks are all performed with 1 to 1.5% lidocaine, 1 to 1.5% mepivacaine (Carbocaine), or 0.5% bupivacaine (Marcaine). Distal blocks (i.e., fingers and toes, wrists and ankles) are never performed with epinephrine because of the risk of prolonged vasospasms. When epinephrine is used for prolongation of peripheral nerve blocks, the optimal concentration is $1:200,000$, which is equivalent to 5 μg epinephrine per ml of local anesthetic. When small amounts of local anesthetics are injected, multiple dose vials are appropriate. When larger amounts of local anesthetics are injected, the single dose vial is used. The difference is that single dose vials contain no preservatives, whereas multiple dose vials do.

Digital Nerve Block

Each finger and toe is innervated by four nerves; two are palmar/plantar and two are dorsal. Block of these four nerves provides adequate anesthesia for minor operations. The injection may be performed at the base of the digit, but an injection about 1 cm further proximal is less painful. Despite anesthesia of half of the two digits next to the anesthetized digit, it is the preferred method (Fig. 4–2).

A 23-gauge 1-in. needle is advanced from the dorsal side to the palmar/plantar fascia so that just the needle tip can be palpated. It is retracted 2 mm, and 3 ml of local anesthetic is injected. The needle is now retracted so that the tip is just below the subcutaneous tissue and another 2 ml is injected. The procedure is repeated on the other side of the digit.

Wrist Block

Blocks of one, two, or all three nerves at the wrist will provide adequate anesthesia of the part of the hand innervated by the blocked nerve(s).

The **median nerve** runs in the wrist between the palmaris longus and flexor carpiradialis tendons. It is blocked approximately 2 cm proximal to the proximal wrist crease. With the hand slightly dorsiflexed, a 23-gauge 1-in. needle is advanced perpendicular to the skin between

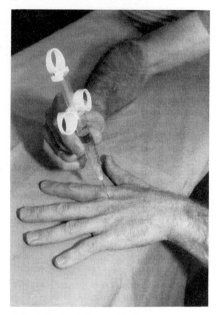

FIG. 4–2   Digital nerve block.

these two tendons, and the area is infiltrated with 5 to 8 ml of local anesthetic (Fig. 4–3). If there is paresthesia, the needle is stopped and the entire volume is injected. If there is no paresthesia, the local anesthetic is deposited with a fan-wise injection. This block is not used in patients with carpal tunnel syndrome and is not performed distally at the level of the carpal tunnel.

The **ulnar nerve** is blocked approximately 6 cm proximal to the proximal wrist crease, to the radial side of the tendon of the flexor carpiulnaris. The nerve is on the ulnar side of the ulnar artery. A 23-gauge 1-in. needle is inserted perpendicular to the skin and 8 to 10 ml of local anesthetic is injected. If the block is performed less than 6 cm proximal to the wrist, it will not include the dorsal branch of the ulnar nerve. A block of this branch must be performed with a subcutaneous ring of anesthesia around the ulnar aspect of the wrist, starting from the flexor carpiulnaris tendon. Five ml of local anesthetic is used for this block.

The **radial nerve** is blocked with infiltration under the brachioradialis tendon 8 cm proximal to the proximal wrist crease. Alternatively, the

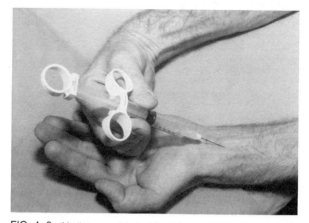

FIG. 4-3 Median nerve block at the wrist.

radial nerve is blocked with a subcutaneous ring of anesthesia. The ring starts at the radial aspect of the wrist at the flexor carpiradialis and continues around the wrist dorsally to the styloid process of the ulna. Either of the two methods requires approximately 5 to 8 ml of local anesthetic.

Elbow block

The **ulnar nerve** is blocked 3 cm proximal to its course in the groove behind the medial epicondyle. A 23-gauge 1-in. needle is advanced at a 45° angle to the course of the nerve either pointed distally or proximally. Five to eight ml of local anesthetic is injected around the nerve.

The **median nerve** lies on a line drawn on the anterior elbow between the two epicondyles on the medial side of the brachial artery and is easily palpated in thin individuals. The block is performed at this level with a 23-gauge 1-in. needle. When paresthesia is encountered, 5 to 8 ml local anesthetic is injected (Fig. 4–4). A subcutaneous infiltration is required to block the cutaneous branches to the forearm.

To find the **radial nerve,** a line is drawn from the most prominent point of the humeral head to the lateral epicondyle. The nerve crosses the humerus one-third of the way up from the lateral epicondyle. It can be palpated on the bone, and the block is performed with a 23-gauge 1-in. needle and 5 to 8 ml of local anesthetic. Alternatively, the radial nerve is blocked with the lateral cutaneous nerve of the forearm as described next.

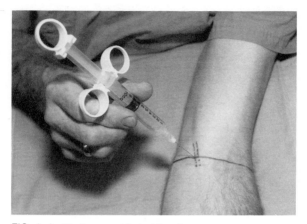

FIG. 4–4 Median nerve block at the elbow.

The **lateral cutaneous nerve of the forearm** is a continuation of the musculocutaneous nerve, and it perforates the deep fascia on the lateral side of the biceps muscle just proximal to the elbow. The lateral cutaneous nerve and the radial nerve can both be blocked with a 23-gauge 1.5-in. needle inserted between the brachioradialis muscle and the biceps tendon (Fig. 4–5). The needle is directed proximal toward the anteriolateral surface of the lateral epicondyle and 3 ml of local

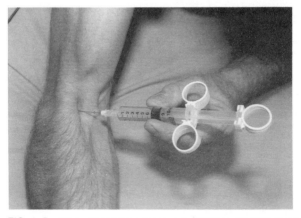

FIG. 4–5 Block of the lateral cutaneous and radial nerves at the elbow.

anesthetic is injected just above the periosteum. Bone contact is made two more times, and 3 ml is injected each time above the periosteum. An additional 5 ml of local anesthetic is injected as the needle is withdrawn. If paresthesia is elicted, 5 to 8 ml of local anesthetic is injected and no further bone contact is necessary. A subcutaneous ring of 5 ml of local anesthetic from the biceps tendon to the brachioradialis muscle will provide anesthesia of the superficial branches of the musculocutaneous nerve.

Ankle Block

Foot operations lasting less than 2 h can be done with an ankle block. The block provides anesthesia for a tourniquet at the level of the malleoli. A common mistake is to block the ankle too distally. An injection 1 to 2 cm above the malleoli provides a more complete block. The block is a conduction block of the five nerves which innervate the foot; three on the dorsal side and two on the plantar side. The block is performed with a 23-gauge 1-in. needle, and 5 to 10 ml of local anesthetic is infiltrated around each of the nerves as described in the following:

The **saphenous nerve** is blocked at the greater saphenous vein 1 to 2 cm above the medial malleolus (Fig. 4–6).

The **deep peroneal nerve** is blocked around and deep to the dorsalis pedis artery. Alternatively, the infiltration is performed between the tibialis anterior and the extensor hallus longus tendons. Flexion of the first and second toes improves visualization of the two tendons (Fig. 4–7).

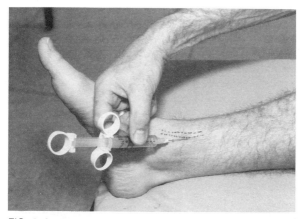

FIG. 4–6   Saphenous nerve block.

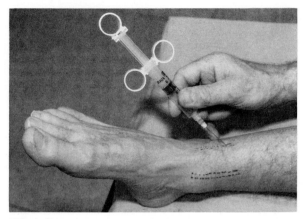

FIG. 4–7 Deep peroneal nerve block.

The **superficial peroneal nerve** is blocked with subcutaneous ring infiltration from the anterior edge of the tibia to the anterior edge of the fibula (Fig. 4–8).

The **sural nerve** is blocked with subcutaneous fan-wise infiltration between the Achilles tendon and fibula (Fig. 4–9).

The **tibial nerve** is blocked with a needle advanced just lateral to the posterior tibial artery toward the posterior surface of the tibia. The

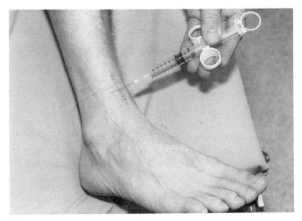

FIG. 4–8 Superficial peroneal nerve block.

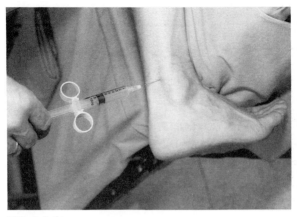

FIG. 4–9 Sural nerve block.

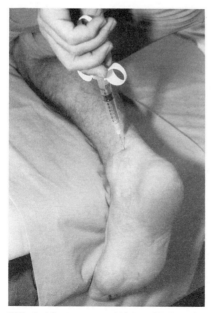

FIG. 4–10 Tibial nerve block.

needle is retracted 1 cm after contact with the tibia and after the anesthetic is injected (Fig. 4–10).

Hematoma Block

Spread of local anesthetic to the nerve fibers, supplying soft tissue and periosteum around a fracture, is obtained with a hematoma block. This technique is contraindicated if there is any risk of contamination of the fracture site from the skin puncture.

A large-bore needle (e.g., a 10-gauge 1.5-in. needle) is used for this block because it is important to withdraw blood from the fracture hematoma and replace it with local anesthetic. This gives better anesthesia, and it also reduces the risk of a high compartment pressure. After aspiration of the hematoma, 10 to 15 ml of 1% lidocaine is injected. When there is an associated distal radioulnar joint injury, 5 to 8 ml of 1% lidocaine is injected in the radioulnar joint in addition to the hematoma.

5 | Fracture Healing and Bone Grafting

Michael E. Joyce   Clayton R. Perry

In this chapter we describe fracture healing at the clinical, radiographic, biomechanical, cellular, regulatory (i.e., growth factors), and biochemical levels. In addition, bone grafting, a surgical procedure that stimulates fracture healing, is described.

FRACTURE HEALING

The **clinical** course of fracture healing is predictable. Failure to progress clinically is an indication of delayed union or impending nonunion. Initially, all fractures are characterized by pain due to disruption of nerve endings in the periosteum and surrounding soft tissue. Other findings at the time of injury include abnormal motion, soft tissue swelling, warmth, and redness. Characteristically, motion through the fracture exacerbates pain. Conversely, immobilization of the fracture with splinting or internal fixation decreases pain. Fractures managed with splinting gradually become less painful as they heal and usually at 2 weeks there is minimal pain. Initially, the patient may have the sensation of a "click" or "pop" as the fractured bone ends move over each other, but this sensation gradually disappears during the next 2 to 4 weeks. Concurrently, a fusiform mass becomes evident around the fracture, representing external callus. When the fracture site is stressed, a feeling of discomfort is elicited, and a "spring" is present (i.e., there is slight motion of the fracture fragments, but they return to their initial position). Gradually, the discomfort and spring decrease and eventually disappear 6 to 12 weeks after injury. At this point, the fracture is clinically healed. Remodeling is a prolonged process resulting in a variable decrease in the size of the external callus mass.

This is the normal healing sequence that is followed when the fracture has been managed with an intramedullary rod. However, when the fracture has been stabilized rigidly (i.e., with a plate and screws), the presence of callus, motion, and pain are signs of failure of fixation.

The rate at which fracture healing proceeds is decreased in elderly patients and increased in children. Medical conditions (diabetes mellitus) or medications (Prednisone) prolong fracture healing. Different bones in the body are known to heal at different rates (e.g., tibia vs. radius). Similarly, different regions of the same bone heal at different rates (e.g., metaphysis vs. diaphysis). The type of injury has a profound effect on the rate of fracture healing. Soft-tissue injury and bone loss are associated with a decreased rate of healing.

29

The initial **radiographic** sign of healing is the appearance of callus. This occurs 2 to 4 weeks following fracture. Initially, ossification is seen at the periphery of the callus, gradually moving centripetally. As the callus matures, it develops trabeculae and a cortex. Necrotic bone becomes relatively radiodense, appearing whiter than surrounding bone. This is due to the hyperemia and resulting osteopenia of living bone. The appearance of callus around fractures that have been rigidly stabilized indicates failure of fixation. Trabeculae crossing the fracture site is the radiographic indication of a healed fracture that has been rigidly stabilized.

The restoration of strength or the **biomechanical** healing of fractures is divided into four stages. The first stage is at the time of injury when the only mechanical strength is due to the stability attributable to the interdigitation of the fracture fragments. The second stage starts with the formation of a soft callus. The soft callus is cartilage and provides only a fraction of the normal strength of the bone. In the third stage, soft callus ossifies and is replaced by a hard callus comprised of woven bone. The hard callus is detectable radiographically and results in full restoration of strength. The fourth stage is remodeling of the hard callus into compact and cortical bone that results in restoration of the architecture.

On the **cellular level,** there are five stages of fracture healing. Stage 1, healing response to injury, occurs immediately after fracture when a hematoma forms at the fracture site. Soft tissue surrounding the fracture is invaded by monocytes and inflammatory cells. Within the first 24 h, cells in the deep layer of the periosteum begin to proliferate.

Stage 2, intramembranous ossification, occurs within 3 days following fracture. New bone matrix is synthesized by osteoblasts located adjacent to the fracture site and below the proliferating periosteal cells. The bone that forms here does so without a cartilaginous intermediate, a process termed intramembranous ossification. The area of subperiosteal bone formation determines the area of hard callus formation.

Stage 3, chondrogenesis, occurs within 7 to 10 days. Chondrocytes appear within the granulation tissue in the immediate vicinity of the fracture gap. Mesenchymal cells, presumably chondrocyte precursors, are found within granulation tissue bordering the advancing chondrogenic front. Chondrogenesis occurs as the newly differentiated chondrocytes mature within the enlarging cartilaginous matrix. This process continues until the fibrous tissue within this soft callus is replaced by cartilage, thereby bridging the fracture gap.

Stage 4, endochondral ossification, takes place within 9 to 14 days. Chondrocytes begin to hypertrophy within the soft callus adjacent to subperiosteal bone. The surrounding extracellular matrix calcifies prior to vascular invasion and repopulation with osteoblasts. This process (identical to that which occurs at the growth plate) continues until the fracture gap has been bridged. Remodeling eventually restores the normal bone architecture.

Stage 5, remodeling, involves the simultaneous removal and replacement of bone. Removal is accomplished by osteoclasts, and replacement is accomplished by osteoblasts. In cortical bone, osteoblasts tunnel through existing bone, followed by blood vessels. Osteoblasts accompanying the blood vessels lay down lamellar bone, forming a new osteon. In trabecular bone, the osteoclasts and osteoblasts line the surface of the trabeculae. Remodeling results in "primary bone healing" (i.e., the bridging of a fracture by osteons) when cortical bone ends are rigidly and anatomically reduced and in "creeping substitution" (i.e., the ingrowth of blood vessels and bony trabeculae) when cancellous bone ends are reduced rigidly.

The **regulation** of cellular proliferation, differentiation, chemotaxis, and the synthesis of extracellular matrix is not fully understood; however, it is clear that a class of peptides, termed **growth factors,** plays a central role. Their role in the regulation of fracture healing has been deduced by their localization within fracture callus by immunohisto-chemistry.

Growth factors arrive at the fracture callus by two pathways. First, they can be delivered by the blood stream (e.g., released by platelets into the fracture hematoma). Second, they can arrive through synthesis by cells within the fracture callus.

Platelet-derived growth factor (PDGF) is released from platelets and macrophages in the earliest stage of wound healing, suggesting an important role for PDGF in the initiation of fracture repair. At the initiation of fracture healing, PDGF acts as a stimulator of mesenchymal cell proliferation and an initiator of new matrix formation during fracture repair. PDGF stimulates type I collagen synthesis and intramembranous bone formation. Other mitogenic factors (e.g., transforming growth factor beta [TGFB] and insulin-like growth factor II [IGFII]) further stimulate the primitive mesenchymal cells to proliferate.

Maturation factors, such as bone morphogenic protein (BMP), TGFB, acidic fibroblast growth factor (AFGF), and basic fibroblast growth factor (BFGF), stimulate differentiation of primitive mesenchymal cells to various specialized cell lines. BMP induces differentiation of osteoblasts. TGFB has a more complex and central role as a modulator of fracture healing. Differing concentrations at different stages of healing stimulate fibrocytes, chondrocytes, or osteocytes. The exclusive intracellular immunostaining of AFGF suggests that its synthesis and action are through autocrine regulatory pathways within the fracture callus. BFGF induces the differentiation of chondrocytes and osteoblasts, as well as neovascularization, by promoting endothelial cell proliferation and capillary cell differentiation.

The **biochemical** composition of the healing fracture evolves as it matures. Collagen synthesized by fibroblasts (types III and V) is replaced by collagen synthesized by chondrocytes (types II and IX) and in turn is replaced by collagen synthesized by osteoblasts (type I). Initially, the proteoglycan composition of the extracellular matrix is primarily dermatan sulfate. By the second week, chondroitin sulfate predominates. As healing progresses, the concentration of proteoglycan in the fracture callus decreases and the proportion of monomeric proteoglycan increases. Activity and concentrations of various enzymes also change throughout the healing process. Enzymes are key in the process of deposition of hydroxyapetite (alkaline phosphatase) and degradation of macromolecules, such as early types of collagen and proteoglycans (collagenase and proteoglycanase). In addition to collagen, proteoglycan, and enzymes, there are numerous other types of molecules that play roles in modulating responses (e.g., enzyme inhibitors or activators), form basic building blocks, perform specialized functions such as acting as a nidus of calcification, or are simply debris.

BONE GRAFT

Bone graft is an avascular source of osteoconductive and osteoinductive matrix. **Osteoconductive** matrix is defined as a material that provides a "scaffold" for bone ingrowth. Allogenic bone grafts are harvested postmortem and preserved by desiccation or freezing. They are used to manage large bone defects, but they are only osteoconductive. **Osteoinductive** matrix is defined as a material that induces mesenchymal cells to differentiate into osteoblasts and chondroblasts. Autologous bone graft is osteoinductive. Bone morphogenic protein is one of the factors present that stimulates bone formation de novo in a variety of mesenchymal-rich tissues, including muscle. Autografts also supply mesenchymal cells which have osteogenic potential. These cells reside in themarrow and surrounding trabecular network of cancellous bone, and although the majority die during the grafting procedure, some remain viable.

Injuries of the
Glenohumeral Joint

John A. Elstrom   Clayton R. Perry

This chapter reviews dislocations of the humeral head from the glenoid fossa and fractures of the humeral head.

ANATOMY

The **proximal humerus** consists of the head, greater and lesser tuberosities, and anatomic and surgical necks. The head is approximately half a sphere and is covered with hyaline cartilage. When the axis of the distal humerus is at $0°$ in the coronal plane, the humeral head is directed posteriorly $15°$. The **greater tuberosity** is the insertion of the supraspinatus superiorly, and the infraspinatus and teres minor posteriorly. It is the most lateral bony projection of the shoulder. The **lesser tuberosity** is anterior and is the insertion of the subscapularis. The long head of the biceps lies in the intertubercular groove between the two tuberosities. The anatomic and the surgical neck refer to the constrictions around the base of the humeral head and the metaphysis just distal to the tuberosities, respectively. The anterior and posterior circumflex humeral arteries and the axillary nerve circle the proximal humerus at the level of the surgical neck. The vascular supply of the humeral head is via the anterior lateral ascending artery which originates from the anterior humeral circumflex artery. The anterior lateral ascending artery runs proximally along the lateral aspect of the intertubercular groove and enters the humeral head through foramina along its course.

The function of the **glenoid** is to serve as a fulcrum against which the muscles of the shoulder work to move the humerus. The glenoid forms a shallow cavity with an articular surface covered with hyaline cartilage. The articular surface of the glenoid is one-third of the area of the articular surface of the humeral head.

The **glenohumeral articulation** is a multiaxial ball-and-socket joint with a remarkable range of motion. Stability is dependent on passive and active mechanisms. Passive mechanisms of stability include the glenoid labrum, the coracoacromial ligament, the capsule, the glenohumeral ligaments, and the coracohumeral ligament. The **glenoid labrum** deepens the glenoid fossa and consists of dense fibrocartilage. It is frequently detached from the rim of the glenoid during an anterior dislocation of the shoulder. The **coracoacromial ligament,** along with the acromion, form the roof of the glenohumeral articulation and prevent proximal migration of the humeral head. The capsule of the glenohumeral articulation is large and redundant. This allows the range of motion of the shoulder, but imparts minimal stability. The three glenohumeral ligaments are intracapsular (i.e., thickenings of the capsule) and are major passive stabilizers of the joint. These ligaments are in the anterior capsule and are called the **superior, middle, and inferior glenohumeral ligaments.** They vary in size and shape, but serve as primary restraints to anterior translation of the humeral head on the glenoid. The **coracohumeral ligament,** also an intracapsular structure, prevents excessive external rotation of the humerus.

Active glenohumeral stability is due to the muscles of the rotator cuff and the long head of the biceps. The muscles of the **rotator cuff** (i.e., the subscapularis, supraspinatus, infraspinatus, and teres minor) function to maintain the humeral head in the glenoid, preventing dislocation, while the deltoid, pectoralis major and minor, teres major, and latissimus dorsi abduct, extend, flex, and rotate the humerus.

DISLOCATIONS OF THE GLENOHUMERAL ARTICULATION

Dislocations of the glenohumeral articulation are classified according to the position of the humeral head in relation to the glenoid, the duration or number of times the glenohumeral joint has been dislocated, and the etiology of the dislocation.

The humeral head is dislocated anteriorly, posteriorly, inferiorly, or superiorly. The majority of glenohumeral dislocations are **anterior.** The humeral head is most commonly subcoracoid, although it may also be subclavicular, subglenoid, or intrathoracic (Fig. 6–1). **Posterior dislocations** are rare, with the humeral head usually subacromial or occasionally subglenoid (Fig. 6–2). Posterior dislocations are difficult to diagnose and may be overlooked without a careful physical examination and axillary radiograph or CT scan of the involved shoulder. **Inferior dislocations** are known as traumatic **luxatio erecta** (Fig. 6–3). **Superior dislocations** are rare and result from a superiorly directed axial load applied to the arm. The humeral head is driven superiorly, disrupting the rotator cuff and often fracturing the acromion.

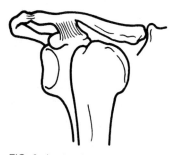

FIG. 6–1 Anterior glenohumeral dislocation.

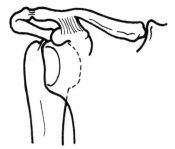

FIG. 6–2   Posterior glenohumeral dislocation.

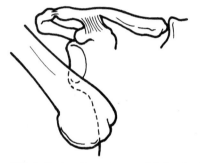

FIG. 6–3   Luxatio erecta, or an inferior glenohumeral dislocation.

Glenohumeral dislocations are further classified as acute, chronic, or recurrent. We arbitrarily define **acute dislocations** as being dislocated 2 days or less and **chronic dislocations** as being dislocated more than 2 days. Most dislocations are acute as the patient immediately seeks attention due to pain. However, occasionally glenohumeral dislocations are neglected, especially by the elderly. A dislocation is defined as **recurrent** when it has occurred previously.

Finally, glenohumeral dislocations are classified according to their etiology as being atraumatic, acquired, or traumatic. The **atraumatic** dislocation is associated with ligamentous laxity and is an ill-defined event in which self-reduction occurs. Management of the initial atraumatic dislocation does not affect the outcome. The **acquired** dislocation results from repeated minor injuries that typically take place in sports such as weight lifting and it occurs during a minor injury that would not dislocate a normal shoulder. Manipulative reduction is required, but initial management with immobilization is not effective in preventing recurrences. This group includes a significant portion of patients with shoulder instability. The **traumatic** dislocation results from a violent injury and requires manipulative reduction. Management of the initial traumatic dislocation by reduction and prolonged immobilization is effective in preventing recurrent injury. We are concerned primarily with traumatic dislocations.

Associated Injuries

Injuries associated with traumatic dislocations include fracture of the glenoid or proximal humerus, injuries of the rotator cuff, arterial disruption, and nerve injuries. Fractures associated with glenohumeral dislocations include fracture of the humeral neck, fracture of the glenoid rim, impaction fracture of the humeral head, and fractures of the greater and lesser tuberosities.

Careful review of the radiographs determines the presence of these fractures. The most clinically significant is an undisplaced fracture of the humeral neck which may displace during attempted reduction of the dislocation. In this situation, to minimize the probability of displacement, reduction is performed under anesthesia and is monitored fluoroscopically. Displaced fractures of the humeral neck associated with glenohumeral dislocation usually require open reduction and internal fixation; these are covered in Fractures of the Proximal Humerus. Fracture of more than 25 percent of the glenoid may result in chronic instability. Impaction fractures of the humeral head are equivalent to fractures of the glenoid rim. These fractures are known as the **Hill-Sachs lesion** and contribute to glenohumeral instability. The Hill-Sachs lesion is seen on the anteroposterior radiograph when the arm is maximally internally rotated. Fractures of the greater and lesser tuberosities are avulsions of the insertions of the subscapularis, infraspinatus, teres minor, and subscapularis muscles. Frequently, these fractures reduce when the glenohumeral joint is reduced. If not, open reduction and internal fixation are indicated.

The presence of a **rotator cuff tear** is determined by physical examination (e.g., inability to initiate abduction of the glenohumeral joint). In questionable cases, arthrography, magnetic resonance imaging (MRI), and electromyograms (EMGs) are helpful in determining the etiology of persistent weakness of the rotator cuff following reduction.

Rupture of the axillary artery is more likely to occur following a high-energy injury, in older patients, and in association with a brachial plexus injury. Physical signs include an expanding hematoma in the axilla and absent pulses at the elbow and wrist. Rupture of the axillary artery is an absolute surgical emergency.

The neurologic injury most frequently associated with glenohumeral dislocation is stretching of the **axillary nerve** resulting in a transient palsy. Injury is ruled out when voluntary contraction of the anterior and middle portions of the deltoid muscle are elicited. This is not

possible until the patient's pain is controlled by reduction of the dislocation. Sensory testing of the axillary nerve is unreliable. The radial,
median, ulnar, and musculocutaneous nerves are examined to determine
if a **brachial plexus injury** is present.

Diagnosis and Initial Management

History and Physical Examination

Determine when the injury occurred and whether it is recurrent. The
traumatic anterior dislocation results from a direct blow, or abduction
and external rotation of the arm. The traumatic posterior dislocation
results from a convulsion or a fall forward onto a flexed arm. There
is no clearly defined injury causing atraumatic dislocation. Acquired
dislocations are characterized by a history of repeated minor injuries.

Traumatic dislocations are painful. Anterior dislocations are characterized by external rotation of the arm. The area beneath the acromion
is hollow due to displacement of the humeral head. The diagnosis of
posterior dislocation is frequently missed because of the rarity of this
injury and its subtle radiographic findings. The physical findings are
key to the diagnosis. Posterior dislocations are characterized by internal
rotation and adduction of the arm. For example, the normal anterior
contour of the shoulder is absent and there is a posterior fullness on
the side of the dislocation, best seen by standing behind the seated
patient. The physical examination of the patient with luxatio erecta is
dramatic, with the humerus locked in greater than 90° of abduction.

Radiographic Examination

Radiographic examination of the injured shoulder confirms the direction
of the dislocation and determines the existence of associated fractures.
Three radiographic projections are essential: the scapular, or true, anteroposterior; the scapular, or true, lateral; and the axillary. The scapular
anteroposterior view is taken with the cassette parallel to the plane of
the scapula and the beam directed perpendicular to the scapula (Fig.
6–4). Normally, this view indicates the parallel articular surfaces of the
humeral head and the glenoid fossa. Following an anterior or posterior
dislocation, the parallelism between the articular surfaces is lost and
they are superimposed (Fig. 6–5). The scapular lateral is taken with the
cassette placed against the lateral surface of the shoulder at a right
angle to the plane of the scapula (Fig. 6–6). The beam is directed from
medial to lateral and parallel to the surface of the scapula (Fig. 6–5).
As seen on the scapular lateral projection, the glenoid is found at the
intersection of the body, spine, and acromion. The axillary view is
taken by placing a rolled cassette in the axilla and directing the beam
distally (Fig. 6–7). Alternatively, the cassette is placed proximally to
the shoulder, the arm is abducted, and the beam is directed through the

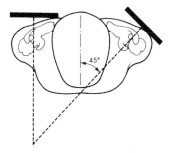

FIG. 6–4   Scapular anteroposterior radiograph and shoulder anteroposterior projections.

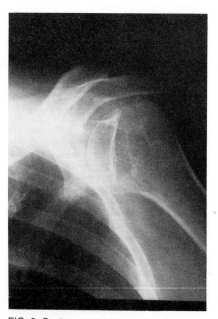

FIG. 6–5   Superimposition of humeral head on glenoid indicates posterior dislocation.

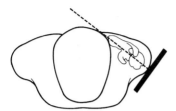

FIG. 6–6   Scapular lateral.

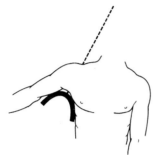

FIG. 6–7   Method of obtaining an axillary radiograph.

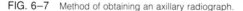

axilla from distal to proximal. The patient requires analgesia to obtain a satisfactory axillary radiograph.

Other radiographic studies of use are an anteroposterior view of the shoulder and a CT scan. CT scans are particularly useful in cases in which an adequate axillary view cannot be obtained (Fig. 6–8).

Initial Management

Chronic dislocations do not require acute reduction and should be reduced only after the patient has been anesthetized. Acute dislocations are reduced closed immediately. Failure to reduce an acute dislocation is a surgical emergency. Prior to reduction, venous access is established, the patient is sedated, and intravenous analgesics are administered as described in Chapter 4. The reduction maneuver used is determined by the type of dislocation. Anterior dislocations are reduced with straight traction in line with the humerus. Gentle internal and external rotation of the arm will relocate the humeral head. Countertraction is applied by an assistant via a sheet wrapped around the chest. The traction is firm and consistent. It is important not to attempt to force the humeral head back into place as this will result in muscle spasm, making reduction more difficult and traumatic. Other methods of reduction of anterior

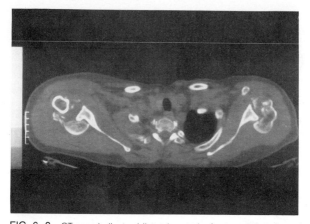

FIG. 6–8   CT scan indicates bilateral posterior fracture dislocations of the shoulder.

dislocations that bear mention include Stimson's method, the Hippocratic method, and Kocher's method. Stimson's method is to hang 5 to 10 lb of weight from the arm of the prone patient. After 10 to 20 min, gentle internal and external rotation of the arm will relocate the humeral head. Stimson's method is useful as a last resort for dislocations that are difficult to reduce by other methods. The Hippocratic method is to apply lateral traction through the arm and countertraction by placing the foot in the axilla. The Hippocratic method is useful if no one is available to assist in the reduction. Kocher's method is to apply traction to the arm, then to adduct and internally rotate the arm, levering the humeral head over the glenoid. This method is no longer used because of the risk of fracturing the proximal humerus. Posterior dislocations are reduced with gentle traction through the arm and application of anteriorly directed pressure to the humeral head. Stimson's method will usually reduce posterior dislocations. Luxatio erecta is reduced with traction along the line of the arm. Countertraction is applied by an assistant.

Following reduction of the shoulder, a focused neurovascular examination is performed, with emphasis on assessment of the axillary nerve and rotator cuff. The shoulder is then immobilized in a stable position. This is usually with the arm held against the body in a sling and swathe. In this position, the arm is internally rotated and adducted. Anterior dislocations are always stable in this position, but a posterior dislocation may not be stable. When the humeral head redislocates, a shoulder spica cast, with the arm abducted and externally rotated, is applied. Axillary and scapular anteroposterior and lateral radiographs are obtained to ensure the adequacy of reduction. Instability or an incongruous reduction may indicate a displaced glenoid rim fracture or a loose body that requires reduction and fixation or removal. A CT scan is useful in determining the cause of instability or an incongruous reduction.

Definitive Management

The definitive management of traumatic dislocation of the glenohumeral joint is based on whether the dislocation is acute, chronic, or recurrent. Management of all acute traumatic dislocations, regardless of the direction of dislocation, has two components: immobilization followed by rehabilitation. There is no benefit achieved from prolonged immobilization of the shoulder following a recurrent dislocation. Patients with recurrent dislocations require a reconstructive procedure to prevent future dislocation.

Acute traumatic dislocation (anterior, posterior, and inferior) is reduced and immobilized as described in the ''Initial Management'' section. Prolonged immobilization (4–6 weeks) reduces the incidence of recurrence. The sling and swathe is loosened for range of motion exercises of the elbow. Isometric exercises in the sling and swathe are begun at 2 to 3 weeks. At 4 to 6 weeks, all immobilization is discontinued and strengthening exercises initiated.

An unstable reduction, or irreducible dislocation, is an indication for immediate surgery. Unstable reduction is due to a glenoid rim fracture, or more commonly, a humeral head defect. Irreducible dislocation is due to soft tissue or bony interposition. The displaced glenoid rim fracture is reduced via an anterior approach for an anterior defect or a posterior approach for a posterior defect, and stabilized with screws. If comminution prevents adequate stabilization, a block of autogenous iliac crest is used to reconstruct the glenoid. Humeral head defects are managed by transferring the subscapularis into the anteromedial defect (posterior dislocation) or infraspinatus into the posteromedial defect (anterior dislocation).

Management of **chronic traumatic posterior dislocation** depends on the activity and health of the patient, length of time that the glenohumeral joint has been dislocated, and size of associated humeral head defect.

Reduction is not attempted if the patient is inactive or a poor surgical candidate.

When the dislocation is less than 4 weeks old and the defect involves less than 20 percent of the articular surface of the humeral head, closed reduction is attempted. If successful, the shoulder is immobilized for

6 weeks as described for acute posterior dislocation. In cases in which closed reduction is not successful, open reduction by an anterior approach and transfer of the lesser tuberosity into the humeral defect is performed.

When the dislocation is more than 4 weeks old, or the defect involves more than 20 percent of the articular surface of the humeral head, open reduction is performed via an anterior approach and the lesser tuberosity transferred into the defect. Postoperatively, the shoulder is immobilized 6 weeks. Very old posterior dislocations, or dislocations associated with large (greater than 50 percent) defects of the humeral head and glenoid are managed with arthrodesis or arthroplasty and bone grafting.

Chronic traumatic anterior dislocation of the shoulder is rare, occurring in the confused elderly or in patients with an impaired level of consciousness. The criteria for attempting a closed reduction include a history of dislocation of less than 4 weeks, the patient's level of activity, and the patient's being healthy enough to undergo general anesthesia. Severe osteoporosis, arteriosclerosis, and other fractures around the shoulder joint are relative contraindications for reduction. If closed reduction is not possible, open reduction is indicated in the appropriate patient with significant disability. Arthrodesis or arthroplasty and bone grafting of a deficient glenoid may be necessary.

Complications

The complications unique to glenohumeral dislocation are recurrent dislocation and adhesive capsulitis. **Recurrent dislocation** is more common in patients who sustained their first dislocation when they were less than 30 years of age, and if there were no associated fractures of the greater and lesser tuberosities of the humerus. Management of recurrent dislocation starts with determining which lesions are contributing to instability. These lesions are then corrected surgically. Procedures have been designed to change the version of the humeral head or glenoid, fill defects of the glenoid rim or humeral head, limit external and internal rotation, and repair and reinforce the anterior capsule.

Adhesive capsulitis of the shoulder (also known as "frozen shoulder") can follow any upper extremity injury. It occurs more frequently in older patients and is marked by painful limitation of motion of the glenohumeral joint. This is a limited process which will spontaneously resolve in 12 to 18 months. Management of adhesive capsulitis is aggressive, employing closed manipulation and expansion of the joint capsule with saline, or conservative, utilizing patience and range of motion exercises.

FRACTURES OF THE PROXIMAL HUMERUS

The proximal humerus is proximal to the insertion of the pectoralis major.

Classification

Fractures of the proximal humerus are classified according to whether there is significant displacement, if there is displacement, the number of fragments, and whether there is an associated dislocation.

Undisplaced fractures are displaced less than 1 cm or angulated less than 45° regardless of the fracture pattern or the number of fragments.

Displaced fractures occur along predictable anatomic lines producing similar patterns of fractures. These anatomic lines are the anatomic neck, the surgical neck, the greater tuberosity, and the lesser tuberosity. Displaced fractures are further classified into three groups according to the number of major fragments present (i.e., two-part, three-part, and four-part fractures).

Two-part fractures occur in four patterns: fracture through either the anatomic or surgical neck, and fracture of either the greater or lesser tuberosity (Figs. 6–9 to 6–12). The vascularity of the head is at risk following a fracture of the anatomic neck. **Three-part** fractures occur in two patterns: fracture of the surgical neck with a fracture of either the greater or lesser tuberosity (Figs. 6–13 and 6–14). Because either the greater or lesser tuberosity remains attached to the head fragment, there is marked rotation of the head due to unopposed muscle pull (i.e., if the greater tuberosity remains attached, the head is abducted and externally rotated; if the lesser tuberosity remains attached, the head is internally rotated). **Four-part** fractures occur in one pattern: fracture of the anatomic neck and fracture of the greater and lesser tuberosities (Fig. 6–15). The vascular supply of the head is disrupted following four-part fracture.

Fracture dislocations are characterized by a dislocation of the glenohumeral articulation and an associated fracture of the proximal humerus. The fracture may be an undisplaced or displaced fracture (Fig. 6–16).

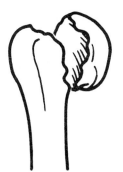

FIG. 6–9   Fracture through the anatomic neck.

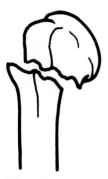

FIG. 6—10   Fracture through the surgical neck.

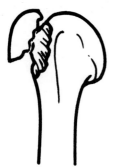

FIG. 6—11   Fracture of the greater tuberosity.

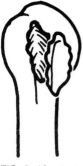

FIG. 6—12   Fracture of the lesser tuberosity.

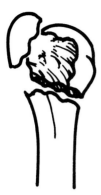

FIG. 6–13 Fracture of the anatomic neck and greater tuberosity.

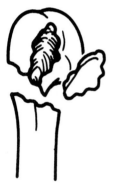

FIG. 6–14 Fracture of the anatomic neck and lesser tuberosity.

The displaced fracture that is most frequently associated with a dislocation is a two-part fracture involving the greater tuberosity.

Associated Injuries

Injuries of the axillary nerve, brachial plexus, and axillary artery and vein are frequently associated with fractures of the proximal humerus. The diagnosis of these injuries is covered in the "Dislocations of the Glenohumeral Articulation" section.

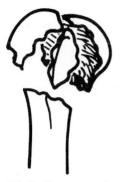

FIG. 6–15   Four-part fracture.

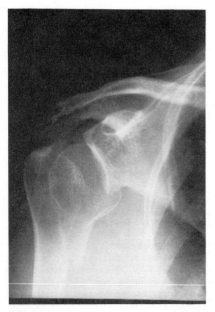

FIG. 6–16   Posterior fracture (two-part) dislocation.

Diagnosis and Initial Management

History and Physical Examination

There is pain that limits motion localized to the shoulder. Acutely, the appearance of the shoulder is relatively normal. It has a normal contour, and because of the overlying muscles there is no discernible swelling or ecchymosis. Within several days, a large ecchymosis appears around the shoulder and distally.

Radiographic Examination

The three essential projections are the scapular anteropostero, the scapular lateral, and the axillary.

Supplemental views (e.g., the anteroposterior projection with the humerus in differing degrees of rotation and the transthoracic lateral) are frequently of value and are obtained at the surgeon's discretion. CT scans are of value in the evaluation of complex fracture dislocations or to assess the glenoid rim.

Initial Management

Initial management of undisplaced fractures consists of immobilization in a sling and swathe. Displaced fractures of the surgical or anatomic neck, regardless of whether there is a fracture of the greater or lesser tuberosities which are to be managed nonoperatively, are placed in a collar and cuff. The collar and cuff is designed to exert constant traction (the weight of the arm) through the fracture. Displaced isolated fractures of the greater or lesser tuberosity managed nonoperatively, are placed in a sling. Fractures that are to be managed operatively are placed in a sling, and ice is applied to minimize swelling. The initial management of fracture dislocations is dependent on the location of the fracture. If there is an isolated fracture of the greater or lesser tuberosity, closed reduction is attempted in the emergency room. If there is a fracture of the anatomic or surgical neck, reduction is performed in the operating room.

Definitive Management

The definitive management is dependent on the type of fracture. Undisplaced fractures are managed as described in the ''Initial Management'' section.

Displaced Fractures

Displaced two-part fractures of the anatomic neck and of the greater tuberosity are managed operatively. Anatomic neck fractures are reduced and stabilized in young patients with high demands. Hemiarthroplasty is performed in elderly patients with osteopenic bone and fewer demands. The fracture is approached through the deltopectoral interval. Screws or screws and plates are used to stabilize the fracture once it has been reduced. Fractures of the greater tuberosity are approached through a deltoid splitting approach, reduced and stabilized with screws and washers.

The majority of displaced two-part fractures of the surgical neck or of the lesser tuberosity are managed nonoperatively. Surgical neck fractures are managed in a collar and cuff. An axillary pad can be added to correct medial displacement of the distal fragment. If the distal fragment cannot be reduced and it remains medially displaced, open reduction via the deltopectoral interval and stabilization with a plate and screws are indicated. Displaced fractures of the lesser tuberosity frequently are associated with an undisplaced fracture of the surgical neck. These fractures are managed with a sling.

Three-part fractures are almost always managed operatively because of the associated rotary deformity. They are approached via the delto-pectoral interval, reduced, and stabilized with screws and plates if possible. Three- and four-part fractures frequently occur in osteopenic bone, and stable fixation is difficult, or impossible, to achieve with screws and plates. Polymethylmethacrylate (PMMA) can be used to supplement fixation in osteopenic bone. When PMMA is used, the fracture is grafted with autogenous cancellous bone to stimulate healing. Alternatively, wires or heavy suture is passed through the tendinous insertions on the greater and lesser tuberosities and is used to stabilize the reduced fragments. With this type of fixation, repair of longitudinal tears in the rotator cuff adds to the stability of fixation and is therefore essential.

The management of four-part fractures is dependent on the demands of the patient and the degree of osteopenia present. These fractures frequently occur through osteopenic bone in sedentary patients with very limited demands. In these cases, four-part fractures are managed nonoperatively in a sling, with the clear understanding that the mobility and strength of the shoulder will be severely limited. In more active patients with osteopenic bone, a hemiarthroplasty is performed. The agoal of hemiarthroplasty is a strong painless shoulder with a relatively limited range of motion. In patients younger than 50 years of age with bone of normal density, open reduction and stabilization are attempted. There is a high incidence of avascular necrosis and nonunion following this procedure but it gives the patient a chance for the best result.

Whether a hemiarthroplasty or reduction and internal fixation is performed, the surgical approach is via the deltopectoral groove. The incision can be extended distally through the midportion and parallel with the fibers of the brachialis. When a hemiarthroplasty is performed, it is key to hold the tuberosities reduced with wires or heavy suture so that healing between them occurs, minimizing the chance of late displacement. The humeral head is used as a source of cancellous graft.

Fracture Dislocation

The most commonly encountered fracture dislocation is an anterior dislocation and a fracture of the greater tuberosity. As described in the "Initial Management" section, a gentle atraumatic reduction is performed in the emergency room. If the greater tuberosity remains displaced it is reduced and stabilized operatively. Two-part fracture dislocations through the anatomic or surgical neck and all three- and four-part fracture dislocations are managed operatively. Closed reduction is not attempted because the brachial plexus and axillary artery may be injured. The fracture is approached through the deltopectoral interval. Two- and three-part fractures are reduced and stabilized with plates and screws (Fig. 6–17). Four-part fractures are managed with a hemiarthroplasty. If open reduction is contraindicated (e.g., an unstable multiply traumatized patient), a large threaded Steinman pin is percutaneously drilled into the head fragment and used to manipulate the head into its reduced position. If the reduction is stable, the pin is removed. If the reduction is unstable, the pin is drilled through the humeral head into the glenoid.

Rehabilitation of the shoulder following fracture is extremely important. Depending on the patient's comfort level and the stability of fixation, pendulum exercises are begun at 2 to 3 weeks. Gentle, passive-assisted abduction and external and internal rotation exercises are added at 3 to 4 weeks. Usually at 6 to 8 weeks enough healing has occurred that active range of motion and strengthening exercises can be initiated.

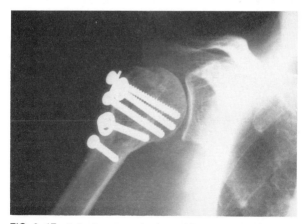

FIG. 6–17   Following open reduction and fixation with screws.

Complications

Avascular necrosis of the humeral head, nonunion, adhesive capsulitis, and posttraumatic arthritis are complications of proximal humerus fractures. Avascular necrosis is not always symptomatic. In cases in which avascular necrosis is symptomatic, it is usually managed with hemiarthroplasty. In very young or active patients, the shoulder is arthrodesed. Nonunion is managed with open reduction, stabilization, and autogenous cancellous bone grafting. The management of adhesive capsulitis is covered in the ''Dislocations of the Glenohumeral Articulation'' section at the beginning of the chapter. Posttraumatic arthritis is managed with arthroplasty or arthrodeses depending on the age and activity of the patient.

SELECTED READINGS

Dislocations of the Humeral Head from the Glenoid Fossa

Gonzalez D, Lopez RA: Concurrent rotator cuff tear and brachial plexus palsy associated with anterior dislocation of the shoulder: A report of two cases. *J Bone Joint Surg* 73A:620–621, 1991.

Rowe CR, Zarins B: Chronic unreduced dislocations of the shoulder. *J Bone Joint Surg* 64A:495–505, 1982.

Fractures of the Proximal Humerus

Bigliani LU: ''Treatment of two- and three-part fractures of the proximal humerus,'' in The American Academy of Orthopaedic Surgeons (ed): *Instructional Course Lectures.* Park Ridge, Illinois, Author, 1989, vol 38, pp 231–244.

Flatow EL, Cuomo F, Maday MG, Miller SR, McIlveen SJ, Bigliani LU: Open reduction and internal fixation of two-part displaced fractures of greater tuberosity of the proximal part of the humerus. *Am J Bone Joint Surg* 73A:1213–1218, 1991.

Neer CS II: Displaced proximal humerus fractures. Part I: Classification and evaluation. *J Bone Joint Surg* 52A:1077–1089, 1970.

Neer CS II: Displaced proximal humeral fractures. Part II: Treatment of three-part and four-part displacement. *J Bone Joint Surg* 52A:1090–1103, 1970.

7 | Fractures and Dislocations of the Clavicle and Scapula

John A. Elstrom

This chapter reviews fractures of the clavicle, injuries of the sternocla-vicular and acromioclavicular joints, and fractures of the scapula. Frac-tures of the glenoid rim occuring during glenohumeral dislocation (e.g., the Hill-Sachs lesion) are not included.

ANATOMY

The clavicle is the strut that connects the upper extremity to the chest. It stabilizes and serves as a fulcrum for the scapula. Without the clavicle, contraction of muscles that cross the glenohumeral joint (e.g., the pecto-ralis major) would pull the proximal humerus to the chest instead of moving the arm.

The **clavicle** is S-shaped when viewed from above. The flat acromial end is covered by the deltoid origin anteriorly and the trapezius insertion posteriorly. The round sternal end gives rise to the origins of the pecto-ralis major anteriorly and the sternocleidomastoid posteriorly.

The **scapula** is a flat triangular bone located on the posterior aspect of the chest. It has three bony processes: the coracoid process; the spine; and the continuation of the spine, the acromion. It has two articulations, the acromioclavicular joint and the glenohumeral joint. The scapula is buried in muscles. The costal, or anterior, surface is covered by the subscapularis muscle. The posterior surface is covered by the supra- and infraspinatus muscles. The spine is the origin of the posterior deltoid and the insertion of the trapezius. The short head of the biceps, the coracobrachialis, and the pectoralis minor originate from, and insert on, the coracoid process. The trapezius and levator scapulae elevate the scapula. The serratus anterior moves the scapula anteriorly holding it against the chest wall. Paralysis of the serratus anterior results in "winging" of the scapula.

The **acromioclavicular joint** is a diarthrodial plane joint. Its articular surfaces are covered by fibrocartilage and separated by a meniscus. The joint is stabilized by weak acromioclavicular ligaments, the deltoid and trapezius muscles, and the coracoclavicular ligaments (i.e., the trapezoid and conoid ligaments). The range of motion through the acromioclavicular joint is 20°, with most of it occurring in the initial 30° of shoulder abduction.

The **sternoclavicular joint** is a diarthrodial saddle joint. Its surfaces are covered with fibrocartilage, and the joint is completely divided by an articular disc. This disc attaches to the articular border of the clavicle, first rib, and joint capsule. The sternoclavicular joint is strengthened by anterior and posterior sternoclavicular ligaments, the interclavicular ligament running between the clavicles behind the sternum, and by the costoclavicular ligament running between the first rib and the clavicle. The clavicle abducts or elevates about 40° through the sternoclavicular joint. This motion occurs throughout shoulder abduction up to 90°. The medial physis of the clavicle fuses around the age of 25; therefore, epiphyseal separations rather than true sternoclavicular dislocations occur in patients younger than 25 years of age. This is important as physeal injuries will remodel: joint dislocations will not.

Behind the sternoclavicular joint are the major blood vessels as well as the trachea and esophagus. The brachial plexus and subclavian artery continue laterally, posterior to the clavicle, passing over the first rib and anterior to the scapula just distal to the coracoid. The costoclavicular space may be decreased by a fracture of the first rib or medial portion of the clavicle resulting in acute neurovascular injury or late compression. The axillary nerve passes below the neck of the glenoid and is frequently injured in shoulder dislocations. The suprascapular nerve passes through the scapular notch just medial to the base of the coracoid under the transverse scapular ligament.

FRACTURES OF THE CLAVICLE

Classification

Clavicle fractures are classified, according to location, as distal, middle, and proximal third fractures. The mechanism of injury is either a direct blow or an axial load resulting from a fall or blow on the lateral aspect of the shoulder.

Distal third fractures are further classified into three types (Fig. 7–1). Type I fractures are the most common and occur between intact coracoclavicular and acromioclavicular ligaments. The ligaments hold the fragments in alignment. Type II fractures are characterized by

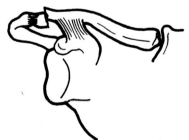

A

FIG. 7–1   The three types of distal clavicle fracture: (a) type I fracture, (b) type II, and (c) type III.

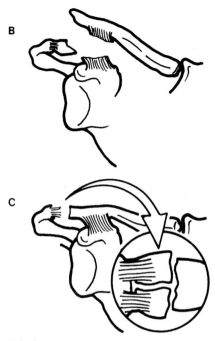

FIG. 7-1 *Continued*

disruption of the coracoclavicular ligaments. The weight of the arm pulls the distal fragment inferiorly and the trapezius and sternocleidomastoid pull the proximal fragment superiorly. Type III are intraarticular, usually undisplaced, and frequently become evident years later as posttraumatic arthritis.

Middle third fractures are the most common type of clavicular fracture. The proximal fragment is displaced superiorly by muscle pull; the distal fragment is displaced inferiorly by the weight of the arm.

Fractures of the proximal third of the clavicle, excluding injuries of the sternoclavicular joint, are uncommon and frequently pathologic.

Diagnosis and Initial Management

History and Physical Examination

The clavicle is subcutaneous; therefore, swelling and deformity are obvious and tenderness on palpation reveals the site of the injury.

Radiographic Examination

Radiographic confirmation and evaluation of fractures of the clavicle are with anteroposterior and 45° cephalic tilt views with the patient upright. Radiographs of proximal third fractures may occasionally have to be augmented with tomograms or a CT scan. In fractures of the distal third of the clavicle anteroposterio, radiographs of both acromioclavicular joints with the use of 5- to 10-lb weights are obtained to determine the presence of ligamentous disruption.

Initial Management

Initial management consists of a sling.

Associated Injuries

Associated injuries to the chest, brachial plexus, and major vessels are ruled out by history and physical examination. Visceral injury is associated with high-energy trauma, an open fracture, and fracture of the first rib or scapula. Scapulothoracic dissociation is a devastating injury associated with clavicle fracture or dislocation. The diagnosis is confirmed by lateral displacement of the scapula with an associated injury of the clavicle, acromioclavicular joint, or sternoclavicular joint. There is frequently an associated injury of the brachial plexus or axillary artery.

Definitive Management

Open reduction and internal fixation of **fractures of the distal third of the clavicle** are indicated if there is superior displacement of the proximal fragment due to disruption of the coracoclavicular ligaments or if there is intraarticular displacement. Type I and undisplaced type III distal clavicle fractures are managed symptomatically with a sling. The figure of eight splint has no value for fractures of the distal third. Type II distal clavicle fractures and the rare displaced type III fractures are managed with open reduction and internal fixation. The distal clavicle is exposed through an incision over its anterior subcutaneous border. The fracture is stabilized with a ''T'', or one-third tubular plate. Fixation is enhanced by passing a lag screw through the plate and clavicle into the base of the coracoid process.

Fractures of the middle and proximal third of the clavicle are treated with manipulative reduction and immobilization with a figure of eight splint which holds the shoulders dorsally. The figure of eight splint is applied and tightened with the shoulders retracted. The splint will stretch and loosen; therefore, it must be tightened every morning for the first few days. A sling supports the arm the first week. After 5 or 6 weeks, the pain diminishes to the point where immobilization is no longer required.

Indications for primary open reduction of middle and proximal third clavicle fractures include: fracture fragments threatening to penetrate the skin, irreducable displacement, neurovascular compromise, open fractures, and fractures associated with other injuries of the shoulder girdle (e.g., scapulothoracic dissociation). Exposure of the clavicle is via an incision just distal to the clavicle. A 3.5-mm reconstruction or dynamic compression plate is contoured and placed on the anteroinferior surface of the clavicle so that the drill is directed superiorly, away from the neurovascular structures and the lung. Autogenous cancellous grafting is required with extensive comminution, devitalization of bone fragments, or loss of continuity. Postoperatively the arm is supported in a sling for a minimum of 6 weeks.

Complications

Complications consist of nonunion, malunion, and neurovascular compromise.

Nonunion of fractures of the middle third of the clavicle occur more frequently following high-energy injuries. Atrophic nonunions are radiographically obvious. Tomography or fluoroscopic examination may be required to demonstrate the more common hypertrophic nonunion. Management of symptomatic nonunions is open reduction, internal fixation, and bone grafting.

Malunion of middle third clavicular fracture is a cosmetic problem. Symptomatic shortening or angulation resulting in tenting of the skin is managed with resection of protruding bone ends or osteotomy, internal fixation, and bone grafting.

Neurovascular complications result from displacement of the fracture fragments at the time of injury, of associated injuries (e.g., first rib fracture), and from late sequalae associated with hypertrophic callus. Subclavian vein obstruction between the clavicle and first rib is characterized by engorgement of the veins in the ipsilateral upper extremity. Angiography, EMG, and MRI are useful in determining the extent of neurovascular compromise. These complications are managed in conjunction with a thoracic surgeon.

FRACTURES OF THE SCAPULA

Fractures of the scapula are rare and often associated with other severe injuries. As a result, they are frequently overlooked.

Classification

The most important factor in classifying a scapular fracture is whether it was caused by high energy (e.g., an automobile accident) or low energy (e.g., avulsion of a muscle insertion). Comminution and displacement, the ''burst fracture,'' indicate high-energy trauma. Scapular fractures are further classified according to location into fractures of the body and spine, the glenoid neck (extraarticular), the acromion, the coracoid process, and the glenoid (intraarticular). Intraarticular fractures of the glenoid are subdivided into undisplaced and displaced fractures. Displaced fractures are simple (i.e., part of the glenoid is intact) or complex (i.e., the entire articular surface of the glenoid is fractured) (Fig. 7–2).

Diagnosis and Initial Management

History and Physical Exam

Pain is localized in the shoulder and back. The arm is adducted and protected against motion. Ecchymosis and swelling are minimal due to the scapula's location beneath layers of muscle. Loss of active abduction and forward elevation of the arm, known as pseudoparalysis of the rotator cuff, is often associated with scapular fracture and is the result of intramuscular hemorrhage and pain.

Radiographic Examination

Radiographic evaluation of the scapula includes a true anteroposterior and lateral view of the scapula and an axillary view. The anteroposterior view of the scapula will show fractures of the glenoid and glenoid neck. Lateral scapular views show fractures of the scapular body and acromion. The axillary view will show fractures of the coracoid and glenoid. Tomograms, CT scans, and anteroposterior and lateral chest radiographs provide additional information.

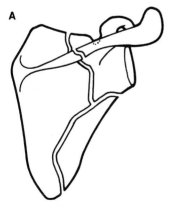

A

FIG. 7–2   The six types of scapular fractures: (a) fracture of the body, (b) extraarticular fracture of the neck of the glenoid, (c) fracture of the acromion, (d) fracture of the coracoid, (e) simple fracture of the glenoid, and (f) complex fracture of the glenoid.

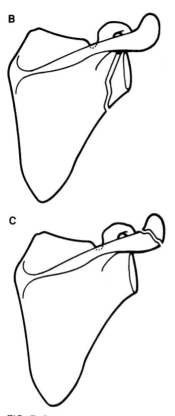

FIG. 7–2 *Continued*

Initial Management

The initial management consists of a sling.

Associated Injuries

The most important factor in the initial management of scapular fractures is that high-energy fractures are associated with life-threatening visceral injuries. The most common associated visceral injuries include pneumo-thorax, pulmonary or cardiac contusion, aortic tear, brachial plexus injury, and axillary artery injury. The most common associated osseous

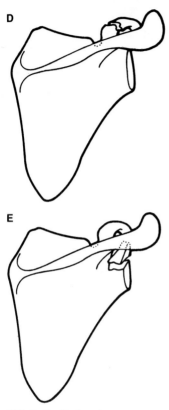

D

E

FIG. 7–2 *Continued*

injuries are fractures of the ribs, clavicle, or humerus, and dislocation of the acromioclavicular joint.

Definitive Management

Management of **fractures of the body and spine** is usually nonoperative. The muscles surrounding the scapula prevent further displacement. A sling and ice are used for the first few days to control pain. As the pain subsides, pendulum exercises in the sling are initiated. Healing is rapid and usually after 4 weeks, active motion can be initiated. Burst fractures with proximal displacement of the lateral margin of the body

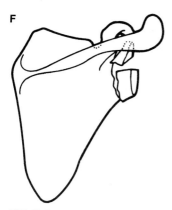

F

FIG. 7–2 *Continued*

may impinge on the glenohumeral joint capsule. When this occurs, the fracture is reduced and stabilized or the offending bony spike is osteotomized.

Extraarticular fractures of the glenoid neck are the second most common type of scapular fracture and occur when the humeral head is driven into the glenoid fossa. A CT scan may be necessary to confirm that the fracture does not involve the joint. Reduction is not attempted. The arm is supported in a sling and management is as described for fracture of the body and spine. The prognosis is good for near full return of function.

Fractures through the scapular spine and base of the neck of the glenoid with an associated clavicular fracture are unstable. The weight of the arm pulls the glenoid fragment distally. Late deformity is prevented by internal fixation of the fractured clavicle.

The **acromion** is fractured by a direct blow from the superior aspect or by superior displacement of the humeral head. Stress fracture results from superior migration of the humeral head due to a long-standing rotator cuff tear. A stress fracture, therefore, is an indication for an arthrogram or MRI to evaluate the rotator cuff. Depression of the acromion is associated with traction injury of the brachial plexus.

Minimally displaced fractures of the acromion are treated conservatively. They are followed closely for the first 3 weeks because they may displace. Significant displacement impairs glenohumeral motion due to impingement on the rotator cuff. Displaced fractures are managed with open reduction and internal fixation with a screw or tension band wire.

Isolated **fracture of the coracoid process** results from a direct blow, avulsion by muscle pull, or is a stress fracture (i.e., ''trap shooter's shoulder''). Fractures occur through the base or the tip. When minimally displaced, they heal uneventfully.

Displaced coracoid fractures occur in combination with an acromioclavicular dislocation. The coracoid is avulsed from the scapula by the coracoclavicular ligaments. Management is open reduction and fixation of the coracoid with a single screw and temporary transarticular fixation of the acromioclavicular dislocation. Displacement of the coracoid can cause compression of the suprascapular nerve and paralysis of the external rotators of the shoulder (i.e., the supraspinatus and infraspinatus). When this occurs, open reduction and fixation of the coracoid and decompression of the nerve is indicated.

The management of **intraarticular fractures of the glenoid** is based on the amount of displacement, the type of fracture, and the presence of glenohumeral instability.

Undisplaced fractures are managed with a sling and immobilization as described for fractures of the body of the scapula. Displaced simple fractures are managed with open reduction and internal fixation if there is a step-off of the articular surface or if there is glenohumeral instability. The degree of congruity of the articular surface is determined by axillary radiographs or CT scan. Instability of the glenohumeral articulation is expected when the fragment is displaced 1 cm and when the fragment comprises one-fourth of the articular surface. Frequently subluxation will be evident on the initial radiographs. An anterior approach through the deltopectoral interval is used to expose fractures of the anterior, superior, and inferior glenoid rim. Posterior glenoid rim fractures are approached posteriorly by reflecting the infraspinatus and posterior capsule medially. Large fragments are reduced and stabilized with screws or plates. Kirschner wires and cerclage wires may break or migrate and are not used. In severely comminuted fractures, the fragments are excised and replaced with an iliac crest bone graft contoured to the shape of the osseous defect and fixed to the glenoid with screws. Alternatively, if the fracture involves the anterior rim, the coracoid process is osteotomized and transferred to the defect.

Complex fractures of the glenoid pose special problems. The surgeon must decide if the extensive surgical procedure will result in a reduced stable glenoid; if not, closed management is indicated. These fractures are difficult to manage surgically because the necessary exposure is so extensive. The fracture is approached anteriorly and posteriorly. In some cases, it is necessary to take down the entire origin of the deltoid to obtain adequate exposure of the glenoid. Once exposed, the fragments are reduced and stabilized as necessary. Postoperative management depends on the stability of fixation and the surgical approach. Ideally, early passive motion is possible.

Closed management consists of an initial period of immobilization followed by early range of motion to mold the articular fragments into as normal a position as possible. The optimal position and type of immobilization is determined by comparing anteroposterior and axillary radiographs of the glenohumeral joint with the arm at the side and in various positions of elevation and rotation. Immobilization may be in the form of a sling and swathe, traction, or an airplane splint. At 3 to 4 weeks, healing has progressed to the point that immobilization can be discontinued. Range of motion is continued in a sling for an additional 3 to 6 weeks. At 6 to 9 weeks, the sling is discontinued and active range of motion is initiated.

Complications

Complications of scapular fractures include chronic glenohumeral instability, posttraumatic glenohumeral arthritis, and rotator cuff injury or impingement.

When these complications occur, the options are conservative management with nonsteroidal anti-inflammatories and occasional intra-articular injection of steroids, arthrodesis, or arthroplasty. Arthrodesis and arthroplasty are last resorts. Arthroplasty is indicated for elderly patients without neurologic injury. Arthrodesis is indicated for all others.

Rotator cuff injury is due to the initial injury or impingement by an unreduced fragment. MRI, arthrogram, and CT scan are used to determine the exact cause of symptoms and the appropriate surgical procedure is performed.

STERNOCLAVICULAR JOINT INJURIES

Classification

Injuries of the sternoclavicular joint are classified as sprains or dislocations. Sprains are undisplaced. Dislocations are anterior or retrosternal.

Diagnosis and Initial Management

History and Physical Examination

A history of injury, pain, and asymmetry of the sternoclavicular joints are the cardinal signs of this injury. The patient supports the injured extremity and tilts his head toward the affected side. Pain and swelling without injury may be signs of septic arthritis or condensing osteitis of the distal end of the clavicle. Spontaneous atraumatic anterior subluxation occurs in young persons with ligamentous laxity and is managed conservatively. In patients younger than 25 years of age, epiphyseal separation must be differentiated from dislocation.

Radiographic Examination

Routine anteroposterior radiographs of the sternoclavicular joint are not diagnostic. Two projections designed to show sternoclavicular joint dislocation are the Hobbs view and the Rockwood view. In the Hobbs view, the seated patient leans forward over a cassette so that the back of his neck is parallel to the table. The beam is directed through the neck onto the cassette. In the Rockwood view, the patient is supine. The beam is titled cephalad 40° and aimed at the sternum. A cassette is placed on the table so that the beam will project both clavicles onto the plate. In an anterior sternoclavicular dislocation, the clavicle appears to be anterior and riding higher than the uninjured side. In a retrosternal dislocation, the clavicle appears to be posterior and is lower than the uninjured side. Tomograms and CT scans differentiate sternoclavicular dislocation from fracture of the medial end of the clavicle and assess the adequacy of reduction.

Initial Management

Initial management consists of a sling. The patient is observed for respiratory and circulatory problems.

Associated Injuries

Compression of the structures of the thoracic inlet may occur with posterior dislocation and should be specifically ruled out. Acutely, this may become life-threatening, and subacutely, it is an indication for surgery. Symptoms of compression of these structures include shortness of breath and hoarseness, dysphasia, paresthesia, or weakness of the upper extremity.

Definitive Management

Sprains of the sternoclavicular joint are treated symptomatically. Anterior dislocations become asymptomatic and reduction (which is usually unstable) is rarely indicated. When reduction is attempted, it is performed in the following fashion. The patient is supine with a bolster between the shoulder blades. A posteriorly directed force is placed on the anterior aspect of both shoulders and the medial end of the clavicle is pressed inferiorly and posteriorly. The shoulders are then held retracted with a figure of eight clavicle strap.

Treatment of a retrosternal dislocation of the clavicle is more important. A thoracic surgeon is consulted if the patient has compression of the structures of the thoracic inlet. The technique of manipulative reduction has been described by Buckerfield and Castle. A bolster is placed between the shoulders. The bolster should be thick enough to elevate both shoulders from the table. With the arm *adducted* to the trunk, caudal traction is applied to the arm while both shoulders are forced posteriorly by direct pressure. Percutaneous manipulation with a towel clip may be required. Reduction is confirmed by lordotic radiographs. Once reduced, the retrosternal dislocation is usually stable. A figure of eight clavicle strap is used to hold the shoulders retracted for 4 to 6 weeks.

If closed reduction fails, open reduction is indicated when there are symptoms of mediastinal compression. Metallic internal fixation is dangerous and should not be used.

Complications

The incidence of complications from retrosternal dislocation of the clavicle is 25 percent. The symptoms associated with these complications are usually corrected with reduction; however, pneumothorax, laceration of the great vessels, and rupture of the trachea and esophagus require emergency intervention. The most serious long-term complications are the result of migration of metallic fixation devices.

ACROMIOCLAVICULAR JOINT INJURIES

Classification

Acromioclavicular joint injuries are classified according to the amount and direction of displacement into seven groups (Fig. 7–3). In type I injuries, the acromioclavicular capsule is stretched, but the coracoclavicular ligaments remain intact. The clavicle is undisplaced. In type II injuries, the acromioclavicular capsule is torn, and the coracoclavicular ligaments are stretched or partially torn. The clavicle is displaced less than one-half of its width. In type III injuries, both the acromioclavicular capsule and coracoclavicular ligaments are torn, the coracoclavicular distance is increased, and the clavicle is completely dislocated from the acromioclavicular joint. The deltoid and trapezius muscles are intact and remain attached to the clavicle. In type IV injuries, the clavicle is displaced posteriorly and is buttonholed through the trapezius, blocking closed reduction. In type V injuries, the trapezius and deltoid are torn, and the distal clavicle is displaced superiorly and is covered only by

A

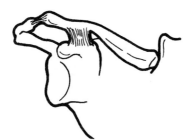

FIG. 7–3   The seven types of acromioclavicular injuries: (*a*) type I, (*b*) type II, (*c*) type III, (*d*) type IV, (*e*) type V, (*f*) type VI, and (*g*) type VII.

B

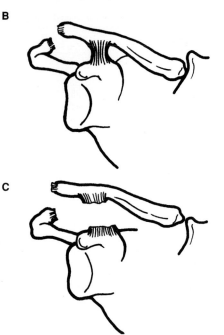

C

D

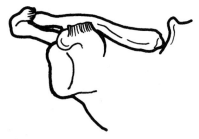

FIG. 7–3 *Continued*

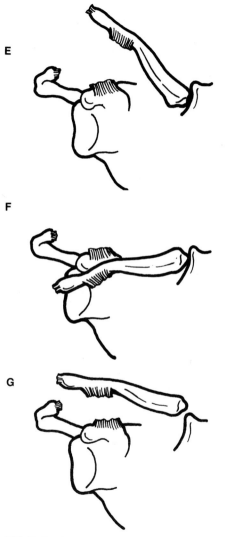

FIG. 7–3 *Continued*

skin and subcutaneous tissue. In type VI injuries, the distal clavicle is dislocated inferiorly and is locked below the coracoid and conjoined tendon. Type VII injuries are panclavicular dislocations.

Diagnosis and Initial Management

History and Physical Examination

There is a history of an axial-loading injury to the lateral aspect of the shoulder, pain, swelling, and tenderness increasing around the acromioclavicular joint. Prominence of the distal end of the clavicle is present on inspection, with the patient sitting and the weight of the arm unsupported, in type III injuries. When the amount of displacement is in question, the integrity of the coracoclavicular ligaments is determined by the patient flexing his elbow against resistance with the arm at the side. When the coracoclavicular ligaments are disrupted, the distal end of the clavicle will seem to rise superiorly as the acromion is pulled distally.

Radiographic Examination

Radiographic confirmation of the acromioclavicular injury and the degree of displacement is obtained with the patient upright and the weight of the arm unsupported. Radiographs taken with the patient supine or with techniques that overpenetrate the acromioclavicular joint obscure displacement. Stress films with the patient holding 5 to 10 lb of weight and comparison films with the opposite side are helpful. An axillary view of the shoulder is obtained to assess displacement in the anteroposterior plane. In type I injuries, there is no displacement of the distal end of the clavicle. In type II injuries, the distal end of the clavicle is slightly elevated but not completely displaced from its articulation with the acromion. In type III injuries, the distal end of the clavicle is displaced superiorly and the coracoclavicular distance is increased. The distance between the coracoid process and the clavicle varies; therefore, it is important to obtain comparison views of the other shoulder. In type IV injuries, the distal end of the clavicle is displaced posteriorly. Displacement is best visualized on the axillary view. In type V, VI, and VII injuries, the amount and direction of displacement indicate the type of injury.

Initial Management

Initial management is a sling.

Definitive Management

Type I and II injuries are treated symptomatically with a sling and ice. The sling is removed daily for range of motion exercises of the shoulder.

The treatment of type III injuries is controversial. The natural history of unreduced type III dislocations is that the pain diminishes and disappears while the deformity persists but improves. Management is closed or open. Closed management consists of maintaining reduction of the acromioclavicular joint with a Kenny Howard shoulder harness. This harness has a strap that runs over the top of the acromioclavicular joint and under the elbow and is tightened sufficiently to reduce the distal end of the clavicle. Most patients find it uncomfortable and compliance is a problem.

Open reduction and internal fixation are performed through a ''saber'' incision. The distal clavicle, acromion, and coracoid are exposed. The joint is debrided, reduced, and stabilized with large, smooth Steinman pins. These pins are left long, brought through the skin, and bent to prevent migration. A heavy nonabsorbable suture is looped under the coracoid, around the clavicle, and then tied. The torn coracoclavicular ligaments are repaired if possible. Postoperatively, the arm is maintained in a sling. The pins are removed at 6 weeks. It is important that the pins do not break. Therefore, physical therapy is not started until the pins have been removed.

Type IV, V, and VI injuries are treated with open reduction and internal fixation of the acromioclavicular joint. Type VII injuries are managed with open reduction and stabilization of the acromioclavicular joint and closed reduction of the sternoclavicular joint. Reduction of the sternoclavicular joint is maintained with a figure of eight splint.

Complications

Complications include shoulder stiffness, deformity, chronic dislocation, and posttraumatic arthritis. Shoulder stiffness is prevented with early range of motion exercises. The deformity diminishes but does not disappear. Symptomatic chronic dislocation and posttraumatic arthritis are managed with resection of the distal 2 cm of the clavicle and transfer of the coracoacromial ligament from its acromial attachment to the distal end of the clavicle.

Complications following open management are more significant. The most frequent is loss of reduction. The most significant is breakage and migration of a pin. This is potentially fatal if the pin migrates to the heart or great vessels.

SELECTED READINGS

Fractures of the Clavicle

Kona J, Bosse MJ, Staeheli JW, Rosseau RL: Type II distal clavicle fractures: a retrospective review of surgical treatment. *J Orthop Trauma* 4:115–120, 1990.

Fractures of the Scapula

Goss TP: Fractures of the glenoid cavity. Current concepts review. *J Bone Joint Surg* 74A:299–305, 1992.

Harris RD, Harris JH Jr: The prevalence and significance of missed scapular fractures in blunt chest trauma. *Am J Rheum* 151:747–750, 1988.

Herscovici D Jr, Fiennes AG, Allgower M, Ruedi TP: The floating shoulder: Ipsilateral, clavicle and scapular neck fractures. *J Bone Joint Surg* 74B: 362–364, 1992.

Sternoclavicular Joint Injuries

Buckerfield CT, Castle ME: Acute traumatic retrosternal dislocation of the clavicle. *J Bone Joint Surg* 66A:379–385, 1984.

Eskola A: Sternoclavicular dislocation: A plea for open treatment. *Acta Orthop Scan* 57:227–228, 1986.

Acromioclavicular Joint Injuries

Bannister GC, Wallace WA, Stableforth PG, Hutson MA: The management of acute acromioclavicular dislocation. A randomised prospective controlled trial. *J Bone Joint Surg* 71B:848–850, 1989.

Weaver JK, Dunn HK: Treatment of acromioclavicular injuries, especially complete acromioclavicular separation. *J Bone Joint Surg* 54A:1187–1194, 1972.

8 | Fractures of the Humeral Shaft

John A. Elstrom

The humeral shaft is the diaphyseal portion of the bone. This excludes the metaphysis proximal to the pectoralis major insertion and distal to the brachialis origin.

ANATOMY

Important anatomic considerations include the deforming forces following fracture and the relationship between the humeral shaft and surrounding neurovascular structures.

The two forces which displace and angulate the fragments following fracture are gravity and unopposed muscle pull. Thin patients' arms hang vertically at their sides and gravity exerts axial traction. Obese patients' fractures develop varus (apex lateral) angulation.

Contraction of the muscles inserting on and originating from the humerus results in deforming forces at various levels of fracture. When fractures occur between the pectoralis major and the deltoid insertions, the proximal fragment is adducted by the pectoralis. The distal fragment is shortened, pulled laterally, and abducted by the deltoid muscle. When the fracture is distal to the deltoid insertion, the proximal fragment is abducted. Contraction of the triceps overcomes that of the biceps and brachialis and results in apex anterior angulation at the fracture site.

The radial nerve is the neurovascular structure most frequently injured when the humeral shaft is fractured. This is because of its close proximity to the shaft of the humerus. As the radial nerve runs distally around the humerus, it lies in the musculoskeletal groove formed by the origin of the brachialis muscle and the cortex of the humerus. Proximally, the radial nerve is cushioned from the humerus by a layer of the medial head of the triceps. Distally, the nerve lies directly on the lateral cortex of the humerus, making its injury more likely with fractures at this level (Fig. 8–1).

The brachial artery runs along the medial border of the biceps giving off nutrient arteries and small arteries supplying the periosteum. Application of a plate disrupts the periosteal circulation. Insertion of an intramedullary nail disrupts the endosteal circulation.

Classification

Humeral shaft fractures are classified according to their location and according to the fracture pattern. Thus, the fracture is described as proximal, midshaft, or distal, and as transverse, oblique, segmental, or comminuted (Fig. 8–2).

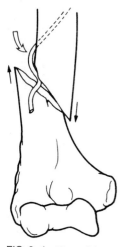

FIG. 8–1 The radial nerve is frequently trapped between the fragments of an oblique fracture of the distal third of the humerus.

Diagnosis and Initial Management

History and Physical Examination

There is evidence of injury, pain, and deformity. The skin is inspected for puncture wounds or lacerations.

Radiographic Examination

The radiographic examination consists of two radiographs of the humerus at right angles. Care is taken to rotate the entire extremity, not the extremity distal to the fracture. Radiographs of the shoulder and elbow are obtained. Other radiographic studies are not necessary to evaluate the fracture.

Initial Management

Initial management consists of splinting the fracture and supporting the arm. This is done as part of the closed management or to temporize until surgery. Hanging the arm at the side reduces oblique and comminuted fractures. A transverse fracture which is displaced and shortened is reduced by gentle axial traction and manipulation. Segmental fractures cannot be adequately reduced by closed methods and are aligned. Once reduction or satisfactory alignment has been achieved, a coaptation splint is applied. The splint starts in the axilla, runs distally along the medial side of the arm around the elbow, and continues up the lateral

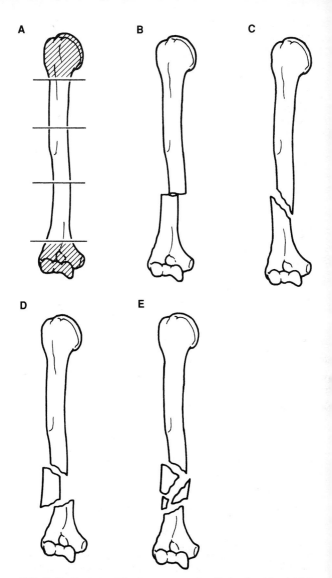

FIG. 8–2 Fractures of the humerus are classified as involving (*a*) the proximal, middle, or distal third; and as (*b*) transverse; (*c*) oblique; (*d*) segmental; or (*e*) comminuted.

side of the arm to the acromion. The splint is held to the arm with a loosely applied elastic bandage. The elbow is flexed 90° and the forearm supported by a sling.

Associated Injuries

The injury most frequently associated with a humeral shaft fracture is a radial neuropraxia. Radial nerve injury, indicated by loss of sensation on the dorsum of the thumb and inability to extend the wrist and metacarpophalangeal joints, is associated with 10 to 20 percent of all humeral shaft fractures. When a radial nerve palsy is identified following a closed fracture, the wrist and dorsum of the thumb are examined at intervals for return of function. If at 3 months, there is no sign of return, an EMG is obtained. If there are no reinnervation potentials, the nerve is assumed not to be in continuity and is explored. If reinnervation potentials are present, the radial nerve is in continuity and exploration is pointless. Two circumstances in which the radial nerve is explored following a closed fracture are when neurapraxia occurs during manipulative reduction and when the fracture is an oblique fracture of the distal humerus (a Holstein-Lewis fracture). In both of these circumstances, there is a high probability that the radial nerve is caught in the fracture site. When there is a radial nerve palsy and an open fracture, the nerve is explored during debridement. If not in continuity, a primary or delayed primary repair is performed.

Associated injuries of the brachial artery, ulnar nerve, median nerve, and musculocutaneous nerve are ruled out by the focused neurovascular examination of the forearm and hand. Associated fractures of the proximal and distal humerus, scapula, clavicle, ulna, and radius are ruled out by radiographs of the shoulder and elbow.

Definitive Management

The most important aspect of the management of humeral shaft fractures is to identify and understand when operative treatment is necessary. Most fractures of the humeral shaft are managed nonoperatively. Relative indications for open management include: open fractures; segmental fractures; multiple trauma; injury of the brachial artery; ipsilateral fractures and dislocations of the elbow, shoulder, and forearm; bilateral humeral shaft fractures; obese or uncooperative patients; pathologic fracture; and failed closed reduction.

Closed Management

The goal of closed management is a united fracture without deformity. Up to 20° of varus angulation and 2 cm of shortening results in minimal functional loss and is acceptable cosmetically. There are four methods of closed management: hanging arm cast, Velpeau dressing, coaptation splint, and functional brace.

The hanging arm cast is basically a way to apply traction. Its disadvantage is that it must be closely monitored and a high degree of patient cooperation is required. Its advantage is that it can be adjusted frequently to improve alignment. Hanging arm cast is contraindicated for obese patients because the arm will not hang vertically at the side and for transverse fractures because of overdistraction. The fracture is not immobilized and, for the first 2 weeks, there is discomfort at the fracture site. The cast is applied so that the proximal end is at the fracture site or slightly higher. The elbow is flexed 90° with the forearm in neutral rotation. The cast is suspended from the wrist by a cuff around the neck. Posterior angulation is corrected with a longer cuff and anterior angulation with a shorter cuff. Lateral angulation (varus) is corrected by attaching the cuff to the dorsum of the wrist; medial angulation (valgus) is corrected by attaching the cuff to the volar side of the wrist. The patient must sleep in a sitting position to maintain alignment. Radiographs are obtained weekly for 4 to 6 weeks. When there is callus on the radiographs, the cast is removed and the arm is examined. If there is clinical union (i.e., no motion or pain at the fracture site with gentle stressing), the hanging cast is discontinued and the arm is protected in a sling. If clinical union is not present, a functional brace is applied for an additional 2 to 6 weeks and active forearm rotation and elbow flexion exercises are initiated.

The Velpeau dressing immobilizes the arm by binding it to the chest. This method is helpful for minimally displaced fractures in elderly patients. The Velpeau dressing is a collar and cuff that suspends the wrist from the neck, and plaster or 6-in. Ace wraps bind the humerus to the chest. It is maintained for 4 to 6 weeks, at which time the arm is protected in a sling and active range of motion exercises of the elbow are initiated.

The coaptation splint is useful for fractures that are angulated because the plaster can be molded to correct varus or valgus deformity. Application of the splint is described in the "Initial Management" section. Three to four weeks postinjury, active forearm rotation and elbow flexion in the splint are initiated. The external support is discontinued when there is clinical union.

The functional brace is a prefabricated polypropylene sleeve that extends from the shoulder to just above the elbow. The fracture is managed initially with a coaptation splint. The functional brace is applied 1 to 2 weeks postinjury. Physical therapy is started at 2 weeks and advanced as tolerated. The brace is discontinued when there is clinical union, usually at 4 to 8 weeks.

Open Management

There are three methods of stabilizing the fracture once it is opened and reduced: external fixation, compression plate fixation, and intramedullary fixation.

External fixation is used for open fractures. The pins placed in the middle and distal third of the humerus are placed under direct vision to avoid radial nerve injury. Early bone grafting and conversion to another type of fixation is done when the wounds are healed to minimize the incidence of nonunion and pin tract infection.

Compression plate fixation of humeral shaft fractures allows rapid return of shoulder and elbow motion and union rates approach 97 percent. The posterior approach is used to expose the fracture. This approach splits the triceps muscle and exposes the radial nerve. Extreme care is used when retracting the radial nerve because it is sensitive to a stretch palsy. A broad 4.5-mm dynamic compression plate is used with a minimum of six cortices above and below the fracture. Bone defects are grafted with autogenous cancellous bone.

Intramedullary fixation of humeral shaft fractures has several advantages including a decreased risk of infection and nerve injury, a higher rate of union, and a lower incidence of implant failure. The primary disadvantage of intramedullary nailing of humeral shaft fractures is insertion site symptoms. The two types of intramedullary nails are flexible (i.e., Ender's nails and Rush rods) and rigid (e.g., the Seidel nail).

Flexible intramedullary nails are inserted antegrade or retrograde. Antegrade insertion is performed through a deltoid splitting approach. The insertion portal is just distal to the greater tuberosity to minimize rotator cuff symptoms. Retrograde insertion is performed through a triceps splitting approach. The insertion portal is 2 cm proximal to the olecranon fossa in the midline of the distal humerus. Whether the flexible intramedullary nails are inserted antegrade or retrograde, they are locked at the insertion portal with screws and the leading ends are flared to give rotational control.

Rigid intramedullary nails can be locked proximally and distally to prevent shortening and rotation through the fracture. Nail insertion is antegrade via a deltoid splitting approach. The insertion portal is the anterior lateral quadrant of the humeral head, through the rotator cuff. When necessary, the medullary canal is enlarged by reaming. Proximal and distal locking are done with an awareness of the location of the surrounding neurovascular structures. The radial and axillary nerves are at particular risk.

Complications

The most significant complication of humeral shaft fracture is nonunion. The diagnosis of nonunion is made at 6 months if there has been no progression of clinical or radiographic healing in the prior 3 months. Methods of management are electrical stimulation, reamed intramedullary nailing, plating and bone grafting, and dynamic external fixation. Electrical stimulation is less successful for humeral nonunions than for

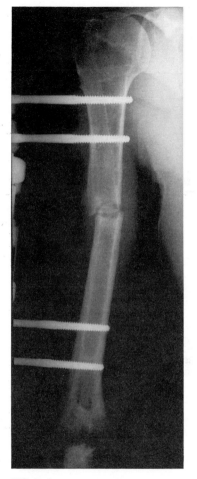

FIG. 8–3   A nonunion of a transverse midshaft fracture managed with a dynamic external fixater.

nonunions of other bones; however, it can be successful and has no surgical risk. Reamed nailing of humeral nonunions is less successful in the management of humeral nonunions than in tibial or femoral nonunions. Plating and autogenous bone grafting has the best chance of success, but also exposes the patient to the risk of infection and implant failure. Dynamic external fixation uses a fixater to compress and distract the nonunion site (Fig. 8–3).

SELECTED READINGS

Bell MJ, Beauchamp CG, Kellam JK, McMurty RY: The results of plating humeral shaft fractures in patients with multiple injuries. *J Bone Joint Surg* 67B:293–296, 1985.

Hall RF, Pankovich AM: Ender nailing of acute fractures of the humerus. *J Bone Joint Surg* 69A:558–567, 1987.

Packer JW, Foster RR, Garcia A, Grantham SA: The humeral fracture with radial nerve palsy, is exploration warranted? *Clin Orthop* 92:34–88, 1972.

Sarmiento A, Kinman PB, Galvin E, Schmitt RH, Phillips JG: Functional bracing of fractures of the shaft of the humerus. *J Bone Joint Surg* 59A:596–601, 1977.

Fractures and Dislocations of the Elbow

Clayton R. Perry

This chapter reviews fractures and dislocations of the elbow or cubital articulation. These injuries include: fractures of the distal humerus (i.e., isolated medial and lateral condylar fractures, transcondylar fractures, supracondylar fractures, and intercondylar fractures), fractures of the radial head and neck, fractures of the olecranon, fractures of the ulna and radius associated with a dislocation, and dislocations of the humeroulnar articulation.

ANATOMY

The cubital articulation consists of the distal humerus, proximal ulna, proximal radius, ligaments, joint capsule, and muscles.

The **distal humerus** is divided into medial and lateral condyles, separated by the olecranon and coronoid fossae. These condyles have articular portions (the capitellum and trochlea) and extraarticular portions (the medial and lateral epicondyles). When viewed from anterior to posterior, the distal humerus is in slight valgus, resulting in cubitus valgus when the elbow is extended. When viewed from the side, the center of the trochlea and capitellum are anterior to the shaft of the humerus and overlay each other, resulting in the cubitus valgus of extension decreasing with flexion.

The **proximal ulna,** or olecranon, has two concavities that articulate with the distal humerus and radial head, the trochlear and radial notches. The trochlear notch forms an arc of 180° and the radial notch forms an arc of 40° to 70°. The brachialis inserts on the coronoid process of the ulna.

The **proximal radius** consists of a head and neck. The head and neck of the radius form an angle of 15° to the radial diaphysis, with the apex directed toward the radial tuberosity. The head of the radius is dish-shaped and its upper surface is concave to articulate with the convex humeral capitellum. The outer circumference, or margin of the radial head, articulates with the radial notch of the ulna. The anterolateral quadrant of the head does not articulate with the radial notch, even in the extremes of pronation and supination, and is a portal for screw or Kirschner-wire placement. The biceps tendon inserts on the radial tuberosity.

The **medial collateral ligament** is the major ligamentous stabilizer of the elbow. It is intracapsular and has two major parts known as the anterior and posterior bands. The anterior band originates from the medial epicondyle and inserts on the medial margin of the coronoid process. The posterior band also originates from the medial epicondyle but attaches to the medial margin of the olecranon. The anterior and posterior bands resist valgus stresses.

The **lateral collateral ligament** is intracapsular and consists of two parts, both of which originate from the lower part of the lateral epicondyle. The radial part inserts on the annular ligament and resists varus stress. The ulnar part inserts on the dorsal surface of the olecranon and resists rotary stress.

The radioulnar joint is stabilized by the **annular ligament,** a fibrous band that encircles the head and neck of the radius keeping it in contact with the radial notch. Anteriorly, the annular ligament is attached to the anterior margin of the radial notch. Posteriorly, it is broader and divided into several bands that attach to a ridge posterior to the radial notch. The superficial surface of the annular ligament blends with the radial collateral ligament of the elbow and gives origin to part of the supinator muscle.

The **capsule** of the elbow joint attaches to the humerus anteriorly and posteriorly above the coronoid and radial fossae. Distally, it attaches to the coronoid process of the ulna and the annular ligament and is continuous with the radial and ulnar collateral ligaments.

Flexion is produced by the brachialis, the biceps, and the brachioradialis. The brachialis is the primary flexor of the elbow. Extension is produced by the triceps and anconeus, supination by the biceps and the supinator, and pronation by the pronator quadratus and pronator teres.

BIOMECHANICS

The elbow is a compound joint consisting of three articulations: the humeroulnar articulation between the trochlea of the humerus and the trochlear notch of the ulna, the humeroradial articulation between the capitellum of the humerus and the head of the radius, and the radioulnar articulation between the margin of the radial head and the radial notch of the ulna.

The humeroulnar and humeroradial articulations form a hinged, or uniaxial, joint through which the forearm moves. The center of rotation is not precisely fixed and moves in the extremes of flexion and extension. The normal extremes of extension and flexion are 0° and 140°. Flexion and extension of the elbow are accompanied by rotation (i.e., the ulna is slightly pronated during extension and slightly supinated during flexion). When fully extended, the elbow is in 15° to 20° of valgus.

The radioulnar articulation is a pivot or trochoid joint around which the forearm rotates. During forearm rotation, the proximal radius rotates around its central axis while the distal radius rotates around the ulna. The normal extremes of pronation and supination are 70° and 85°.

The radial head has two primary functions. It is a restraint to valgus stresses across the elbow by acting as a fulcrum for the medial collateral ligament, and it transfers stresses from the hand and wrist to the distal humerus. As forces are applied in a proximal direction axially along the shaft of the radius, the central tendinous portion of the interosseous membrane tightens. These forces are then transmitted from the radius through the interosseous membrane to the ulna and eventually to the trochlea. When the radial head has been removed, proximally directed stresses result in ulnar shift of the radius as opposed to tightening of the interosseous membrane, thus altering the method of stress transmission to the ulna and the mechanics of the distal radioulnar joint.

SUPRACONDYLAR FRACTURES OF THE HUMERUS

Supracondylar fractures are characterized by dissociation between the diaphysis and the condyles of the distal humerus. The fracture frequently extends distally and involves the articular surface.

Classification

The classification is based on the presence of supracondylar comminution, intercondylar extension, and intercondylar comminution. There are four types of supracondylar fractures: fractures without intercondylar extension (type I); fractures with intercondylar extension, but no comminution (type II); fractures with intercondylar extension and supracondylar comminution (type III); and fractures with intercondylar comminution (type IV) (Fig. 9–1). Type IV fractures frequently have supracondylar comminution.

Diagnosis and Initial Management

History and Physical Examination

There is pain and instability of the elbow. The fracture may have been caused by a fall on the outstretched hand or by a direct blow. On physical exam there is deformity, instability, and crepitation. The normal relationship of the epicondyles to the tip of the olecranon is not present in fractures with intercondylar involvement (types II, III, and IV).

Radiographic Examination

Anteroposterior, lateral, and oblique radiographs determine the extent of injury. Tomograms, CT scans, and special views are not necessary.

Initial Management

Initial management consists of alignment, immobilization in a long arm splint, and application of ice. Reduction is unstable; therefore, repeated attempts are not indicated. The fracture is aligned by hanging the arm

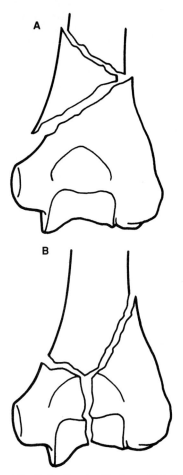

FIG. 9–1 The classification system of supracondylar fractures of the distal humerus: (*a*) type I fracture, (*b*) type II fracture, (*c*) type III fracture, and (*d*) type IV fracture.

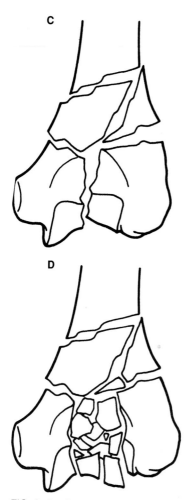

FIG. 9–1 *Continued*

at the side with the elbow flexed 90°. The fracture is splinted with a single posterior slab of plaster extending from the shoulder to the wrist. The upper part of the splint is reinforced with a sugar tongs splint, but a circumferential cast is not used because there may be significant swelling.

Associated Injuries

Associated injuries of the brachial artery, median, ulnar, and radial nerves are common. The patient must be specifically examined for these injuries. If undetected, compartment syndrome of the forearm may develop. The physical signs of compartment syndrome include pain at rest, pain with passive stretch of the muscles in the compartment, palpably tense compartments, and paresthesia. Radiographs of the shoulder, humeral diaphysis, forearm, and wrist are obtained, although there are no specific associated bony injuries.

Definitive Management

The goal of management is a healed fracture with a functional range of elbow motion. Usually, the best way to achieve this goal is anatomic reduction of the fracture, stabilization of the fragments with plates and screws, and early motion of the elbow. Extensive comminution, loss of the humeral condyles, massive soft tissue injury, or an injury of the brachial artery that requires rapid stabilization precludes plate fixation. In these cases, the fracture is managed with an external fixater.

External fixater half pins are inserted laterally in the humerus and, if the elbow is spanned, dorsally in the ulna. Pin insertion in the humerus is via incisions adequate in size to visualize the radial nerve, if it is encountered. To prevent the ulnar pins from blocking forearm rotation, they are inserted with the forearm in 30° of supination. The postoperative management is tailored to suit each patient. Consideration must be given to repeat debridements, delayed closure, bone grafting, free tissue transfer, delayed fixation, and arthrodesis.

Open reduction, stabilization, and early motion result in the greatest return of function. The surgical approach and technique of fixation depend on the type of fracture.

Fractures without intercondylar extension (type I) are exposed through straight medial and lateral approaches and stabilized with medial-lateral and posterolateral plates. Bone grafting is not required.

Fractures with involvement of the distal articular surface of the humerus (types II, III, and IV) are exposed through the transolecranon approach. The articular surface of the distal humerus is exposed by osteotomizing the olecranon and reflecting it with the attached triceps tendon proximally. The olecranon is "predrilled" so it can be stabilized with a single 6.5-mm cancellous screw. The osteotomy is V-shaped with the apex distal. After the fracture is adequately exposed, the intercondylar component is reduced and then stabilized with screws and Kirschner-wires. In fractures with intercondylar comminution (type IV), it is important not to lag the fragments together as this will decrease the medial-lateral diameter of the articular surface resulting in joint incongruity. After the intercondylar fracture is reduced and stabilized, the supracondylar component is reduced and stabilized with medial and lateral plates. If there is supracondylar comminution (all type III and most type IV fractures), autogenous cancellous bone graft is used.

Postoperatively, the elbow is immobilized at 90° in a splint extending from the wrist to the shoulder. When incisional pain becomes tolerable, active range of motion is initiated. This is done several times a day. At all other times, the splint is worn. At 4 to 6 weeks, the splint is discontinued and a sling is worn. At 8 to 10 weeks, all immobilization is discontinued and passive range of motion and strengthening is initiated.

Complications

Complications of supracondylar fractures of the humerus include loss of fixation, nonunion, and posttraumatic arthritis.

Loss of fixation occurs because of inadequate stabilization of the fragments or overenthusiastic physical therapy. Once fixation has been lost, revision and bone grafting are necessary. Immobilization is not an option when fixation has been lost because it results in loss of motion of the elbow.

Nonunion usually involves the supracondylar component of the fracture; the intercondylar component heals. If elbow motion is severely restricted, the prognosis is poor. Management is rigid stabilization and bone graft.

Posttraumatic arthritis is more common in fractures with intercondylar involvement, especially those with intercondylar comminution (type IV). Management options employ conservative therapy with nonsteroidal anti-inflammatories and occasional steroid injections; joint debridement, including resection of the radial head to improve motion; arthrodesis in younger patients; or arthroplasty in elderly patients.

TRANSCONDYLAR FRACTURES

The primary fracture line of a transcondylar fracture is intracapsular and transverse, passing through the epicondyles, olecranon, and coronoid fossae. These low-energy fractures occur in older, more osteopenic patients than supracondylar fractures.

Classification

Classification is based on the presence of displacement, the presence of a vertical fracture line in T-type fractures, and dislocation of the humeral condyles from the trochlear notch (Fig. 9–2). Based on these

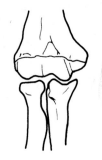

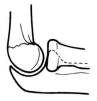

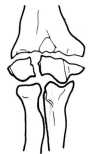

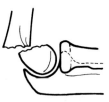

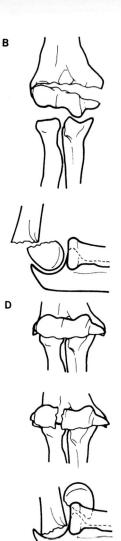

FIG. 9–2 The classification system for transcondylar fractures of the distal humerus: (*a*) type I fracture, (*b*) type II fracture, (*c*) type III fracture, and (*d*) type IV fracture.

parameters, transcondylar fractures are classified into one of four basic patterns: undisplaced (type I), simple displaced (type II), T-type (type III), and fracture dislocation (type IV).

The transverse fracture line is the only fracture line present in undisplaced (type I) and simple displaced fractures (type II). T-type fractures (type III) have, in addition to the transverse fracture line, a vertical fracture line separating the capitellum from the trochlea. In fracture dislocations (type IV), the humeral condyles are dislocated anteriorly from the trochlear notch and the distal metaphysis of the humerus articulates with the trochlear notch. Fracture dislocations may be T-type or simple.

Diagnosis and Initial Management

History and Physical Examination

Physical findings other than pain are not remarkable. The epicondyles and the tip of the olecranon can be palpated and their relationship is normal in all but fracture dislocations (type IV). When this relationship is normal, it distinguishes a transcondylar fracture from an elbow dislocation, an isolated fracture of an epicondyle, an olecranon fracture, and a displaced supracondylar-intercondylar fracture.

Radiographic Examination

The diagnosis is confirmed by anteroposterior and lateral radiographs.

Special views, tomograms, and CT scans are not necessary.

Initial Management

Initial management is immobilization in a long arm splint and sling.

Associated Injuries

Associated injuries are uncommon. The routine focused neurovascular exam is performed and radiographs of the shoulder, humerus, forearm, and wrist are obtained.

Definitive Management

Undisplaced fractures are managed with a long arm cast and a sling. The cast is removed at 3 to 4 weeks and gentle range of motion exercises are initiated. The arm is protected in a splint for a total of 6 to 8 weeks. In simple displaced fractures, closed reduction and casting will not be successful because of fracture instability. Reduction and stabilization are via medial and lateral surgical approaches. Reduction and stabilization of T-type or fracture dislocations are via the transolecranon approach. Stable fixation is difficult to achieve because the distal fragments are small and a large percentage of the fragment surface is covered with articular cartilage. Ulnar nerve transposition allows the cubital tunnel to be used as an additional point of fixation. Laterally, the posterior distal extraarticular portion of the capitellum is the preferred point of fixation. Simple displaced fractures are stabilized with screws inserted from the cubital tunnel and distal capitellum, across the fracture, and up the medial and lateral columns, and one-third tubular or reconstruction plates may be used. In T-type fractures, the distal fragments are first lagged together and then fixed to the proximal humerus. Because there is no bone loss, lagging the distal fragments will not result in a discongruous joint.

Postoperatively, supervised active motion is started when incisional pain allows. When the patient is not undergoing physical therapy, the fixation is protected in a long arm splint. At 6 to 8 weeks, the splint is discontinued.

Complications

All patients lose elbow motion, particularly extension. Loss of motion is less significant in undisplaced fractures than it is in T-type or fracture dislocations.

The complication unique to transcondylar fractures is loss of fixation. This is due to the small size of the distal fragments and their osteopenia. Patients are followed at biweekly intervals with radiographs. If loss of fixation is starting to occur, the elbow is immobilized until healing of the fracture has occurred. If loss of fixation has already occurred, the fixation can either be revised or active range of motion exercises can be continued. Revision of the fixation is difficult and stabilization of the fracture may not be possible. Active range of motion is encouraged with the expectation that the fracture will go on to nonunion but a functional range of motion will be maintained.

FRACTURES OF MEDIAL AND LATERAL CONDYLES OF THE HUMERUS

Isolated fractures of the medial or lateral condyle of the humerus are rare. The fragment includes the entire condyle (the epicondyle and either the capitellum or trochlea) or just the articular portion of the condyle (capitellum or trochlea).

Classification

Isolated fractures of the medial or lateral condyle of the humerus are first classified according to whether they involve the entire condyle or just the articular portion of the condyle. The distinction between these two types of fractures is important because fractures involving only the trochlea or capitellum are avascular with no soft tissue attachments. Fractures of the entire condyle occur in a younger age group than fractures of the capitellum and trochlea.

Milch divided **fractures of the entire condyle** into two groups: avulsion fractures and compression fractures (Fig. 9–3).

Avulsion fractures are the result of a varus (lateral condyle fracture) or valgus (medial condyle fracture) stress across the elbow. Radiographically, they are recognized by distal displacement of the fracture fragment. **Compression fractures** are produced by impaction of the trochlea or radial head into the distal humerus. This impaction can be the result of a longitudinal force or a varus (fracture of the medial condyle) or valgus (fracture of the lateral condyle) force across the elbow. Radiographically, compression fractures are recognized by proximal displacement of the fragment.

Compression fractures are further divided into stable fractures and fracture dislocations. The key to stability is the status of the trochlea. In the case of lateral condylar fractures, if the lateral wall of the trochlea is disrupted, the fracture is unstable; if it is intact, the fracture is stable. In the case of medial condylar fractures, if the medial wall of the trochlea is disrupted, the fracture is unstable; if it is intact, the fracture is stable. The olecranon subluxes laterally or medially if the fracture is unstable.

Fractures involving only the articular portion of the condyle are the result of the radial head or coronoid process impacting the **capitellum or trochlea.**

Fractures of the capitellum are divided into three groups (Fig. 9–4): the **Hahn-Steinthal** fracture, in which the fragment includes the entire

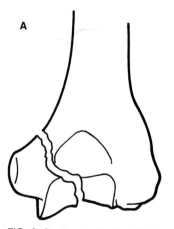

FIG. 9–3 The classification of isolated fractures of the humeral condyles: (*a*) avulsion fracture of the medial condyle, (*b*) avulsion fracture of the lateral condyle, (*c*) unstable compression fracture of the medial condyle, and (*d*) stable compression fracture of the lateral condyle.

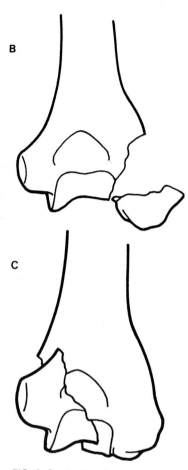

FIG. 9–3   *Continued*

capitellum (Fig. 9–5); the **Kocher-Lorenz** fracture, in which the fragment includes only subchondral bone and the articular surface; and the **compression** fracture of the capitellum with comminution of the articular surface. Isolated fractures of the trochlea are rare, and usually are associated with a fracture of the capitellum. Their management is covered under transcondylar fractures.

D

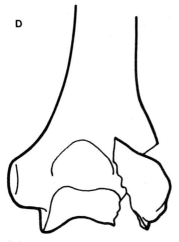

FIG. 9–3 *Continued*

A

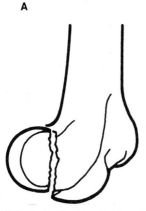

FIG. 9–4 The classification of isolated fractures of the capitellum: (*a*) Hahn-Steinthal fracture, (*b*) Kocher-Lorenz fracture, and (*c*) compression fracture of the capitellum.

B

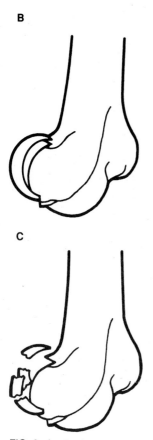

C

FIG. 9–4   *Continued*

Diagnosis and Initial Management

History and Physical Examination

The physical findings other than pain and limitation of motion are not remarkable, unless there is an associated dislocation. Occasionally, when the capitellum is fractured, the fragment can be palpated laterally.

Radiographic Examination

Anteroposterior and lateral radiographs confirm the diagnosis.

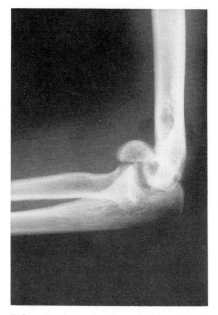

FIG. 9–5   A lateral radiograph of the elbow. There is a Hahn-Steinthal fracture of the capitellum.

Initial Management

The elbow is splinted at 90° and iced.

Associated Injuries

Other than sprain of the contralateral collateral ligament, there are no specific injuries associated with fractures of the humeral condyles. The focused neurovascular exam is performed, and radiographs of the shoulder, humerus, forearm, and wrist should be obtained.

Definitive Management

Definitive management of displaced fractures of the humeral condyles is operative. The two options are reduction and stabilization, or excision of the fragments. Excision is only an option for fractures of the capitellum.

Open Reduction and Internal Fixation

Fractures of the entire lateral condyle are approached through the interval between the extensor carpi ulnaris and the anconeus (the Kocher J approach) or through the anconeus approach as described by Pankovich. Flexion of the elbow and extension of the wrist relaxes the extensor muscles inserting on the fragment, thus aiding reduction. Usually there is a large spike of epicondyle that can be fixed to the humeral metaphysis with screws or a plate. Fractures of the capitellum are exposed through the anconeus approach. The Hahn-Steinthal fracture is stabilized with Herbert screws, small countersunk bone screws, or with threaded Kirschner wires directed anterior to posterior and buried below the articular surface. In Kocher-Lorenz and compression fractures, the fragment may be excised.

Fractures of the medial condyle are approached through a straight medial incision taking care to protect the ulnar nerve. Like fractures of the lateral condyle, these usually are easily reduced and stabilized. Flexion of the elbow and wrist relaxes the flexor mass which is attached to the fragment. Fractures of the trochlea, unstable condylar fractures, and isolated fractures of the trochlea are approached through a transolecranon exposure. Fixation is according to the surgeon's preference, but should be strong enough to allow early motion and a low profile to minimize irritation of surrounding tissues with motion.

Postoperatively, the arm is protected in a splint and sling. When incisional pain has decreased, supervised range of motion is begun. At 6 weeks, the fracture is healed enough to discontinue the sling.

Complications

The complications of isolated condylar fractures include arthritis, loss of motion, and subluxation of the elbow joint. **Arthritis** is managed as described in the supracondylar fracture of the humerus section.

Loss of motion may occur because of failure to realign the centers of rotation of the capitellum and trochlea. Theoretically, revision of the reduction in an unhealed fracture, or osteotomy and realignment in a healed fracture, would increase the range of motion. Resection of the radial head is a more practical solution.

Subluxation occurs most frequently following fracture of the entire lateral condyle in which the lateral wall of the trochlea is involved. The tendency to sublux is an indication for open reduction and rigid stabilization.

RADIAL HEAD FRACTURES

Radial head fractures involve the proximal intraarticular portion of the radius.

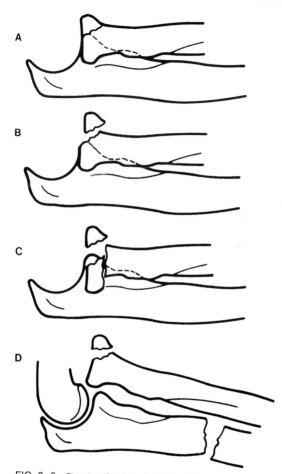

FIG. 9-6   The classification of radial head fractures: (*a*) type I, (*b*) type II, (*c*) type III, and (*d*) type IV. In this drawing, a Monteggia fracture dislocation is illustrated.

Classification

Fractures of the radial head are classified according to displacement, extent of involvement, and associated dislocations (Fig. 9-6). Type I are undisplaced. Type II are displaced fractures involving only part of the head. Type III involve the entire head and are frequently comminuted. Type IV are radial head fractures associated with elbow instability or radioulnar dissociation (i.e., the Essex-Lopresti lesion or Monteggia equivalent).

Diagnosis and Initial Management

History and Physical Examination

There is pain localized to the radial head. The mechanism of injury is usually a fall forward with the elbow extended and the forearm pronated. The necessity for operative or closed management is determined clinically. The two important indications for operative intervention are a block to forearm rotation and ligamentous instability. The hematoma is aspirated and the elbow injected with local anesthetic. The forearm is passively rotated with the elbow in different degrees of flexion. Ligamentous instability is due to disruption of the medial collateral ligament. Stability is assessed with the arm externally rotated and the elbow flexed 15°, relaxing the anterior capsule and removing the olecranon from the olecranon fossae. A gentle valgus stress is applied to the elbow. If the elbow ''books'' open, the medial collateral ligament is torn.

Radiographic Examination

Anteroposterior and lateral views confirm the diagnosis. The radiocapitellar view may provide additional information. The forearm is placed in neutral rotation, and the elbow is flexed and positioned on the cassette as for a routine lateral. The x-ray tube is angulated 45° toward the humeral head. Other radiographic projections, tomograms, and CT scans are not necessary.

Initial Management

The elbow is splinted at 90° and placed in a sling. In cases in which the radial head is dislocated, open reduction is performed emergently.

Associated Injuries

Associated neurovascular injuries are uncommon but must be ruled out. Radiographs of the humerus shoulder and wrist are obtained. The distal radioulnar joint is examined for tenderness, instability, and prominence of the distal ulna. If these are present, there may be an associated Essex-Lopresti lesion. The distal humerus is examined for associated fractures of the capitellum and avulsion fractures of the medial epicondyle (indicative of a medial-collateral ligament avulsion).

Definitive Management

Management is based on the type of fracture. Type I fractures (undisplaced) and type II and III fractures without a mechanical block are managed nonoperatively. The patient is placed in a sling for 3 weeks and gentle active range of motion is encouraged. At 3 weeks, the sling is discontinued and more aggressive physical therapy is initiated.

Fractures associated with elbow instability or with a mechanical block to elbow motion are managed operatively. The decision to reduce and internally fix the fracture or to excise the radial head, with or without prosthetic replacement, is made once the fracture is exposed. Circumstances that mitigate against fixation of the radial head are: an elderly patient, injury of the capitellum, and preexisting osteoarthritis. Circumstances that mitigate for fixation include: a young patient, experienced surgeon, involvement of only part of the radial head (i.e., a type II), and associated dislocation of the radial head (i.e., a type IV). In cases with associated ligamentous injuries, there are three alternatives: reduction and fixation of the head, excision and replacement of the head with a silastic spacer, or ligament repair.

Exposure is via the anconeus approach. The interval between the anconeus and flexor carpi ulnaris is developed. The insertion of the anconeus is reflected from the ulna and joint capsule by blunt dissection. If the capsule and synovium are not torn, they are incised longitudinally. We do not hesitate to incise up to two-thirds of the annular ligament to obtain wider exposure. In addition, the proximal or distal portion of the capsular incision can be T'ed. As the forearm is pronated and supinated, the entire radial head is visualized. Associated fractures of the ulna are reduced and stabilized through the same approach.

Fragments are reduced and fixed with cortical screws, Herbert screws, or Kirschner wires. Ideally, the implants are buried below the articular cartilage. It is important to remember that the anterolateral quadrant of the radial head does not articulate with the ulna and is, therefore, the optimum location for fixation. If depression of the articular surface is present, reduction and bone grafting are performed. If the radial head is resected, the neck is preserved. The edges of the metaphysis are smoothed and any bony spikes are removed. If a silastic spacer is inserted, the largest size possible is used. The wound is closed over a small drain.

After fixation or radial head excision, the elbow and forearm are put through the range of motion. If the elbow subluxes, the medial collateral ligament or anterior capsular structures are repaired through a medial incision. In addition to elbow stability, the stability of the distal radioulnar joint is assessed. If radioulnar dissociation is present the distal ulna will sublux dorsally with pronation of the forearm.

Postoperatively, the arm is placed in a sling. A splint is added if there is associated ligamentous injury. The sling or splint is removed three times a day for supervised active range of motion exercises. At 3 to 4 weeks, the sling and splint are discontinued. Patients with associated radioulnar dissociation present a unique set of problems. In these injuries, the interosseous membrane and distal radial ulnar joint capsule are disrupted and pronation and supination exercises may result in displacement. Therefore, after open reduction and internal fixation of the radial head, the distal radioulnar joint is pinned with the forearm in neutral rotation. Four weeks postinjury the pin is removed. The splint is continued but is removed three times a day for active range of motion. At 6 weeks the splint is discontinued. In cases in which a prosthesis has been used, consideration is given to removal of the prosthesis 1 year postinjury in young patients. The concept is that the complications of implant breakage and silicone synovitis are minimized, and that at 1 year postinjury, the radius will not migrate proximally.

Complications

The complications following radial head fracture include loss of motion, posttraumatic arthritis, and shortening of the radius with resultant wrist pain.

Loss of motion is a difficult problem for which there is frequently no solution. Intensive physical therapy, removal of implants or debridement of the joint, and possible excision of the radial head are methods of management.

Posttraumatic arthritis is managed with excision of the radial head, or with nonsteroidal anti-inflammatories and occasional local steroid injections.

Radial shortening follows excision of the radial head. The patient complains of pain at the distal radioulnar joint. In many cases, there is obvious proximal migration of the radius in relation to the ulna. In questionable cases, the diagnosis is confirmed radiographically by obtaining anteroposterior views of the distal radioulnar joint with the forearm relaxed and with the patient making a fist. In symptomatic cases in which conservative therapy has failed, the management of radial shortening is ulnar shortening, or fusion of the distal radioulnar joint and resection of 1 cm of the distal ulnar diaphysis to produce a nonunion.

OLECRANON FRACTURES

Olecranon fractures involve the ulna proximal to the coronoid process. The majority of olecranon fractures are intraarticular. There may be an associated fracture of the radial head, or anterior displacement of the distal ulna with an anterior dislocation of the radiocapitellar articulation. The absence of a diastasis distinguishes olecranon fractures from other injuries (e.g., Monteggia fracture) which also involve the proximal ulna.

Classification

Olecranon fractures are classified into six types based on the presence of displacement, intraarticular involvement, comminution, radial head fracture, and radiocapitellar dislocation (Fig. 9–7). Type I fractures are displaced less than 2 mm, without an intraarticular stepoff. Type II

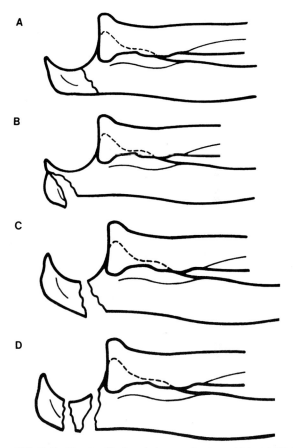

FIG. 9–7 The classification of olecranon fractures: (*a*) type I, (*b*) type II, (*c*) type III, (*d*) type IV, (*e*) type V, and (*f*) type VI.

fractures are extraarticular, and involve the proximal portion of the olecranon. These fractures are an avulsion of the triceps from the proximal ulna. Type III fractures are simple intraarticular fractures with a transverse or oblique pattern. Type IV fractures are comminuted. The fracture lines may extend distal to the olecranon, and there may be depression of an intraarticular segment. Type V and VI fractures are an olecranon fracture with either an associated anterior dislocation of

E

F

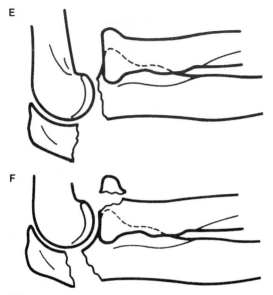

FIG. 9–7 *Continued*

the radiocapitellar articulation or an associated radial head fracture. The olecranon fracture in a type V or VI fracture is invariably displaced and intraarticular (i.e., a type III or IV fracture).

Diagnosis and Initial Management

History and Physical Examination

There is pain localized to the elbow and a history of trauma. Type II fractures are caused by indirect trauma, while type III and IV fractures are caused by direct trauma. Type V and VI fractures are high-energy injuries caused by a combination of direct and indirect forces. The physical findings are ecchymosis swelling and, if the fracture is displaced, a palpable gap at the fracture site. A break in the skin is assumed to communicate with the fracture.

Radiographic Examination

Lateral and anteroposterior views of the elbow are obtained. The lateral indicates the location and direction of the fracture line, the degree of comminution, and whether there is an associated radiocapitellar dislocation. The anteroposterior indicates the presence of an associated radial head fracture. Oblique views and tomograms are not helpful in determining if surgery is necessary or how the fracture should be stabilized.

Initial Management

The arm is placed in a sling for comfort. A splint is not required. If there is an associated anterior subluxation, a closed reduction will not be successful due to instability, and the fracture should be stabilized as soon as possible.

Associated Injuries

Associated neurovascular injuries are rare but must be ruled out. Radiographs of the humerus, shoulder, forearm, and wrist are obtained.

Definitive Management

The goal of management is an elbow with a functional, painless range of flexion and extension. It is important to preserve flexion even at the cost of losing extension; therefore, prolonged splinting of the elbow in extension is seldom indicated. The articular surface must be anatomically reduced to minimize the incidence of posttraumatic arthritis.

Undisplaced fractures (type I) are managed by splinting the elbow at 90° for 3 weeks. The splint is removed once a day for active range of motion. Radiographs are obtained at weekly intervals to confirm that the fragments have not displaced. At 3 weeks, the splint is discontinued and a sling is used for the next 3 weeks.

Type II, III, IV, V, and VI fractures are managed surgically. Type II through V fractures are approached by way of a straight posterior incision over the subcutaneous border of the olecranon. Type II and transverse type III fractures can be stabilized using the tension band technique with 2.0-mm Kirschner wires and an 18-gauge wire. A 6.5-mm cancellous screw and washer can be substituted for the Kirschner wires. Oblique type III fractures and all type IV and V fractures are stabilized with a plate and screws. A semitubular or 3.5-mm dynamic compression plate is used. Fixation with a plate as opposed to a tension band wire is indicated for two reasons: first, to prevent shortening of axially unstable fractures (i.e., oblique type III fractures and type IV fractures); and second, to provide rigid stabilization of the olecranon and prevent anterior subluxation of the radial head in patients with type V fractures. Type VI fractures have an associated fracture of the radial head. The radial head fracture is reduced and stabilized or the radial head is excised via the anconeus approach.

Postoperatively, early active motion is encouraged after incisional pain has become tolerable (usually by the third postoperative day).

Complications

Complications include loss of fixation, nonunion, infection, posttraumatic arthritis, and radioulnar synostosis.

Loss of fixation is managed either by revising the fixation or by excising the proximal fragment and attaching the triceps tendon to the remaining olecranon. Before the fragment is excised, it must be confirmed that the elbow is stable without the fragment (i.e., that the radial head and remaining olecranon will not sublux anteriorly once the fragment is removed). If a minimum of 30° of the trochlear notch remains, the elbow will probably be stable, but this must be confirmed intraoperatively by removing all fixation, flexing the elbow to 90°, and gently stressing the elbow.

Nonunion may be asymptomatic due to fibrous tissue between the fragments. Symptomatic nonunions are managed with reduction, plate fixation, and autogenous cancellous bone grafting.

Infection is a common occurrence because of the subcutaneous location of the fracture. It is to be managed aggressively because it involves the elbow joint. Fixation is removed to gain access to the joint that is debrided and irrigated. Necrotic bone is debrided, and the fracture stabilized. Systemic antibiotics are continued a minimum of 6 weeks.

Posttraumatic arthritis is managed conservatively if possible with nonsteroidal anti-inflammatories or steroid injections. Surgical alternatives include arthrodesis and arthroplasty.

Radioulnar synostosis occurs most frequently following type IV, V, or VI fractures. Management alternatives include doing nothing, resection of an osseous bridge, or osteotomy to place the hand in a more functional position.

ELBOW DISLOCATIONS

This section reviews elbow dislocations, excluding Monteggia fractures and isolated dislocations of the radial head.

Classification

Elbow dislocations are classified according to the position of the radius and ulna in relation to the distal humerus. The types of elbow dislocations are posterior, medial, lateral, anterior, and divergent.

Posterior dislocations are by the far the most common type of elbow dislocation. In addition to being posteriorly displaced, the radius and ulna may be displaced slightly laterally or medially. The presence of medial or lateral displacement does not affect the management or the prognosis; therefore, we classify all posterior dislocations together.

Medial and lateral dislocations are rare injuries. These have a poorer prognosis than the more common posterior dislocation. Frequently, a medial or lateral dislocation is, in reality, a subluxation (i.e., in a medial dislocation, the trochlear notch articulates with the medial epicondyle and the radial head articulates with the trochlea; in a lateral dislocation, the trochlear notch articulates with the capitellum) (Fig. 9–8).

Anterior dislocations of the elbow are extremely rare injuries. The mechanism of injury is either traction on the forearm with the elbow extended or a blow to the posterior aspect of the flexed elbow.

Divergent dislocations are also rare injuries. They are distinct from other types of elbow dislocations because there is dissociation of the radius and ulna. The annular ligament and interosseous membrane must be torn for a divergent dislocation to occur. There are two varieties, anteroposterior and medial lateral. In anteroposterior divergent dislocations, the radial head is dislocated anteriorly into the coronoid fossa and the ulna is dislocated posteriorly with the coronoid process in the olecranon fossa. In medial-lateral divergent dislocations, the radial head articulates with the trochlea and the trochlear notch articulates with the capitellum.

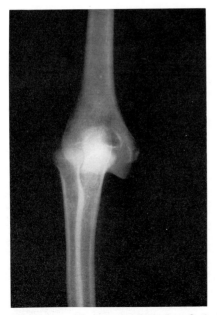

FIG. 9–8   Lateral dislocation of the elbow. On the lateral projection (not shown), the olecranon articulates with the capitellum.

Diagnosis and Initial Management

History and Physical Examination

The patient presents with pain and swelling of the elbow. All elbow dislocations are characterized by loss of the normal relationship of the epicondyles to the tip of the olecranon. This physical finding may be obscured by swelling. However, if present, it distinguishes elbow dislocation from other injuries such as extra articular supracondylar and transcondylar fracture of the humerus. Posterior dislocations are further characterized by apparent shortening of the forearm and the elbow's being fixed in 45° of flexion. In medial and lateral dislocations, the elbow appears wider than normal, and there may be some active and passive motion of the elbow. In anterior dislocations, the elbow is fixed in extension, the forearm is usually supinated, and the capitellum and trochlea are palpable posteriorly. In divergent dislocations, the forearm appears shortened and the elbow is fixed in varying amounts of flexion.

Radiographic Examination

The diagnosis of elbow dislocation is confirmed by anteroposterior and lateral radiographs. Oblique views are helpful to further define the relationship between the distal humerus and the radius and ulna. Special views, tomograms, and CT scans usually do not help to define the injury further.

Initial Management

The elbow is splinted or held in a sling until radiographs are obtained and a closed reduction can be performed.

Associated Injuries

Associated injuries of the surrounding neurovascular structures occur. The most clinically significant is injury of the brachial artery. Associated injuries of the median, ulnar, and radial nerves occur with relative frequency. Therefore, a careful neurologic exam is performed. Associated bony injuries are also common. The most clinically significant is fracture of the radial head or neck. An undisplaced fracture of the radial head or neck may displace during closed reduction. In addition to radial head and neck fractures, there frequently are fractures of the medial or lateral epicondyles. These become clinically significant when they prevent a concentric reduction, or if they remain displaced and nonunion is likely. The distal humerus is examined for evidence of osteochondral fractures that increase the likelihood of posttraumatic osteoarthritis and prevent concentric reduction. Radiographs of the shoulder, humerus, forearm, and wrist are obtained.

Definitive Management

In most cases, management is closed reduction under local anesthesia followed by splinting. Regional or general anesthesia with fluoroscopic monitoring of the reduction is indicated if there is an associated undisplaced radial head or neck fracture. Open reduction is indicated if there are any of the following: interposed osteochondral fragment preventing concentric reduction, irreducible dislocation, operative fracture of the radial head or neck, or ligamentous instability.

Closed reduction is performed as atraumatically as possible. This requires adequate analgesia and muscle relaxation. Analgesia is achieved by aspirating the hematoma and injecting local anesthetic. Muscle relaxation is obtained by intravenous administration of a sedative. The specific reduction maneuver depends on the type of dislocation.

Posterior dislocation is reduced by traction in line with the deformity for several minutes, allowing the coronoid process to slip distally past the humerus, and the elbow is flexed to 90°. There should be immediate relief of pain and increased motion. If this maneuver fails, the patient is placed prone on a stretcher with the arm and forearm hanging over the edge. Five to ten pounds of weight are suspended from the wrist. After 5 min, the arm is lifted, flexing and reducing the elbow. If these maneuvers are not effective, the dislocation is considered irreducible and open reduction is performed.

Medial and lateral dislocations are reduced by traction and medial or lateral pressure.

Anterior dislocations are reduced by applying longitudinal traction to the forearm. Pressure is applied to the anterior aspect of the forearm, while counterpressure is applied to the posterior aspect of the humerus.

Anteroposterior divergent dislocations are reduced by first reducing the ulna and then the radius. The ulna is reduced as if it were a posterior dislocation. The radial head is reduced by direct pressure and supination of the forearm. Medial-lateral dislocations are reduced with traction and by pressing the radius and ulna together.

Surgical exposure for **open reduction** is via the anconeus approach. The appropriate debridement or repair of lateral structures is performed. If there is marked medial instability, the medial side is approached through an incision over the cubital tunnel. The ulnar nerve is transposed anteriorly, exposing the medial capsule and intracapsular ligaments which are repaired.

Complications

Complications of elbow dislocations include posttraumatic arthritis, loss of motion, chronic instability, and heterotopic ossification. The management of **posttraumatic arthritis** and **loss of motion** has been described.

Chronic instability results in arthritis, pain, and loss of motion. It can take the form of redislocation or inability to resist a valgus stress. If it is discovered within 4 weeks of injury, an open reduction is performed and the anterior capsular structures and medial-collateral ligament are repaired primarily. In cases in which the elbow has redislocated, it is necessary to pin the humeroulnar and radiocapitellar joint in order to maintain the reduction. Chronic instability is managed conservatively with a brace and activity modification, a ligamentous reconstruction, or arthrodesis of the elbow.

Heterotopic ossification usually involves the collateral ligaments, capsule, or brachialis. Initially, it is managed by discontinuing all passive motion exercises and administering indomethicin. After the heterotopic bone has matured, as indicated by a cold bone scan and normal serum alkaline phosphatase levels, it can be excised. Preoperatively, CT scans and MRIs help to delineate the relationship of the heterotopic ossification to surrounding nerves and arteries.

SELECTED READINGS

General

Cassebaum WH: Operative treatment of T and Y fractures of the lower end of the humerus. *Am J Surg* 83:265, 1952.

Morrey BF: Anatomy and kinematics of the elbow, in Tullos HS (ed): *Instructional Course Lectures*. Park Ridge, Illinois, The American Academy of Orthopaedic Surgeons, 1991, vol XL, pp 11–16.

Pankovich AM: Anconeus approach to the elbow joint and the proximal part of the radius and ulna. *J Bone Joint Surg* 59A:124–126, 1977.

Supracondylar Fractures of the Humerus

Niemann KMW: Condylar fractures of the distal humerus in adults. *South Med J* 70:915–918, 1977.

Riseborough EJ, Radin EL: Intercondylar T fractures of the humerus in the adult. A comparison of operative and non-operative treatment in twenty-nine cases. *J Bone Joint Surg* 51A:130–141, 1969.

Transcondylar Fractures

Grantham SA, Tietjen R: Transcondylar fracture-dislocation of the elbow: A case report. *J Bone Joint Surg* 58A:1030–1031, 1976.

Perry CR, Gibson CT, Kowalski MF: Transcondylar fractures of the distal humerus. *J Orthop Trauma* 3:98–106, 1989.

Fractures of the Medial and Lateral Condyles of the Humerus

Fowles JV, Kassab MT: Fracture of the capitellum humeri: Treatment by excision. *J Bone Joint Surg* 56A:794–798, 1974.

Milch H: Fractures and fracture dislocations of the humeral condyles. *J Trauma* 4:592–607, 1964.

Radial Head Fractures

Mason ML: Some observations on fractures of the head of the radius with a review of one hundred cases. *Br J Surg* 42:123–132, 1954.

Morrey BF, Askew L, Chao EY: Silastic prosthetic replacement for the radial head. *J Bone Joint Surg* 63A:454–458, 1981.

Morrey BF, Chao EYS: Passive motion of the elbow joint. A biomechanical analysis. *J Bone Joint Surg* 58A:501–508, 1992.

Olecranon Fractures

Hume MC, Wiss DA: Olecranon fractures: A clinical and radiographic comparison of tension band wiring and plate fixation. *Clin Orthop* 285:229–235, 1992.

Elbow Dislocations

Durig M, Muller W, Ruedi TP, Gauer EF: The operative treatment of elbow dislocation in the adult. *J Bone Joint Surg* 61A:239–244, 1979.

Linscheid RL, Wheeler DK: Elbow dislocations. *J Am Med Assoc* 194:1171–1176, 1965.

10 | Injuries of the Forearm

Clayton R. Perry

This chapter reviews diaphyseal and metaphyseal fractures of the radius and ulna and radioulnar diastasis.

ANATOMY

Important anatomic features of the forearm include: the radius, the ulna, the proximal and distal radioulnar articulations, the interosseous membrane, muscles, nerves, and arteries. The proximal and distal radio-ulnar articulations are described in Chapters 9 and 11.

The **radius** is an extension of the hand. Straightening of its apex lateral bow results in loss of forearm rotation. The shaft of the radius is triangular in cross section with its ulnar corner, serving as the attachment of the interosseous membrane. The blood supply of the diaphyseal cortex of the radius is via periosteal and intramedullary vessels. The intramedullary vessels originate from a single nutrient artery that enters the radius via a foramina on the anterior surface of the radius in its proximal third.

The **ulna** is an extension of the arm; it has a slight apex posterior curve. The proximal half of the ulna has an apex lateral curve, and the distal half has an apex medial curve. The radial border of the ulna serves as the attachment of the interosseous membrane. The posterior, or subcutaneous, surface is the origin of the deep fascia of the forearm. The blood supply of the ulna is via periosteal and intramedullary vessels. The intramedullary vessels originate from a single nutrient artery that enters the ulna via a foramina located on the anterior surface of the ulna just proximal to its midpoint.

The **interosseous membrane** is a fascial sheet whose fibers are directed fan-wise from the radius to the ulna. A condensation of fibers in its midsubstance is termed the **interosseous ligament.** Gaps in the interosseous membrane transmit the anterior and posterior interosseous vessels. The interosseous membrane separates the flexor and extensor compartments and serves as the origin of both flexor and extensor muscles. It also dampens the transmission of proximally directed forces along the radius to the capitellum. An intact interosseous membrane is strong enough to resist proximal migration of the radius, making possible resection of the radial head.

The **muscles** of the forearm are divided into flexor and extensor compartments. The **flexors** are further divided into superficial flexors which originate from the humerus and deep flexors which originate from the radius, ulna, and interosseous membrane. The superficial group includes the pronator teres, flexor carpi radialis, palmaris longus, flexor carpi ulnaris, and flexor digitorum superficialis. The deep flexor group includes the flexor digitorum profundus, the flexor pollicis longus, and the pronator quadratus. All the flexors are innervated by the median nerve or its terminal muscular branch, the anterior interosseous nerve, except the flexor carpi ulnaris and the ulnar side of the flexor digitorum profundus. These are innervated by the ulnar nerve.

The **extensor** compartment is divided into superficial and deep groups. The muscles of the superficial group originate from the humerus and common extensor tendon. The superficial group includes the brachioradialis, the extensor carpi radialis longus and brevis, the extensor digitorum, the extensor digiti minimi, and the extensor carpi ulnaris. The deep extensor group includes the supinator, abductor pollicis longus, the extensor pollicis longus and brevis, and the extensor indicis. The muscles of the deep extensor group, with the exception of the supinator, originate from the radius, ulna, and interosseous membrane. The muscles of the extensor compartment are innervated by the radial nerve or its terminal muscular branch, the posterior interosseous nerve.

Three muscles span the radius and ulna: the pronator teres, the pronator quadratus, and the supinator. Following a forearm fracture, they narrow the interosseous space, resulting in loss of forearm rotation.

The **brachial artery** divides into the **radial and ulnar artery** a centimeter distal to the elbow joint. The radial artery runs along the radial side of the forearm to the wrist, where it lies between the flexor carpi radialis tendon and the radius. It is most easily palpated here. The radial artery terminates in the deep palmar arch. The ulnar artery runs along the ulnar side of the forearm until it reaches the wrist. Along the way, it gives off several branches, the most important of which is the common interosseous artery. The common interosseous artery in turn gives off the anterior and posterior interosseous arteries. The anterior interosseous artery runs on the anterior surface of the interosseous membrane with the anterior interosseous branch of the median nerve. It gives off muscular branches and the nutrient arteries supplying the radius and the ulna. The posterior interosseous artery traverses the interosseous membrane proximally to reach the extensor compartment, where it runs between the superficial and deep groups of muscles, giving off numerous muscular branches.

Classification

Injuries of the forearm are broadly classified into two groups: simple and complex. **Simple** injuries are fractures without associated ligamentous disruption. Included in this group are isolated fractures of the radius and ulna (the ''nightstick'' fracture), and fractures of both the radius and the ulna (the ''both-bone'' fracture) (Figs. 10–1 to 10–5). Simple injuries are the result of direct trauma (e.g., a blow to the forearm).

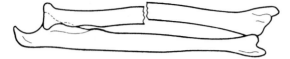

FIG. 10–1   Nightstick fracture of the radius.

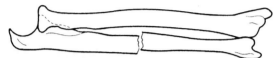

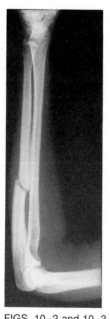

FIGS. 10–2 and 10–3   Nightstick fractures of the ulna.

They are described as being open or closed; simple or comminuted; and displaced, shortened, or angulated.

Complex injuries are characterized by ligamentous disruption. These injuries disrupt either the proximal, distal, or both radioulnar articulations and part, or all, of the interosseous membrane. The soft tissue

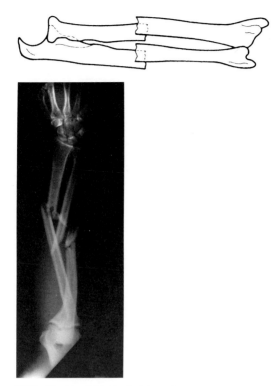

FIGS. 10–4 and 10–5 Both-bone fractures.

component of these complex injuries, in many cases, is more significant than the fracture.

The **Monteggia** fracture is usually a fracture of the mid- or proximal ulna with an anterior dislocation of the radial head (Fig. 10–6). The mechanism of injury can be either forced pronation or result from a direct blow to the dorsum of the ulna. This injury includes a tear of the annular ligament and disruption of the interosseous membrane from its most proximal extent to the fracture of the ulna.

The **Galeazzi fracture** and **fracture of the distal ulna with ligamentous disruption** are fractures of the distal third of the radius or ulna and a dislocation of the distal radioulnar articulation (Figs. 10–7 to 10–9). Both of these fractures are short oblique fractures occurring at the distal metaphyseal diaphyseal junction. The mechanism of injury

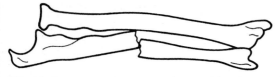

FIG. 10–6   Monteggia fracture, or a fracture of the ulna, associated with a dislocation of the proximal radius.

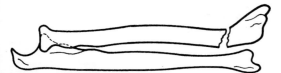

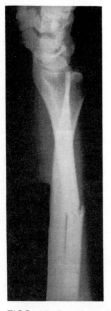

FIGS. 10–7 and 10–8   Galeazzi fracture or a fracture of the distal radius, associated with disruption of the distal radioulnar articulation.

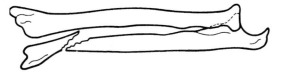

FIG. 10–9   Fracture of the ulna associated with disruption of the distal radioulnar articulation.

of the Galeazzi fracture is forced pronation (usually during a fall on the outstretched hand) or from a direct blow. The mirror injury, fracture of the ulna with dislocation of the distal radioulnar articulation, has been described recently and is not well understood. Both injuries include disruption of the distal radioulnar joint (either tear of the triangular fibrocartilage or avulsion of the ulnar styloid) and a tear of the interosseous membrane from its most distal extent to the fracture of the radius or ulna.

Essex-Lopresti's injury is a fracture of the radial head with disruption of the distal radioulnar articulation and tearing of the entire interosseous membrane. Attention focuses on the radial head fracture, but the major component of the injury is the radial ulnar diastasis. The mechanism of injury has not been adequately described.

Associated Injuries

Injuries associated with fractures of the forearm include fractures and dislocations of the elbow and wrist, neurovascular injuries, and compartment syndromes.

Radiographs of the wrist and elbow determine whether there are associated fractures or dislocations.

Laceration compression or stretching of arteries and nerves frequently occurs at the time of the injury. The greater the initial displacement, the greater the chance of an associated neurovascular injury. The presence of pulses distal to the fracture and capillary refill of the nail beds indicates adequate vascularity. In questionable cases, an arteriogram makes the definitive diagnosis.

The nerve most frequently injured in association with a forearm injury is the posterior interosseous nerve. This is particularly true of Monteggia fractures. Neurologic injury is identified by a focused neurologic examination of the radial ulnar and median nerves.

Compartment syndrome most frequently involves the flexor compartment, but the extensor compartment can also be involved. The patient complains of severe pain. The compartments are tense and any attempt at passive stretch of the muscles in the compartment exacerbates the pain. Measurement of the compartment pressure yields the definitive diagnosis. The management is emergent surgical decompression, including the bicipital aponeurosis proximally and the carpal tunnel distally.

Diagnosis and Initial Management

History and Physical Examination

There is pain and a history of trauma. There may be obvious deformity. The skin is examined for wounds that may communicate with the fracture. The elbow and distal radioulnar articulation are examined to determine whether they have been injured.

Radiographic Examination

Radiographs in the anteroposterior and lateral projections of the forearm, wrist, and elbow are adequate to evaluate most injuries of the forearm. Occasionally, comparison views of the opposite wrist, or CT scans of both wrists, are helpful in evaluating the relative positions of the distal radius and ulna. Stress views obtained by radially deviating the wrist may be diagnostic of Essex-Lopresti's injury.

Initial Management

Initial management is aligning and splinting the forearm. Displaced or angulated fractures are aligned by administering a hematoma block and applying traction across the forearm by suspending the hand from fingertraps and hanging 5 to 20 lb of weight from the arm. Anatomic alignment of fractures that will be managed operatively is not necessary. Some shortening or angulation is acceptable because it will be corrected at surgery. A splint extending from the proximal humerus across the elbow to the metacarpophalangeal joints is applied. The elbow is flexed to 90° with the forearm in neutral rotation. If the radial head cannot be reduced with closed methods following a Monteggia fracture, open reduction and stabilization are performed within 24 h of injury to minimize the incidence of neurovascular compromise.

Isolated fractures of the radius or ulna (nightstick fractures) are managed nonoperatively if displaced less than 50 percent and angulated less than 15°. A splint is applied that extends from the elbow to metacarpophalangeal joints. The splint is on the ulnar side of the forearm for ulnar fractures and on the volar side of the forearm for radial fractures.

Definitive Management

Simple Injuries of the Forearm

Isolated fractures of the radius and ulna that are displaced less than 50 percent, angulated less than 15°, and in which the interosseous space is maintained are managed nonoperatively. These fractures are splinted as described in the "Initial Management" section. At 1 week, the splint is removed. If the radius is fractured, the forearm is placed in a short arm cast that is molded to maintain the interosseous space. If the ulna is fractured, the forearm is lightly wrapped in a compression bandage. Radiographs are obtained at 1, 3, and 6 weeks to confirm that alignment has not changed and the fracture is healing.

Isolated fractures of the radius and ulna that are displaced, angulated, or in which the interosseous space is compromised are reduced and stabilized. Fractures of the proximal half of the radius are approached dorsally; fractures of the distal half of the radius are approached volarly. Fractures of the ulna are approached along the subcutaneous border. The fracture is reduced and stabilized with a dynamic compression plate. If more than half the cortex is comminuted, the fracture is grafted with autogenous cancellous bone.

Intramedullary nailing is indicated for segmental fractures and for fractures of the proximal radius in which the posterior interosseous nerve is vulnerable to injury during the exposure. The nails are inserted ulnar to Lister's tubercle for fractures of the radius and via the olecranon for fractures of the ulna. The nails are bent to restore the normal bow of the radius and ulna, reestablishing the interosseous space.

Postoperatively, active range of motion of the forearm, wrist, and elbow is encouraged. If the fracture has been plated, it is assessed as being healed when trabeculae cross the fracture radiographically. This may take up to 6 months. Callus, displacement, or angulation indicate loss of fixation. Healing of fractures that have been stabilized with an intramedullary nail is easier to assess because fixation is not rigid and the patient's symptoms correlate with the amount of healing.

Complex Injuries

An important part of management of complex injuries is postoperative immobilization to allow healing of ligamentous disruptions.

Monteggia's fracture is managed operatively. The ulna is reduced anatomically and plated. Surgical exposure is via an incision along the subcutaneous border of the ulna. Failure to obtain anatomic reduction of the fracture indicates that the radial head is not reduced. The skin incision is extended proximally along the lateral border of the triceps and the anconeus is elevated, as described in Chapter 9, to expose the radial head and annular ligament. Usually, the block to reduction is an intact annular ligament which must be incised to reduce the radial head. The radial head is reduced and the ulna is plated with a dynamic compression plate. It is not necessary to repair a torn annular ligament. Intraoperative radiographs are obtained to confirm that the reduction is anatomic and that the radial head is reduced. Postoperatively, a long arm splint is applied with the elbow in 90° of flexion and the forearm in neutral rotation. The radial head will remain located with the elbow immobilized in this position.

Galeazzi's fracture and fracture of the distal ulna with radioulnar disruption are managed with rigid plating of the fracture. The surgical exposure is via a volar approach for the radius and for the ulna via a skin incision parallel with its subcutaneous border. When the ulnar styloid is avulsed by the triangular fibrocartilage, it is reduced and stabilized with Kirschner wires or a screw. The distal radioulnar joint is reduced by supinating the forearm. A long arm splint is applied.

Essex-Lopresti's injury is managed with closed reduction and stabilization of the radius to the ulna with percutaneous Kirschner wires. Fractures of the radial head are exposed via the anconeus approach and are either reduced and stabilized or excised and replaced with a radial head implant. Fractures of the ulnar styloid are reduced and stabilized. Postoperatively, a long arm splint is applied with the elbow flexed 90°.

Postoperative management of indirect injuries is similar. The splint is changed to a long arm cast at 2 days. Radiographs every 2 weeks confirm maintenance of reduction. The cast is changed at 2 weeks to remove skin sutures. At 6 weeks, the cast is removed and active range of motion is initiated. Kirschner wires, used to maintain the relationship between the radius and ulna, are removed when the cast is discontinued.

Complications

The complications of injuries of the forearm include malunion, non-union, heterotopic ossification, and subluxation or posttraumatic arthritis of the distal or proximal radioulnar joints.

Malunion of the radius and ulna are managed by osteotomy at the site of the malunion and stabilization with dynamic compression plates.

Asymptomatic **nonunions** do not require treatment. Symptomatic nonunions are reduced, stabilized with a dynamic compression plate, and grafted with autogenous cancellous bone.

Heterotopic ossification is most frequently encountered following forearm injuries resulting from high-energy trauma, or when the patient has a concomitant head injury. It may affect any soft tissue structure, and it becomes symptomatic when it results in loss of motion. When heterotopic ossification is initially noticed, physical therapy is stopped for 1 to 2 weeks. The forearm is maintained in 10° to 20° of supination with a splint, and the arm is rested. At 2 weeks, active range of motion is initiated. Passive range of motion or excision of the bony mass before it is mature is contraindicated. Indications of maturity are a well ossified mass with corticalized margins, a cold bone scan, and a normal serum alkaline phosphatase. Once the heterotopic ossification is mature, it can be excised with the goal of increasing the range of motion. Alternatively, osteotomies of the radius and ulna are performed to place the forearm in the position of maximum function.

Painful **subluxation** and **posttraumatic osteoarthritis** of the radioulnar articulations are managed with nonsteroidal anti-inflammatories and local steroid injections. If these measures fail, proximal radioulnar subluxation is managed by reconstructing the annular ligament with a strip of triceps fascia. Proximal radioulnar arthritis is managed with radial head excision. When there is associated axial instability of the radius, a silastic prosthesis is inserted to prevent proximal migration of the radius. Distal radioulnar subluxation and arthritis are managed by arthrodesing the distal radius and ulna, and resection of a 1-cm section of the distal ulnar metaphysis to produce a nonunion, thus preserving forearm rotation.

SELECTED READINGS

Grace TG, Eversman Jr WW: Forearm fractures: Treatment by rigid fixation with early motion. *J Bone Joint Surg* 62A:433–438, 1980.

Pollock FH, Pankovich AM, Prieto JJ, Lorenz M: The isolated fracture of the ulnar shaft. Treatment without immobilization. *J Bone Joint Surg* 65A:339–342, 1983.

Reckling FW: Unstable fracture-dislocations of the forearm (Monteggia and Galeazzi lesions). *J Bone Joint Surg* 64A:857–863, 1982.

Trousdale RT, Amadio PC, Cooney WP, Morrey BF: Radio-ulnar dissociation. A review of twenty cases. *J Bone Joint Surg* 74A:1486–97, 1992.

Fractures of the Distal
Radius and Distal Radioulnar
Joint Injuries

Donald L. Pruitt

This chapter reviews fractures of the distal radius (within 5 cm of the articular surface) and dislocations of the distal radioulnar joint.

ANATOMY

Important anatomic considerations are the bones, joints, their x-ray appearance, and surrounding soft-tissue structures.

The **distal radius** is fan-shaped when viewed from anterior. The styloid projects past the ulna. On the dorsal surface of the radius is Lister's tubercle which is grooved on its medial side for the tendon of the extensor pollicis longus. The volar surface of the radius is the insertion of the pronator quadratus. Elevation of this muscle gives access to the volar side of the radius. The sigmoid notch articulates with the distal ulna.

The **distal ulna** is made up of the head and styloid. It is grooved dorsally for the extensor carpi ulnaris. The distal portion of the head of the ulna is separated from the lunate and triquetrum by the articular disk, or triangular fibrocartilage. One hundred and eighty degrees of the ulnar head is covered with articular cartilage and articulates with the sigmoid notch of the distal radius. The volar surface of the distal ulna is the origin of the pronator quadratus.

The **wrist joint** is biaxial (i.e., it moves along two axes), and consists of two lesser articulations: the radioscaphoid and radiolunate joints. The radial portion of the radioscaphoid joint is the scaphoid fossa. This part of the radius is fractured in a Chauffer's fracture. The lunate fossa is separated from the scaphoid fossa by a small ridge. The lunate fossae is known as the "die-punch fragment" when fractured and depressed. The normal range of motion is 80° of palmar and 70° of dorsiflexion.

The **distal radioulnar joint** is a uniaxial pivot joint. The radius rotates around a fixed axis, the ulnar attachment of the triangular fibrocartilage. The triangular fibrocartilage complex binds the distal ulna and radius together. It is attached to the ulnar side of the distal radius and to the base of the ulnar styloid. The normal range of motion of the distal radioulnar joint is 80° of supination and 70° of pronation.

Important features of the **radiographic appearance** of the distal radius include radial length, radial angle, and volar tilt. **Radial length** is measured from a line perpendicular to the radial shaft drawn through the lunate fossa to the tip of the radial styloid (normally 12 to 15 mm) (Fig. 11–1). **Radial angle** is the angle between a line drawn through

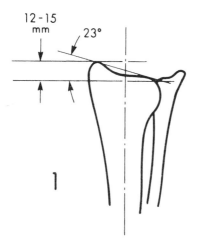

FIG. 11–1   Radial length and radial angle.

the distal radioulnar joint and the radial styloid and a line perpendicular to the radial shaft through the lunate fossa (normally 23°) (Fig. 11–1). **Volar tilt** is measured on the lateral film and is the angle between a line drawn through dorsal and volar rims and a line drawn perpendicular to the radial shaft (normally 15°) (Fig. 11–2).

Surrounding **soft tissue** structures are an important consideration in distal radial fractures. Strong ligaments surround the volar aspect of the radiocarpal joint. The dorsal radiocarpal ligaments are not as stout

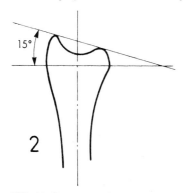

FIG. 11–2   Volar tilt of the distal radius.

as the volar. Extensor tendons travel through retinacular compartments on the dorsal aspect of the wrist. Although rarely injured acutely, attritional ruptures may occur when a malunion is present. Volar to the distal radius is the carpal tunnel, containing nine tendons and median nerve. Symptoms of median nerve dysfunction are checked for in all distal radial fractures. Guyon's canal, containing the ulnar artery, ulnar nerve, and flexor carpi ulnaris tendon, lies volar to the distal radioulnar joint. The radial artery and the flexor carpi radialis tendon are found on the radial side of the volar distal radius.

FRACTURES OF THE DISTAL RADIUS

Classification

Distal radial fractures are classified into three major groups: nondisplaced, displaced extraarticular, and displaced intraarticular.

Nondisplaced fractures are extra- or intraarticular.

Displaced extraarticular fractures either do not involve the radiocarpal or radioulnar articulation, or have an undisplaced extension into one of these joints. They are further classified according to the direction of displacement: dorsally, Colles' fracture; or volarly, Smith's type I or II (Fig. 11–3). Displaced comminuted extraarticular fractures are high-energy injuries.

A

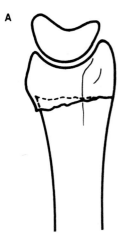

FIG. 11–3   The three types of extraarticular fractures of the distal radius: (*a*) a dorsally displaced, or Colles', fracture; (*b*) a volarly displaced metaphyseal, or Smith's type I, fracture; and (*c*) a volarly displaced fracture that starts at the dorsal rim, or Smith's type II fracture.

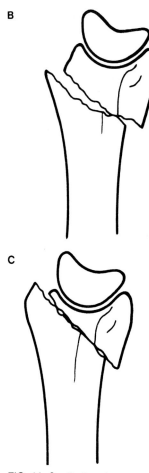

FIG. 11–3   *Continued*

Displaced intraarticular fractures involve the radiocarpal joint, the distal radioulnar joint, or both. Uncorrected articular step-off has a bad prognosis, especially in younger patients. Most often, the articular incongruity involves the lunate fossa (die-punch fragment). Displaced intraarticular fractures are further classified according to whether they are simple or comminuted. Eponyms for these displaced intraarticular fractures are dorsal Barton's, volar Barton's, and Chauffeur's fracture (Fig. 11–4).

Diagnosis and Initial Management

History and Physical Examination

There is pain, swelling, and deformity of the wrist. There are two patient populations that sustain distal radial fractures. The first includes older patients with osteopenic bone who have sustained the fracture during relatively minor trauma (e.g., a fall from a standing position onto an outstretched hand). In this group, the fracture is usually metaphyseal and extraarticular. The second group of patients is younger and sustained the fracture as a result of a high-energy injury (e.g., a fall from a height). Most of these patients have dense bone, and the fracture is often intraarticular and comminuted with associated injuries. A focused neurovascular exam is performed, and the wrist is examined for the presence of open wounds.

Radiographic Examination

The wrist is splinted and anteroposterior, lateral, and oblique radiographs are obtained. Prereduction films are helpful in assessing fracture stability. Further radiographic studies that help in determining the extent of injury are tomograms and CT scans. These studies are performed

A

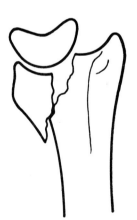

FIG. 11–4   The four types of intraarticular fractures of the distal radius: (a) a dorsal Barton's fracture; (b) a volar Barton's fracture; (c) a fracture of the radial styloid, or Chauffer's fracture; and (d) a compression of the lunate fossa, or die-punch fracture.

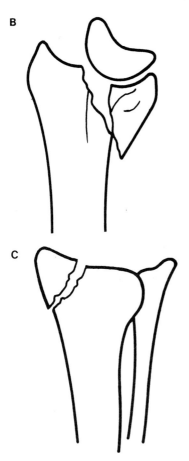

FIG. 11–4 *Continued*

after initial reduction and are particularly useful in studying displaced intraarticular fractures.

Initial Management

Displaced fractures are reduced. This frequently is the definitive management, but even in fractures that will require surgery, early reduction will reduce swelling and decrease the incidence of subacute neurovascular compromise.

D

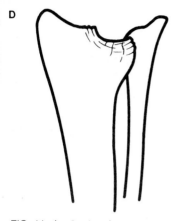

FIG. 11–4 *Continued*

Patients with severely displaced or comminuted fractures are admitted overnight and the arm is elevated and iced. The neurovascular status is checked frequently. Compartment syndrome or acute carpal tunnel syndrome may occur and is managed aggressively.

Associated Injuries

Injuries to the neurovascular structures around the wrist and bony or ligamentous injuries of the elbow are associated with fractures of the distal radius. The neurovascular status of the hand is carefully examined. Median nerve compression is the most common neurovascular injury and is indicated by loss of palmar abduction of the thumb and by decreased sensation on the palmar aspect of the thumb, index, and long fingers. Injury of the ulnar nerve is indicated by the inability to abduct the fingers and loss of sensation on the ulnar border of the hand. The superficial radial nerve is seldom injured. Good capillary refill of the nailbeds indicates adequate perfusion of the hand.

High-energy fractures of the distal radius are associated with injuries of the elbow joint, including fracture of the radial head and dislocation of the elbow. The elbow is examined for pain and swelling, and radiographs are obtained routinely. Associated injuries distal to the radial fracture include scaphoid fracture; scapholunate dissociation; and other carpal, metacarpal, and phalangeal fractures. Displaced radial styloid fractures are frequently associated with scapholunate dissociation. Anteroposterior and lateral radiographs of the hand and wrist are obtained.

Definitive Management

The definitive management is primarily based on the type of fracture. Other factors that are considered include the patient's age, occupation, degree of osteopenia, and associated medical conditions.

Nondisplaced fractures are managed with a short arm cast, unless considerable swelling is present, in which case a sugar tongs splint is applied. The patient returns in 7 to 10 days for a follow-up radiograph. The cast is changed as swelling decreases and is removed between 4 and 6 weeks. A wrist cock-up splint is worn for an additional 2 weeks, after which range of motion exercises are initiated. The majority of these fractures unite without difficulty.

Displaced extraarticular fractures are displaced dorsally (Colles') or volarly (Smith's). The definitive management is based on the direction of displacement.

Indications for reduction of a **Colles' fracture** are greater than 5 mm loss in radial length and 10° or more of dorsal tilt. A hematoma block, IV regional, or axillary block is administered for anesthesia. The thumb and index fingers are suspended in finger traps, with a roll of 3-in. webril placed between them to keep the first web space open and place the wrist in ulnar deviation. Countertraction is provided with 10 to 20 lb of weight draped over the arm in a padded stockinette. A preliminary period of traction of 5 to 10 min disimpacts the fragments. Reduction is carried out by first reproducing the injury with hyperextension and then flexing the wrist. The distal radius is molded with the surgeon's thumbs on the dorsal and radial surfaces in order to push the distal fragment back onto the metaphysis. The distal fragment is pushed volarly to oppose the volar cortices. Palpation along the dorsal and radial surfaces, looking for any evidence of a step-off, confirms when reduction is adequate. While the wrist is being palmar flexed about 20 to 30° with traction maintained, a short arm plaster cast or a sugar tongs splint is applied. Once the short arm portion of the cast has set, traction is released and the cast extended above the elbow. Postreduction x-rays are obtained. If a circular cast has been applied, it is split with a cast saw and the webril is cut to allow for swelling. All patients are instructed on cast care, elevation of the arm, warning signs of excessive swelling, and asked to return the next day for a cast check.

Postreduction films are evaluated for reestablishment of radial length, radial angle, volar tilt, and the presence of intraarticular step-off. Factors that are associated with instability include excessive comminution, initial loss of radial length of more than 15 mm, initial dorsal tilt over 20°, or comminution of both the dorsal and volar cortex seen on the postreduction films. In general, any fracture that requires a manipulative reduction is carefully followed for potential loss of reduction. Weekly films are obtained for at least the first 3 weeks after a fracture. If alignment is unchanged 3 weeks postreduction, the patient is placed in a short arm cast and started on elbow range of motion exercises. At 6 weeks, the cast is removed, a removable wrist splint is placed on the wrist, and range of motion exercise is started. Emphasis is on regaining range of motion for the first 3 weeks; strengthening is started later. If the patient is not recovering a reasonable range of motion within 3 weeks after cast removal, dynamic splinting is started.

Criteria indicating the need for remanipulation and possible fixation are loss of radial length or angle and dorsal tilt greater than 15°. It is difficult to obtain good anesthesia in the office 5 days postfracture, so we prefer to treat patients with loss of reduction in the operating room. Fractures can be remanipulated for up to 3 weeks after fracture. Beyond this time, open reduction is necessary.

Remanipulation is carried out as described for fresh fractures and an image intensifier is used to check the adequacy of reduction. Kirschner wires are inserted percutaneously into the fracture site in order to gently free up the fracture. After alignment has been restored, the fracture is stabilized with percutaneous pins. A 0.062 Kirschner wire is inserted into the radial styloid and driven across the fracture site coming through the proximal metaphysis. A second wire is inserted from the dorsal ulnar corner of the distal fragment to the volar radial metaphysis. Two wires are usually enough, but additional wires may be added as necessary. Percutaneous pins are not firm fixation and a cast is still necessary to maintain reduction. The pins are cut off beneath the skin and can be removed in the office under local anesthesia.

Smith's fractures are unstable. The pull of the flexor muscles across the wrist exerts shear forces across the fracture site, resulting in redisplacement after closed reduction. If the fracture is displaced on the initial films, internal fixation is indicated. In younger patients, these fractures can be reduced closed and percutaneously pinned. In older patients or those with osteopenic bone, the fracture is managed with a volar buttress plate. A short arm cast is applied and the postoperative management is as described for Colles' fractures.

Open or severely comminuted Colles' and Smith's fractures present a different set of management priorities. Open distal radial fractures are managed with emergent irrigation and debridement of the fracture site. After debridement, grade I and II fractures are treated as a closed fracture. Grade III fractures are managed with external fixation.

Comminution causes instability and frequently, reduction is impossible to maintain in a cast alone. In general, if the metaphyseal comminution is not extensive and the patient has dense bone, the fracture can be stabilized with percutaneous pins (Figs. 11–5 to 11–7). Otherwise, the fracture is managed with external fixation.

Prior to application of the **external fixater,** the fracture is reduced in the operating room with sterile finger traps and brachial countertraction. An image intensifier is used to confirm reduction. Metacarpal pins are placed through incisions that are large enough to retract the soft

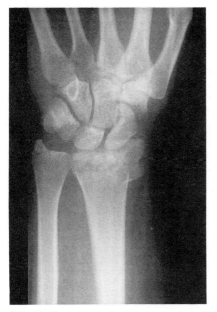

FIG. 11–5   A dorsally displaced extraarticular fracture. Volar tilt is minus 30°. Radial length is 4 mm. The radial angle is 5°.

tissues out of the way. Radial pins are placed through an incision that is long enough to adequately visualize the superficial radial nerve and safely retract it out of harm's way. In the metacarpals, 2.5-mm pins are used, and in the radius, 3.0-mm pins. Fixaters are kept on for 6 to 8 weeks until there should be callus formation. Cancellous bone grafting allows earlier fixater removal.

Displaced intraarticular fractures have a poorer prognosis than equivalent extraarticular fractures and demand more aggressive management. The two types of displaced intraarticular fractures are simple fractures and comminuted fractures.

Simple intraarticular fractures involve the radial styloid (Chauffeur's fracture), the dorsal rim (dorsal Barton's), and the volar rim (volar Barton's).

Chauffeur's fractures usually go from the radial metaphysis into the radiocarpal joint between the scaphoid and lunate fossa. Nondisplaced radial styloid fractures are managed with cast immobilization; displaced fractures are reduced and pinned.

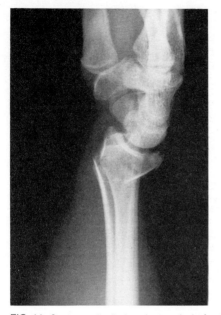

FIG. 11–6 A dorsally displaced extraarticular fracture. Volar tilt is minus 30°. Radial length is 4 mm. The radial angle is 5°.

Volar Barton's fractures are unstable due to the pull of the flexor muscles, resulting in volar subluxation of the carpus. They are managed with a volar buttress plate. The radius is approached through a volar incision parallel to and over the flexor carpi radialis tendon. Dissection proceeds between the flexor carpi radialis tendon and the radial artery to the pronator quadratus muscle which is detached sharply from its insertion on the radius. The fracture is exposed, reduced, and a volar buttress plate is applied. The distal screw holes in the plate may be left unfilled, especially in osteopenic patients. Postoperatively, a short arm cast is maintained for 4 weeks.

Management of dorsal Barton's fractures varies depending on the size of the fragment. Small dorsal fragments are managed with closed reduction and cast immobilization with the wrist in extension. Careful follow-up is necessary to ensure that subluxation does not occur. For larger fragments, or those with comminution, either percutaneous pin fixation or a dorsal buttress plate is used. Postoperatively, a short arm cast is applied for 4 weeks.

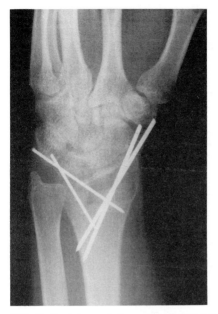

FIG. 11–7 Anteroposterior radiograph after closed reduction and pinning. The radial length has been restored to 15 mm. The radial angle is 25°.

Comminuted displaced intraarticular fractures are the most difficult distal radial fractures to manage. If the fracture can be reduced closed, management is with an external fixater. An external fixater is used because the reduction is unstable and will be lost in a cast. If the fracture cannot be reduced closed, an open reduction is performed.

First, the fracture is reduced, then the **external fixater** is applied as described previously. Final adjustments in fracture position are made, and the frame is tightened. Percutaneous Kirschner wires or plates and screws are added to secure major fragments. Practically, with external fixation alone, the best the dorsal tilt can be reestablished is to neutral. Factors that make external fixation alone unreliable include extensive dorsal comminution, interposition of soft tissues between fracture components, depression of the lunate fossa (die-punch fragment), and rotation of fragments.

The primary indication for **open reduction** of comminuted, intraarticular distal radial fractures is displacement that cannot be reduced by closed manipulation. The articular incongruity most commonly involves the lunate fossa. External fixation, along with a limited operative exposure of the lunate fossa, has been a useful technique in these die-punch fractures. The lunate fossa is elevated by means of a limited dorsal incision, supported with Kirschner wires and autogenous iliac crest bone graft. Open reduction is necessary when there is soft-tissue interposition or malrotation. Application of an external fixater at the beginning of the case helps in maintaining alignment and holds the fragments apart. Postexposure, fragments are stabilized using a combination of Kirschner wires, screws, and plates. Kirschner wires, placed just beneath the subchondral bone, help support the restored articular surface.

Postoperatively, the arm is placed in a long arm splint, elevated, and early finger and shoulder motion is encouraged. Most fractures involve the distal radioulnar joint, so the long arm splint is continued for several weeks for comfort. The fixater is removed when there is callus formation. Aggressive physical therapy is necessary, including the use of dynamic splints. Even with optimal surgical treatment, some degree of residual pain, loss of motion, and grip strength is inevitable.

Complications

Acute complications include carpal tunnel syndrome, reflex sympathetic dystrophy, loss of reduction, and instability of the distal radioulnar joint. Transient neuropathy can occur with the original injury, due to the initial trauma and displacement of the fracture. If the neuropathy does not improve after reduction, all circumferential dressings are loosened and the wrist is placed in neutral position. If sensory changes persist, operative decompression of the carpal canal and the distal forearm fascia is performed. Increasing pain, swelling, progressive stiffness of the fingers, and dysethesia raise the suspicion of a developing reflex sympathetic dystrophy. Early, aggressive physical therapy and stellate ganglion blocks are the mainstays of treatment. Loss of reduction is common after distal radius fractures. Frequent x-ray follow-up is necessary in order to catch a loss of reduction early, while it can still be treated.

Late complications include malunion; posttraumatic arthritis; and residual stiffness of the fingers, hand, or shoulder.

DISLOCATIONS OF THE DISTAL RADIOULNAR JOINT

Isolated dislocations of the distal radioulnar joint are rare injuries. Dislocations associated with a distal radial fracture (i.e., Galeazzi's fracture) are covered in Chapter 10.

Classification

Dislocations of the distal radioulnar joint are classified according to the direction of displacement of the ulna in relation to the radius as either volar or dorsal.

Initial Diagnosis and Management

History and Physical Examination

There is pain on the ulnar side of the wrist, accompanied by snapping and crepitation with forearm rotation or by the inability to rotate the forearm. The history of injury frequently includes forced pronation or supination. Physical findings of a dorsal dislocation include a prominent ulnar head, increased mobility of the ulnar head, and limited supination. Physical signs of a volar dislocation include an apparently absent ulnar head, narrowing of the wrist, and limited pronation.

Radiographic Examination

Radiographically, the anteroposterior and lateral projections may not be diagnostic unless compared with the identical views of the opposite wrist. Tomograms and CT scans confirm the diagnosis.

Initial Management

Once the diagnosis has been made, a closed reduction is attempted. A hematoma block is used for analgesia. Dorsal dislocations are reduced with supination and immobilized in a long arm splint or cast. Volar dislocations are reduced with pronation. If closed reduction is not possible, open reduction is required.

Definitive Management

Factors that mitigate for surgical management include a dislocation that cannot be reduced with closed methods and a fracture of the ulnar styloid and base, indicating an easily repaired avulsion of the triangular fibrocartilage. Volar dislocations are approached from the volar side and the head of the ulna is levered from under the volar surface of the radius. Dorsal dislocations are approached from the dorsal side. Usually an osteochondral fragment or tendon in the sigmoid notch is blocking reduction. If the ulnar styloid is to be repaired, it is reduced and held in place with a small screw and washer, or with Kirschner wires. This is done through a separate incision if a volar approach has been used or by extending the dorsal incision. Once reduction has been achieved, the forearm is held in neutral rotation and the ulna is pinned to the radius. A long arm cast is maintained 6 weeks. At 6 weeks, the cast is taken off and the pin is removed.

If closed management is chosen, a long arm cast in supination (dorsal dislocation) or pronation (volar dislocation) is maintained for 6 weeks.

Complications

Complications unique to this injury include chronic radioulnar instability and arthritis. Management consists of excision of the ulnar head, or, preferably, fusion of the ulnar head to the radius and extraperiosteal resection of 2 cm of the distal ulnar diaphysis to produce a nonunion.

SELECTED READINGS

Clancey, GJ: Percutaneous Kirschner wire fixation of Colles' fractures. A prospective study of thirty cases. *J Bone Joint Surg* 66A:1008–1014, 1984.

Cooney WP: External fixation of distal radius fractures. *Clin Orthop* 180:44–49, 1983.

Fernandez DL: Correction of post-traumatic wrist deformity in adults by osteotomy, bone-grafting, and internal fixation. *J Bone Joint Surg* 64A:1164–1178, 1982.

Knirk JL, Jupiter JB: Intra-articular fractures of the distal end of the radius in young adults. *J Bone Joint Surg* 68A:647–659, 1986.

Leung KS, Shen WY, Tsang KH, Chiu KH, Leung PC, Hung LK: An effective treatment of comminuted fractures of the distal radius. *J Hand Surg* 15A:11–17, 1990.

Louis DS: Barton's and Smith's fractures. *Hand Clin* 4:399–402, 1988.

12 | Fractures and Dislocations of the Wrist

Donald L. Pruitt

This chapter reviews dislocations and fractures of the carpus.

ANATOMY

The eight **carpal bones** are divided into a proximal row—scaphoid, lunate, triquetrum, and pisiform—and a distal row—trapezium, trapezoid, capitate, and hamate. The proximal row has no tendon insertions and functions as an intercalated segment between the forearm and hand. The shape of the carpal bones and their ligamentous connections maintain stability; however, they are predisposed to collapse.

Articular cartilage covers 80 percent of the **scaphoid's** surface. The proximal pole is intraarticular with no independent blood supply. Two vessels supply the scaphoid, both at the distal end. Thus, fractures of the middle third interfere with the blood supply of the proximal pole causing a high incidence of avascular necrosis and nonunion.

The two types of **ligaments** in the wrist are intrinsic and extrinsic. Intrinsic ligaments, also known as interosseous ligaments, connect two or more carpal bones and lie within the synovial cavity. The **scapholunate** and the **lunotriquetral** ligaments are the most important interosseous ligaments. Extrinsic ligaments are specialized thickenings of the wrist capsule and lie outside of the synovial cavity. The major extrinsic ligaments are the **radioscaphoid, radiocapitate,** and **radiotriquetral** ligaments, all of which are located on the volar surface.

The neck of the capitate gives origin to the **intercarpal deltoid** ligament, which fans out toward the scaphoid and triquetrum in an inverted "V" configuration. This leaves a space between the head of the capitate and the lunate, known as the **space of Poirier,** through which dislocations occur.

Biomechanically, the carpus is a link joint, with the lunate acting as a potentially unstable segment between the distal row and the radius. The scaphoid functions as a bridge, providing stability to an otherwise unstable intercalated segment (Fig. 12–1).

DISLOCATIONS OF THE WRIST

Classification

Dislocations of the wrist are classified as perilunate, lunate, transscaphoid perilunate, radiocarpal, and radioulnar translocation. Less severe stages of perilunate dislocation present as scapholunate dissociation.

Perilunate, lunate, and transscaphoid perilunate dislocations are variations of the same injury and are caused by hyperextension of the

131

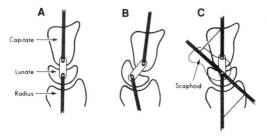

FIG. 12–1   Link joint concept of carpal stability: (*a*) the lunate acts as an intercalated segment between the capitate and radius; (*b*) the segment is unstable, tending to collapse; and (*c*) the scaphoid acts as a stabilizing link to prevent collapse.

wrist. The five stages of injury are: I, tearing of the scapholunate and volar radioscaphoid ligaments, resulting in **scapholunate dissociation,** or rotary subluxation of the scaphoid; II, dislocation of the capitate head through the space of Poirier; III, tearing of the lunotriquetral ligament, resulting in separation of the lunate and triquetrum; IV, disruption of the dorsal ligaments, and dislocation of the carpus dorsally (the lunate remains in the lunate fossa of the radius), resulting in a **perilunate dislocation;** and V, the carpus drives the lunate volarly and articulates with the radius, resulting in a **lunate dislocation.**

Variations in the path of force transmission result in a variety of related injuries. For example, if the path goes through the body of the scaphoid, a **transscaphoid-perilunate-fracture dislocation** results.

Radiocarpal dislocation, or dislocation of the entire carpus from the radius, is often associated with a radial styloid fracture (Fig. 12–2).

Ulnar translocation is another form of a radiocarpal dislocation in which the ligaments between the radius and proximal carpal row are disrupted, allowing the carpus to slide ulnarly on the radius (Fig. 12–3).

Diagnosis and Initial Management

History and Physical Examination

There is pain localized to the wrist, usually after falling onto an outstretched hand. Swelling varies from barely perceptible to significant in the case of a major dislocation. Begin the clinical examination by noting areas of ecchymosis, active range of motion, and neurovascular status. Pinpoint sites of tenderness. When dislocated, the wrist appears shortened, with a fullness over its dorsum or in the carpal tunnel. Any movement produces pain. Determine if there are signs of median nerve compression.

Scapholunate dissociation is difficult to diagnose clinically. In many cases, no specific traumatic incident can be recalled. There is an area

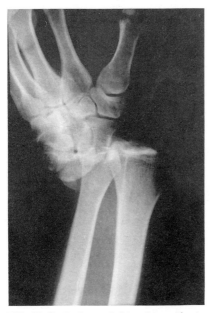

FIG. 12–2   Radiocarpal dislocation and fracture of the radial styloid.

of point tenderness dorsally over the scapholunate joint. Motion may not be restricted by pain. In the **"clunk test,"** the examiner's thumb is placed against the volar aspect of the scaphoid (distal pole), while the other hand is used to move the wrist from ulnar to radial deviation. If there is scapholunate dissociation, this maneuver forces the proximal pole of the scaphoid dorsally out of the scaphoid fossa of the radius eliciting a painful clunk.

Radiographic Examination

A minimum of four views of the wrist is obtained: an anteroposterior view in neutral, an anteroposterior view in ulnar deviation, an oblique view, and a true lateral view.

A series of arcs that are helpful in detecting carpal instabilities is seen on the anteroposterior projection (Fig. 12–4). Arc I is formed by the proximal borders of the scaphoid, lunate, and triquetrum; arc II, by the distal borders of the same three bones; and arc III, by the proximal ends of the capitate and hamate. Normally, the arcs form smooth lines. A break in the arc is a sign of fracture, dislocation, or instability.

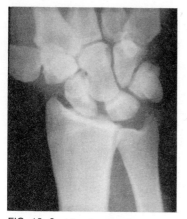

FIG. 12–3   Ulnar translocation.

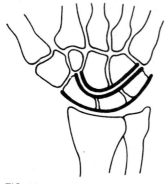

FIG. 12–4   Carpal arcs.

If carpal instability is suspected, the scapholunate (S-L), and capito-lunate (C-L) angles are measured. These are determined on the lateral radiograph (Fig. 12–5). To determine the **scapholunate angle,** one line is drawn along the longitudinal axis of the scaphoid and a second line at a right angle to a line connecting the dorsal and volar poles of the lunate (essentially bisecting the lunate). The angle between the two lines normally ranges from 30° to 60°. Angles above 60° indicate a dorsal intercalated segmental instability (DISI), and angles less than 30° indicate a volar intercalated segmental instability (VISI) (Fig.

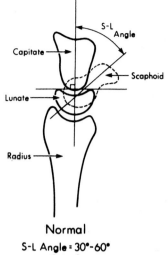

Normal

S-L Angle = 30°-60°

C-L = 0

FIG. 12-5 The scapholunate (S-L) angle and capitolunate (C-L) angles.

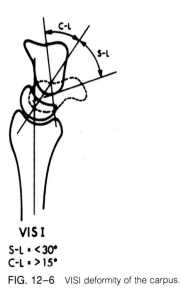

VIS I

S-L = <30°

C-L = >15°

FIG. 12-6 VISI deformity of the carpus.

12–6). The **capitolunate angle** is formed by a line along the capitate axis and the line bisecting the lunate. This should normally be less than 15°. If it is greater and pointing dorsally, DISI is present; if it is pointing volarly, VISI is present.

Radiographic findings of a perilunate dislocation are triangular-shaped lunate on the anteroposterior view, loss of parallelism between adjacent articular surfaces of the radius and proximal carpal row, and the head of the capitate dorsal to the lunate on the lateral view. A lunate dislocation is characterized by absence of the lunate from its fossa on the anteroposterior radiograph and displacement of the lunate volarly on the lateral radiograph. A transscaphoid perilunate dislocation is characterized by the signs of a lunate or perilunate dislocation, along with a fracture of the scaphoid. Distraction films separate the fragments, making the diagnosis more obvious.

The key finding of scapholunate dissociation is a widened space between the scaphoid and lunate as seen on the anteroposterior view (Fig. 12–7). On the lateral view, there is a more horizontal orientation to the scaphoid and the scapholunate angle is greater than 70°. Comparison views of the uninjured side help in making the diagnosis. When the clinical exam points to a scapholunate dissociation but radiographic signs are equivocal, cineradiographs and arthrography are obtained.

The diagnosis of radiocarpal dislocation is obvious on the lateral view as illustrated in Fig. 12–2. The lunate and entire carpus are displaced off the radius. On the anteroposterior radiograph, there is often a fracture of the radial styloid and the carpus overrides the distal radius.

The diagnosis of ulnar translocation is made from the anteroposterior radiograph (Fig. 12–3). The carpus is displaced ulnarly or the scaphoid remains in place and the rest of the carpus has shifted ulnarly.

Initial Management

Perilunate, lunate, and transscaphoid perilunate dislocations are reduced as soon as possible to minimize the incidence of median nerve injury. Axillary block or IV regional anesthesia provides adequate muscular relaxation; IV sedation or local injection will not. A preliminary period of traction (10 to 15 lb) relaxes the muscles. This is an excellent time to take radiographs because the carpal bones are distracted and additional injuries are easier to pick up. After 5 to 10 min of traction, the finger traps are removed and the surgeon maintains traction. One thumb is placed over the carpal tunnel to push the lunate back into the lunate fossa. Extension of the wrist, followed by gradual palmar flexion, allows the head of the capitate to slip back into the concavity of the lunate. A thumb spica plaster splint is applied with the wrist in neutral or slight palmar flexion. Postreduction films are obtained and the patient admitted overnight with hourly neurovascular checks while the arm is elevated and iced.

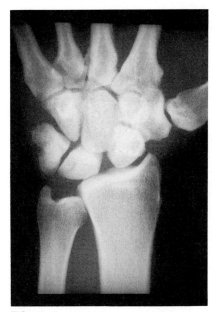

FIG. 12-7 Scapholunate dissociation.

Closed reduction of a **scapholunate dissociation** is usually not possible. The wrist is splinted for comfort until surgery is performed.

Radiocarpal dislocation and radioulnar translocation are reduced using the same technique employed for fractures of the distal radius. Plaster splints are applied and the patient observed for signs of median nerve compression. Postreduction films are examined for signs of concomitant injuries, especially carpal instability.

Associated Injuries

The most frequent associated injury is median nerve compromise. This is indicated by loss of sensation on the palmar surface of the thumb, index, and long fingers, and, occasionally, inability to oppose the thumb. Loss of median nerve function is an indication for immediate reduction dislocations or fractures.

Other less common associated injuries include disruption of the radial or ulnar arteries and injury of the ulnar nerve. These are ruled out by a focused neurovascular examination.

Definitive Management

Most **perilunate and lunate dislocations** are percutaneously pinned using fluoroscopy because of the high likelihood of late collapse. A short arm thumb spica cast is applied. The pins are removed at 8 weeks and an orthoplast splint is worn for an additional 4 weeks. Range of motion exercises are started at 8 to 10 weeks, but strengthening is delayed until 3 months.

When anatomic reduction is not achieved by closed means, open reduction and internal fixation are indicated via an extended carpal tunnel approach. The lunate is located in the carpal tunnel and reduced through the rent in the volar capsule. Percutaneous pin fixation of the scaphoid and lunate is carried out using fluoroscopy. If an anatomic reduction is not achieved, a dorsal exposure is employed to visualize the scaphoid and lunate. Pins are placed between the scaphoid and lunate, the scaphoid and capitate, and the radius and lunate. The rent in the volar capsule is repaired.

Postoperatively, the wrist is immobilized in a thumb spica sugar tongs plaster splint. The plaster splint is changed to a short arm thumb spica cast at 1 week. The Kirschner wires are kept in place for 8 to 10 weeks. Range of motion and strengthening exercises are begun after removal of the Kirschner wires.

Transscaphoid perilunate dislocation is reduced as described in initial management. Postreduction radiographs are taken after the splint is applied. The adequacy of reduction of the scaphoid fracture is assessed. If there is doubt, tomograms or a CT scan is obtained. Pay special attention to DISI instability or a dorsal "humpback" deformity. If the reduction is acceptable, a thumb spica cast is applied. Follow-up radiographs are taken weekly for the first 3 weeks. Cast immobilization is maintained until healing of the scaphoid fracture occurs (often several months).

If the scaphoid fracture is displaced over 1 mm or angulated, open reduction is performed through a modified Russe approach that can be extended to allow access to the volar wrist capsule. The fracture is stabilized with either Kirschner wires or a Herbert screw. Radiographs are obtained and the relationship of the scaphoid and lunate is evaluated. If there is residual malalignment, the Russe approach is extended into a carpal tunnel approach. Kirschner wires are used to stabilize the lunate, capitate, and scaphoid in their normal relationship. When open reduction is performed late, bone grafting of the scaphoid fracture is necessary.

Postoperatively, a sugar tongs thumb spica splint is applied after wound closure. The postoperative splint is changed to a short arm thumb spica cast at 1 week. Patients are followed at 4 to 5 week intervals, the cast is changed, and radiographs obtained. If there is no progression toward healing 4 to 6 months after injury, bone grafting is indicated. Kirschner wires are removed after healing of the scaphoid fracture.

Physical therapy, including the use of dynamic splints, is usually necessary following cast removal.

Closed reduction and pin fixation of **scapholunate dissociations** are performed under image intensification. Permanent films are obtained and if the relationship between the scaphoid and lunate is not anatomic, open reduction is undertaken.

If the injury is acute, the scapholunate ligament is repaired through a dorsal approach. The ligament is usually found to be torn off the scaphoid. Nonabsorbable sutures are placed into the ligament and attached through drill holes to the scaphoid after the bones are reduced and stabilized with Kirschner wires.

Postoperatively, a short arm thumb spica is applied. The wires are removed 8 to 10 weeks after surgery and a removable splint is worn for another 4 weeks.

Radiocarpal dislocation is managed closed unless there is associated carpal instability, in which case open reduction, pinning, and possible ligament repair are performed.

Treatment options of ulnar translocation are reduction and ligament repair, or radiocarpal fusion.

Complications

The complication unique to dislocations of the carpal bones is late instability. After the lunate is reduced, DISI may occur due to the loss of the stabilization provided by the scaphoid and/or scapholunate ligament. Left uncorrected, a DISI pattern leads to progressive intercarpal arthritis. A similar instability pattern, VISI, is seen on the ulnar side of the wrist. Here, forces first destabilize the lunotriquetral articulation. This less common form of wrist instability also results in arthritis, but not as rapidly as with a DISI deformity.

FRACTURES

Fractures of the wrist occur in isolation or in combination with other fractures or dislocations. The scaphoid is the most commonly fractured carpal bone, followed in order of frequency by the triquetrum, lunate, capitate, pisiform, and the other carpal bones.

Classification

Scaphoid fractures are classified according to whether they are displaced and by the location of the fracture. Therefore, there are displaced and undisplaced fractures of the proximal pole, waist, and distal pole. Displaced fractures include any fracture with greater than 1 mm stepoff on the anteroposterior view, an intrascaphoid angle greater than 45° on lateral tomograms (normal is 30° or less), or the presence of an associated carpal instability pattern. The mechanism of injury is that during wrist hyperextension, the dorsal rim of the radius is driven into the scaphoid waist and, simultaneously, tensile stresses are developed on the volar surface of the scaphoid, resulting in a fracture. The scaphoid tends to open dorsally and compress the volar surfaces together, gradually assuming the humpback deformity that is associated with an increased likelihood of nonunion.

Triquetral Fractures

The most common triquetral fracture is an avulsion fracture off the dorsal surface. These are best seen on the lateral view.

Lunate Fractures

Fractures of the lunate are uncommon unless associated with Kienböck's disease. There are two types of acute lunate fractures: lunate body fractures and rim fractures. Lunate body fractures are either the result of a compression force applied to the wrist or of the normal compressive forces from the capitate head pressing on an avascular lunate in Kienböck's disease. It is often difficult to assess displacement on plain radiographs, and tomography is recommended.

Dorsal and volar rim fractures of the lunate occur in association with other wrist injuries, especially perilunate dislocations. If the fracture involves a significant portion of the lunate articular surface, open reduction and internal fixation is considered.

Capitate Fractures

Fractures of the neck of the capitate occur in isolation or in association with other injuries. They are undisplaced or displaced.

Pisiform Fractures

The pisiform is a sesamoid bone located within the FCU tendon and has an articulation with the hamate. Fractures of the pisiform occur due to direct trauma, usually from a fall. These fractures are best visualized radiographically on the oblique. Displaced fractures of the articular surface may lead to painful arthritis of the pisohamate joint surface.

Other Carpal Fractures

Fractures have been described for all of the carpal bones. In general, fractures that involve significant portions of the body of a bone or articular surface should be carefully evaluated for displacement. Fractures of the hook of the hamate are rare injuries that are frequently the result of repetitive trauma (e.g., using a jackhammer).

Associated Injuries

Intercarpal dislocations and ligamentous injuries are frequently associated with displaced fractures of the carpus. These are ruled out with the appropriate radiographic studies. Neurovascular injuries are rare, but are ruled out with a focused examination.

Diagnosis and Initial Management

History and Physical Examination

There is wrist pain with point tenderness directly over the involved bone. The scaphoid is the most commonly fractured carpal bone. Scaphoid fractures are usually seen in young adult males. The physical finding unique to scaphoid fractures is pain upon thumb pinch, upon palpation of the proximal pole in the snuffbox, and upon palpation of the distal pole on the volar side of the wrist.

Radiographic Examination

A minimum of four views is obtained: an anteroposterior view with the wrist in neutral deviation, an anteroposterior view with the wrist in yulnar deviation, an oblique view, and a lateral view. Special scaphoid views are obtained by progressive tilting of the x-ray beam to elongate the scaphoid. Other tests that are useful in establishing the diagnosis of a fracture of a carpal bone are tomograms, CT scans, and MRIs.

Nonunions are distinguished from acute fractures on plain films by resorption or cyst formation, sclerosis at the fracture site, displacement of the fracture, and dorsal angulation.

Initial Management

The key initial decision is whether the fracture will be managed with closed methods or surgery. If closed methods are to be used, the initial management is the definitive management. If the fracture is to be managed with surgery, a long arm thumb spica splint is applied, and the wrist is elevated and iced.

Definitive Management

Scaphoid Fractures

Nondisplaced scaphoid fractures are managed with a long arm thumb spica cast, with the wrist in neutral for the first 4 weeks, followed by a short arm thumb spica cast until healing occurs. The only exception is a tuberosity fracture which will heal in a short arm cast. The cast is changed every 4 weeks, and radiographs are obtained out of plaster. Immobilization is continued until there is bony bridging across the fracture. Tomograms or CT scans are helpful when there is any question about union.

When initial radiographs are negative but the clinical exam is suspicious for a fracture, the wrist is immobilized in a plaster thumb spica splint and repeat radiographs are obtained in 10 to 14 days. If the radiographs are still negative, and the clinical exam is still suspicious for a fracture, a bone scan is obtained.

Open reduction via a Russse approach and fixation with Kirschner wires or a Herbert screw is indicated for displaced fractures. Bone grafting is not necessary in acute fractures unless there is comminution. The wrist is immobilized in a short arm thumb spica cast until union occurs. Wires are removed in the office; screws are removed only if they become symptomatic.

Triquetral fractures are managed with a short arm cast until asymptomatic, usually 2 to 4 weeks. Fractures of the triquetral body occur with more extreme trauma. If significantly displaced, body fractures are managed with open reduction and fixation.

Displaced **lunate body fractures** are managed with open reduction and fixation. Fractures of the dorsal or volar rim, if small and not associated with other injuries such as a perilunate dislocation, are managed for 4 to 6 weeks with a short arm cast extending to the metacarpophalangeal joints. Rim fractures involving a significant portion of the articular surface are managed with open reduction and fixation.

Nondisplaced **capitate** neck fractures are managed with cast immobilization, but are to be followed with frequent radiographs to ensure that displacement does not occur. Displaced neck fractures are managed with anatomic reduction and fixation, usually via a dorsal approach.

Pisiform fractures are initially managed with splinting. If symptomatic, due to nonunion or pisohamate arthritis, the pisiform is excised.

Other **carpal fractures** with significant displacement of the articular surface are managed with open reduction and internal fixation. Avulsion fractures indicate ligament injury and are managed with immobilization until healed. Symptomatic fractures of the hook of the hamate are excised.

Complications

The complications most frequently encountered following fracture of one of the bones of the carpus are arthritis, nonunion, and avascular necrosis.

Arthritis is initially managed conservatively with activity restriction, splinting, and nonsteroidal anti-inflammatories. If arthritis is sufficiently symptomatic, management with arthrodesis of the joint involved (i.e., a limited intercarpal arthrodesis), or of the entire wrist, may salvage the situation.

Nonunion and avascular necrosis are not uncommon problems following a fracture of the scaphoid (Fig. 12–8). Ten percent of all acute scaphoid fractures will go on to a nonunion. Factors associated with increased likelihood of nonunion include delayed initial diagnosis, initial displacement or angulation, and proximal pole fractures. Important considerations in the treatment of scaphoid nonunion include preservation of blood supply, bone grafting of the nonunion site, internal

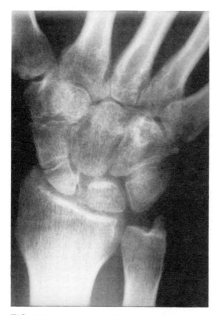

FIG. 12–8 Nonunion of the scaphoid.

fixation for stability, correction of humpback deformity, and associated carpal instability.

Symptomatic scaphoid nonunion associated with arthritis has no management option that will restore normal function and is best treated with a salvage procedure. Options include a fascial interposition arthroplasty, four-corner fusion with scaphoid excision, proximal row carpectomy, and wrist fusion.

SELECTED READINGS

Adkison JW, Chapman MW: Treatment of acute lunate and perilunate dislocations. *Clin Orthop* 164:199–207, 1982.

Gelberman RH, Menon J: The vascularity of the scaphoid bone. *J Hand Surg* 5:508–513, 1980.

Gilford WW, Bolton RH, Lambrinudi C: The mechanism of the wrist joint with special reference to fractures of the scaphoid. *Guy's Hosp Rep* 92:52–59, 1943.

Gilula LA, Destouet JM, Weeks PM, Young LV, Wray RC: Roentgenographic diagnosis of the painful wrist. *Clin Orthop* 187:52–64, 1984.

Mayfield JK, Johnson RP, Kilcoyne RK: Carpal dislocations: Pathomechanics and progressive perilunar instability. *J Hand Surg* 5:226–241, 1980.

Taleisnik J: Wrist: Anatomy, function and injury, in American Academy of Orthopaedic Surgeons (ed): *Instructional Course Lectures,* 27d ed. St. Louis, Mosby, 1978, pp. 61–87.

13 | Fractures and Dislocations of the Metacarpals and Phalanges

Mark Gonzalez

This chapter reviews fractures and fracture dislocations of the metacarpals and phalanges

ANATOMY

The **metacarpals 2 through 5** have an expanded cuboidal base with facets for articulation with the carpus and neighboring metacarpals. Dorsal and palmar intermetacarpal ligaments and interosseous ligaments stabilize these articulations. The first **carpometacarpal joint** (CMC) is a biconcave saddle joint stabilized primarily by the anterior oblique ligament and the intermetatarsal ligament.

The **metacarpal phalangeal joints** (MCP) are complex hinge joints which allow medial and lateral movement in full extension. The volar aspect of the joints is supported by a volar plate. The collateral ligaments are lateral to the joints and are the primary medial and lateral stabilizers. The metacarpal head is cam-shaped and the collaterals are under maximal stretch in flexion. The MCP is safely splinted in 70 to 90° of flexion. The cam effect of the metacarpal head maintains collateral ligament length and prevents an extension contracture (Figs. 13–1 and 13–2). The MCP of the thumb is structurally similar to the other MCPs, but its intrinsic muscles (adductor pollicis, abductor pollicis brevis, and flexor pollicis brevis) and three extensor tendons (flexor pollicis longus, extensor pollicis brevis, and extensor pollicis longus) are dynamic stabilizers. The thumb is splinted to avoid contracture of these intrinsic muscles (i.e., the first web space).

Proximal and middle phalanges have a slight apex dorsal curve. The **proximal and distal interphalangeal joints** (PIPs and DIPs) are true hinge joints. Stabilizing ligaments are similar to those of the MCP, but there is no rotatory or side-to-side motion. The PIP joints are splinted in 0 to 10° flexion preventing the development of checkrein ligaments about the volar plate and a flexion contracture.

The **extensor hood** is dorsal to the PIP. Its central slip inserts on the middle phalanx and the lateral bands form the DIP extensor. The flexor digitorum sublimis (FDS) inserts on the middle phalanx, and the flexor digitorum profundus (FDP) on the distal phalanx.

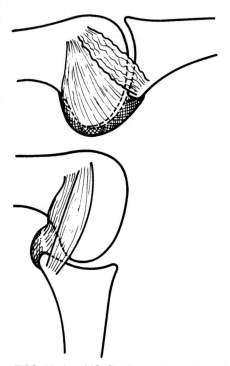

FIGS. 13–1 and 13–2 The cam shape of the metacarpal head results in the collateral ligaments being stretched maximally when the MCP joint is flexed.

FRACTURES OF THE METACARPALS

Classification

Fractures of the metacarpals are classified as involving the base, the diaphysis, the neck, or the head. Additional factors which influence management are whether the fracture is open, closed, or the result of a high-energy injury, and whether more than one metacarpal is fractured.

Fractures of the **metacarpal bases** are frequently associated with dorsal subluxation of the CMC (Fig. 13–3). This is particularly true of fractures of the base of the fifth metacarpal, which are displaced proximally by the extensor carpi ulnaris (Fig. 13–4).

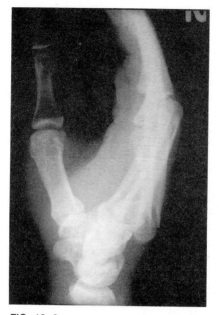

FIG. 13–3 Dorsal dislocation of the fifth MCP joint and a fracture of the base of the fourth metacarpal.

Metacarpal neck fractures, also known as ''**Boxer's fractures,**'' are due to a volarly directed force to the metacarpal head. The intrinsics maintain the fracture in a flexed position.

Fractures of the **metacarpal head** are due to avulsion of a collateral ligament or impaction from a longitudinal blow. Fracture of the metacarpal head due to impaction of a tooth during a fist fight, is also known as a ''fight bite.''

Diagnosis and Initial Management

History and Physical Examination

There is pain and a history of trauma. Deformity and swelling may be present.

Radiographic Examination

Anteroposterior, lateral, and oblique views of the hand are obtained. A CT scan may help in the evaluation of the CMC.

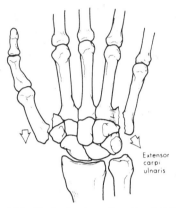

FIG. 13–4 Fracture with subluxation of the base of the fifth metacarpal and Bennet's fracture of the first metacarpal.

Initial Management

Initial management of metacarpal fractures is reduction of displaced fractures and immobilization in a splint. The splint extends from the DIPs to the elbow. In the immobilization position, MCPs are flexed to 90°, PIPs are extended, and the wrist is dorsiflexed 20°. In cases in which reduction is required, a hematoma block is administered.

Fracture dislocations of the **base of the metacarpals** are reduced by longitudinal traction and pressing the metacarpals volarly. Fractures of the metacarpal diaphysis and neck are angulated with the apex dorsal. **Diaphyseal fractures** are reduced with longitudinal traction and application of pressure to the apex of the deformity. **Boxer's fractures** are reduced by flexing the MCP and PIP joints, and pushing the proximal phalanx dorsally while maintaining volar pressure on the metacarpal. Fractures of the **metacarpal head** usually do not require closed reduction and are splinted.

Associated Injuries

There are no injuries specifically associated with metacarpal fractures and dislocations of the metacarpals.

Definitive Management

Most metacarpal fractures are managed with splinting for 3 to 6 weeks. Immobilization is discontinued when there are clinical (i.e., absence of pain at the fracture site) and radiographic signs of healing. There are specific indications for surgery for each type of metacarpal fracture.

Unstable and less than anatomic reduction of fractures of the **metacarpal bases** are indications for operative reduction and pinning. The fracture is surgically exposed through a dorsal incision or reduced with the aid of fluoroscopy. Pins are driven across the fracture into an adjacent metacarpal or into the carpus. Postoperatively, the hand is splinted for 3 to 6 weeks at which time the pins are removed. During this time, the splint is removed daily for range of motion exercises of the PIPs and MCPs.

Indications for internal fixation of fractures of the **metacarpal diaphysis** include more than 3 mm of shortening, rotation resulting in digital scissoring when the MCPs are flexed, angulation of the fourth and fifth metacarpals greater than 30°, angulation of the second and third greater than 10°, multiple metacarpal fractures (because of instability), and gunshot wounds or crush injuries with comminution or loss of bone. The fracture is reduced closed under fluoroscopy or exposed via a dorsal incision. Fractures reduced closed are stabilized with percutaneous Kirschner wires. Screws, plates, cerclage wires, interosseous wires, and intramedullary wires are used to stabilize fractures which have been opened and reduced. Fractures with a deficient or contaminated soft tissue envelope are managed with external fixation, wires, or polymethylmethacrylate spacers prior to the definitive reconstruction. Postoperatively, simple fractures are immobilized 6 weeks, the splint is removed daily for range of motion exercises, and the pins are removed at 6 to 8 weeks. Postoperative management of fractures with loss of bone and severe soft tissue injury is individualized.

Indications for internal fixation of fractures of the **metacarpal neck** are rotational deformity, resulting in digital scissoring, and excessive apex dorsal angulation. Up to 40° of angulation in the fourth and fifth metacarpals and up to 10° in the second and third metacarpals is acceptable. More angulation is acceptable in the fourth and fifth metacarpals because the second and third CMC joints are more rigid and significant angulation results in a prominent metacarpal head and painful grasp. The fracture is reduced closed under fluoroscopy and stabilized with percutaneous Kirschner wires driven into an adjacent metacarpal or used as intramedullary rods and inserted through the MCP. When inserted through the MCP, they are left long and the MCP is maintained in flexion until the fracture heals (usually 4 to 6 weeks) at which time the pins are removed.

Undisplaced fractures of the **metacarpal head** are splinted as described in the "Initial Management" section for 3 weeks. Fractures with large displaced intraarticular fragments are exposed via a dorsal incision, and reduced and stabilized with Kirschner wires, a Herbert screw, or intraosseous wires. Comminuted fractures that cannot be reduced are managed with distraction in an external fixater.

Ligamentous avulsions of the collaterals are managed with buddy taping. Collateral avulsion with bony displacement greater than 5 mm is managed with open reduction and pinning. **Fight bites** are always opened through a dorsal incision, debrided, and irrigated. Postoperatively, systemic antibiotics are administered for a minimum of 2 weeks.

Complications

Complications include malunion, nonunion, and tendon adhesions. **Malunion** is managed with osteotomy and internal fixation. **Nonunion** is managed with stable fixation and bone grafting. **Adhesions** are managed initially with intensive physical therapy, then surgical release, if necessary. Silicone arthroplasty and MCP fusion are salvage procedures and are only considered if there are no alternatives.

FRACTURES AND DISLOCATIONS OF THE PHALANGES

Fractures of the phalanges are classified as involving the base of the proximal phalanx, the diaphysis of the proximal or middle phalanx, the PIP joint, the DIP joint, or the distal phalanx. Dislocations are of the MCPs, PIPs, or DIPs.

Fracture of the **base of the proximal phalanx** is due to avulsion of the collateral ligament or impaction by the metacarpal head. Fracture of the **diaphysis of the proximal or middle phalanx** is caused by a direct blow or torsion.

Fractures of the proximal phalanx have apex volar angulation secondary to the interossei. Deforming forces on the middle phalanx are the FDS tendon and the long extensor tendon. Distal fractures have apex volar angulation. Proximal fractures have apex dorsal angulation.

Fractures of the **PIP** involve the proximal or middle phalanx. Fractures of the proximal phalanx are undisplaced, unicondylar, or bicondylar and comminuted.

Fractures of the base of the middle phalanx are undisplaced fractures, volar or dorsal lip fractures, lateral avulsions, or comminuted.

Fractures of the **DIP** involve either the head of the middle phalanx or the base of the distal phalanx. Fractures of the dorsal lip of the distal phalanx, or ''mallet finger,'' are caused by avulsion of the extensor tendon. Fractures of the volar lip of the distal phalanx are caused by avulsion of the FDP tendon or volar plate during hyperextension. FDP avulsions occur in contact sports, such as rugby or football, and most often involve the fourth finger.

Distal phalangeal fractures are caused by a direct blow and are longitudinal, transverse, or comminuted. Dislocations of the **MCP, PIP, and DIP** are usually dorsal and caused by hyperextension.

Diagnosis and Initial Management

History and Physical Examination

There is a history of trauma and pain. There may be swelling and deformity. Dimpling of the skin associated with a dislocation indicates that reduction may not be possible by closed means.

Radiographic Examination

Anteroposterior and lateral radiographs define the injury. Other studies are not necessary.

Initial Management

The majority of fractures of the phalanx are managed with closed methods. Buddy taping is used for fractures of the proximal and middle phalanx that do not require reduction. Reduction is performed with a hematoma block. Immobilization of reduced fractures of the proximal phalanx is with a splint extending from the metacarpal heads to the elbow and an alumafoam extension for the involved digit. The wrist is immobilized in 20° of dorsiflexion, the MCP in 90° of flexion, and the PIPs and DIPs in extension. Fractures of the PIP and distal phalanx are immobilized in an alumafoam splint.

Definitive Management

Small **avulsion** fractures of the **base of the proximal phalanx** are managed with buddy taping and early protected motion. Fragments comprising more than 30 percent of the articular surface are exposed via volar or dorsal incisions, depending on location, and fixed with small Kirschner wires, interosseous wires, or screws. **Impaction** fractures are managed with reduction of the joint surface, bone grafting to elevate depressed articular segments, and fixation of the joint surface to the diaphysis. The MCP is immobilized at 90° to "mold" the fracture to the shape of the metacarpal head. Motion is started at 3 to 5 weeks. When a comminuted impaction fracture cannot be reduced and stabilized, traction through the proximal phalanx maintains reduction and allows motion.

Undisplaced fractures of the **diaphysis of the proximal and middle phalanx** are managed with buddy taping.

Displaced fractures are managed with closed reduction and splinting. Up to 15° of angulation in the plane of motion is well tolerated. Rotational deformity results in digital scissoring. Angulation in the medial-lateral plane results in spaces between the fingers when cupping the hand. "Bayoneting" of the fragments results in a prominent spike, causing soft tissue impingement and limiting motion.

Failure to maintain reduction, open fractures, and injuries with multiple fractures are indications for operative reduction and stabilization. Reduction is open via a dorsal incision or closed with fluoroscopy. Fixation is with Kirschner wires, interosseous wires, screws, plates, or external fixaters. Postoperatively, immobilization is maintained for 3 to 5 weeks, when vigorous range of motion exercises are initiated.

Undisplaced fractures of the **PIP** (proximal or middle phalanx) are managed with buddy taping. Displaced unicondylar or bicondylar fractures of the proximal phalanx are reduced open and stabilized. The surgical exposure splits the extensor tendon, preserving the attachment of the central tendon on the middle phalanx. Stabilization is with Kirschner wires, interosseous wires, or screws. Comminuted fractures are managed in an external fixater or with dynamic traction.

Displaced **volar lip** fractures involving more than 30 percent of the joint surface are often associated with joint instability. They are exposed via a volar incision, the pulley is opened, flexor tendons are retracted, and the fragment is reduced and stabilized with Kirschner wires. Alternatively, comminuted fragments are excised and the volar plate advanced into the defect. The joint is pinned for 3 weeks, when protected motion is begun. Agee has described a force-coupling device for maintaining joint reduction while allowing motion. Fractures of the **dorsal lip** are rare and represent avulsion of the central slip of the extensor tendon. Displacement greater than 2 mm results in an extensor lag or boutonniere deformity. If more than 30 percent of the articular surface is involved, the joint may be unstable. Exposure is via a dorsal approach and stabilization is with Kirschner wires or a pullout stitch tied over a volar button. Displaced lateral avulsion fractures are the result of collateral ligament avulsion. They are opened, reduced, and stabilized with Kirschner wires.

The **comminuted** fracture of the middle phalangeal base is similar to a pilon fracture. Up to four fragments can be reduced and stabilized with Kirschner wires or screws. Collapse of the joint surface requires elevation and bone graft. Severely comminuted fractures are managed with an external fixater or dynamic skeletal traction.

Fractures of the **DIP** involve the head of the middle phalanx or the base of the distal phalanx. Intraarticular fractures of the head of the middle phalanx are similar to condylar fractures of the proximal phalanx. Undisplaced fractures of the head of the middle phalanx are managed with splinting or buddy taping. Displaced fractures are pinned percutaneously, or reduced open and pinned. The DIP is immobilized for 6 weeks, but the PIP is left unsplinted. Fractures of the **dorsal lip of the distal phalanx,** or "**mallet finger,**" is an avulsion of the extensor tendon. Most are managed with immobilizing the DIP in hyperextension for 4 weeks. Fragments greater than 30 percent of the joint have associated joint instability and are reduced and stabilized with Kirschner wires or a pullout wire. Postoperatively, they are splinted in hyperextension for 3 weeks. Volar lip fractures that are FDP avulsions are explored and the tendon repaired or fragment of bone stabilized. A pullout wire or small diameter Kirschner wire is used to maintain the reduction.

Undisplaced transverse tuft fractures of the **distal phalanx** are splinted. Displaced fractures are often associated with a soft tissue laceration and, if unstable, are pinned. Longitudinal fractures may be intraarticular and, when displaced are pinned percutaneously or open.

Dislocation of the MCPs, PIPs, and DIPs that cannot be reduced by closed means are exposed via a dorsal incision. The head of the metacarpal is buttonholed through volar soft tissue preventing reduction.

This tissue is incised if necessary and slipped around the head, resulting in reduction. The head of the proximal (PIP dislocation) or middle phalanx (DIP dislocation) is buttonholed beneath the flexor tendons, or soft tissue is interposed between the articular surfaces. If the collateral ligaments are torn, they are repaired through midlateral incisions. All of these reductions are stable. Following reduction, the joint is immobilized for 2 weeks, when motion is initiated.

Complications

Complications of phalangeal fractures and dislocations include malunion, nonunion, and stiffness. These are managed with osteotomy, stabilization with bone grafting, and aggressive physical therapy. Occasionally, symptomatic loss of motion will require a soft tissue release.

FRACTURES OF THE THUMB

There are two injuries unique to the first ray or thumb: fractures of the base of the metacarpal and gamekeeper's thumb. Other fractures of the first ray are managed as their counterparts in the second through fifth rays.

Fractures of the base of the first metacarpal are classified as a Bennet's fracture, Rolando's fracture, or extraarticular fracture. **Bennet's fracture** is a fracture dislocation. The volar lip fragment is held by the anterior oblique ligament and varies in size. The metacarpal is subluxed radially, proximally, and dorsally by the pull of the adductor pollicus brevis and the abductor pollicus longus (Fig.13–4). **Rolando's fracture** is a comminuted fracture of the base of the first metacarpal. **Extraarticular fractures** of the base of the first metacarpal are usually transverse fractures within 1 cm of the articular surface.

Gamekeeper's thumb is an avulsion of the ulnar collateral of the first MCP. The collateral often is torn in midsubstance allowing the adductor to become interposed between the ends. This produces the Stenner lesion (Figs. 13–5 and 13–6). Less commonly, the collateral is avulsed from the proximal phalanx with an osteocartilaginous fragment of articular surface.

Diagnosis and Initial Management

History and Physical Examination

There is a history of injury to the thumb and pain localized to the area of injury. Stressing of the MCP joint may reveal instability in equivocal cases of gamekeeper's thumb.

Radiographic Examination

Anteroposterior and lateral radiographs are obtained. Stress views of the first MCP joint are diagnostic of gamekeeper's thumb.

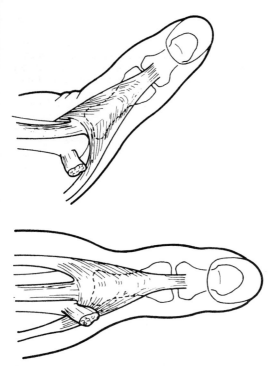

FIGS. 13–5 and 13–6 Gamekeeper's thumb and the Stenner lesion.

Initial Management

Initial management is splinting.

Definitive Management

Bennet's fracture is reduced closed under fluoroscopy with longitudinal traction, abduction, and pronation. Reduction is stabilized with percutaneous pinning. The first metacarpal is pinned to the carpus or to the second metacarpal. It is not necessary to transfix a small fragment as long as reduction is maintained. Fragments comprising more than 30 percent of the articular surface are reduced and pinned to ensure maintenance of reduction of the articular surface. Postoperatively, the hand is casted from the first DIP to the elbow for 4 weeks, when the pins are removed.

Rolando's fracture is reduced open via a hockey stick incision on the volar side of the MCP. The fracture is reduced and Kirschner wires or small screws are used to stabilize the fragments. Comminuted Rolando's fractures are not amenable to open reduction. A well-molded cast or percutaneous pinning of the metacarpal shaft to the second metacarpal can maintain length and an approximate reduction. Postoperatively, the hand is casted from the first DIP to the elbow for 4 weeks.

Extraarticular fractures are managed with closed reduction and casting for 4 to 5 weeks. Reduction is obtained by longitudinal traction and pronation of the distal fragment. Fifteen degrees of angulation is acceptable.

Gamekeeper's thumb is managed with open repair of the ulnar collateral ligament via an ulnar incision. The ligament is repaired, and bony avulsions are reduced and stabilized with Kirschner wires, a pullout wire, or screws. Postoperatively, the hand is casted from the DIP to the elbow for 4 weeks for bony avulsions and 6 weeks for ligament repairs.

Complications

Complications include CMC arthritis and instability of the MCP due to failure of repair. CMC arthritis is managed conservatively with nonsteroidal anti-inflammatories and local steroid injections. If these measures fail, the joint is arthrodesed. Failure of repair of the ulnar collateral ligament is managed with revision, if possible, or ligamentous reconstruction, if necessary.

SELECTED READINGS

Agee JM: Unstable fracture dislocation of the proximal interphalangeal joint of the fingers: A preliminary report of a new treatment technique. *J Hand Surg* 3:386–389, 1978.

Bora FW, Didzian NH: The treatment of injuries of the carpometacarpal joint of the little finger. *J Bone Joint Surg* 56A:1459–1463, 1974.

Burkhalter WE: Closed treatment of hand fractures. *J Hand Surg* 14A:390–393, 1989.

Eaton RG, Malerich MM: Volar plate arthroplasty for the proximal interphalangeal joint. A ten year review. *J Hand Surg* 5:260–268, 1980.

Gonzalez MH, McKay W, Hall RI Jr: Low velocity gunshot wounds of the metacarpal: Treatment by early stable fixation and bone grafting. *J Hand Surg* 18A:267, 1993.

Hastings H II, Carroll C IV: Treatment of closed articular fractures of the metacarpophalangeal and proximal interphalangeal joints. *Hand Clin* 4:503–527, 1988.

Lubahn JD: Mallet finger fractures: A comparison of open and closed technique. *J Hand Surg* 14A:394, 1989.

Mueller JJ: Carpometacarpal dislocations: Report of five cases and review of the literature. *J Hand Surg* 11A:184–188, 1986.

Parsons SW, Fitzgerald JAW, Shearer JR: External fixation of unstable metacarpal and phalangeal fractures. *J Hand Surg* 17B:151–155, 1992.

Pellegrini VD Jr: Fractures at the base of the thumb. *Hand Clin* 4:87–102, 1988.

Schneider LH: Fractures of the distal phalanx. *Hand Clin* 4:537–547, 1988.

Stern PJ, Roman RJ, Kiefhaber TR, McDonough JJ: Pilon fractures of the proximal interphalangeal joint. *J Hand Surg* 16A:844–850, 1991.

14 | Fractures and Dislocations of the Spine

*Lawrence G. Lenke   Michael F. O'Brien
Keith H. Bridwell*

Spinal trauma includes injuries occurring in the axial skeleton from the occipital-cervical junction to the coccyx. The anatomic classification of spinal trauma is organized into upper cervical, subaxial cervical, thoracic and lumbar, and sacral injuries. The pathophysiology of spinal trauma, as well as the initial assessment of a patient with a suspected spinal injury, is similar for all patients.

When presented with a spinal injury, the key questions are: What is the mechanism of injury? Are there other injuries, including life-threatening injuries? What are the injured anatomic structures of the spine? Is there actual or impending neurologic damage? Can the spine function as a weight-bearing column? What is the best treatment method (operative or nonoperative) for the particular fracture? The most important decision initially is whether definitive management should be operative or nonoperative.

ANATOMY

The function of the spine as a support column is broken down into the four anatomical segments: cervical, thoracic, lumbar, and sacrococcygeal. Normally, these segments align in a linear fashion in the coronal or frontal plane. However, in the sagittal plane, there is approximately 25° of cervical lordosis, 35° of thoracic kyphosis, and approximately 50° of lumbar lordosis allowing the skull to align directly over the midportion of the top of the sacrum.

The cross-sectional anatomy of the spine is organized into **three columns** (Fig. 14–1). The **anterior column** consists of the anterior longitudinal ligament, anterior half of the vertebral body, annulus fibrosis, and disc. The **middle column** consists of the posterior one-half of the vertebral body, annulus, disc, and posterior longitudinal ligament. The **posterior column** includes the facet joints, ligamentum flavum, posterior elements, and interconnecting ligaments.

The three-column theory of the spine produces a basic classification system of spinal injuries. Thus, spinal injuries are classified into four different categories dependent on the specific column(s) injured: compression fractures, burst fractures, seat belt type flexion-distraction injuries, and fracture-dislocations (Table 14–1). **Compression fractures** are characterized by failure of the anterior column under compression with an intact middle and posterior column. When the anterior and middle column fail under axial loading forces, a **burst fracture** is

157

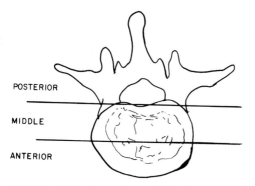

POSTERIOR

MIDDLE

ANTERIOR

FIG. 14–1 The three columns of the spine.

produced. Distraction of the middle and posterior column produces a seat belt type of **flexion-distraction** injury. **Fracture-dislocations** are characterized by involvement of all three columns in compression, distraction, rotation, and/or shear.

Although the three-column theory of the spine provides an excellent model to describe the individual spinal segments injured, it is essential to determine the overall structural stability of the spine. For example, compression injuries to the anterior and/or middle column may cause kyphosis. Because spinal injuries result from a combination of various forces acting on the spinal column, including compression, distraction, axial load, rotation, torsion, or shear, careful attention is paid to alignment in the coronal and sagittal plane to identify potential subluxation or dislocations of the spine.

Osseous Anatomy

The **cervical spine** comprises the first seven vertebrae and connects the skull to the thoracic spine. The cervical spine functions to protect the spinal cord and nerve roots while supporting the skull and allowing flexibility to position the head. Approximately one-half of the neck

TABLE 14–1 Classification of Spinal Injuries

Type of injury	Columns injured		
	Anterior	Middle	Posterior
I Compression fractures	yes	no	no
II Burst fractures	yes	yes	no
III Flexion-distraction injuries	yes/no	yes	yes
IV Fracture-dislocations	yes	yes	yes

flexion-extension occurs between the base of the skull and C1. Similarly, half of the rotation of the head on the neck occurs at the C1 to C2 articulation. The remaining motions of flexion, extension, rotation, and side-bending occur between the C2 to T1 articulations.

The atlas (C1) and the axis (C2) differ markedly in structure from the lower five cervical vertebrae (C3 through C7). The atlas is unique among vertebrae in that it has no vertebral body but a thick anterior arch which has two bulky lateral masses and a thin posterior arch. The axis has the odontoid process or dens, which is the fused remnant of the body of the first cervical vertebra. The odontoid process sits cephalad on the body of C2 and rests just posterior to the anterior arch of the atlas, where it is held tightly by ligaments. The remaining lower cervical vertebrae (C3 through C7) have small vertebral bodies which are convex on the superior surface and concave on the inferior surface. Arising anterolaterally from the bodies are transverse processes which have both an anterior as well as posterior tubercle. The foramen transversarium is located between the posterior tubercle and the lateral part of the vertebral body. The vertebral artery passes through this foramen entering at C6 and exiting at C2. The exiting nerve roots pass just posterior to the vertebral arteries at the level of the disc space.

Posterior to the vertebral foramina are the lateral masses which comprise that portion of bone between the superior and inferior facets. The lateral masses are important anatomic structures for the placement of screws in posterior plating procedures of the cervical spine. The cervical facet joints are oriented more in a horizontal than vertical plane with the superior facet sitting anterior to the inferior facet of the level above. This allows for a great amount of flexion and extension of the neck but limits side-bending. The remainder of the posterior elements of the cervical spine include the lamina and spinous processes which are posterior and medial to the facet joints and lateral masses.

There are 12 vertebrae of the **thoracic spine.** The differential features of thoracic vertebrae are thin pedicles which connect the vertebral body to the posterior elements; the transverse processes which project superolaterally from the posterior part of the pedicle and are larger in size than the cervical transverse processes; and the ventral surface of the transverse process which has a costal articulation. The thoracic spine is a more rigid column than the cervical or lumbar spine because of the rib cage. As in the cervical spine, the facets of the thoracic spine are oriented in the coronal plane with the superior facet anterior to the inferior facet. At the thoracolumbar junction, the facet joints change gradually from a coronal to a more sagittal orientation.

The vertebrae of the **lumbar spine** are larger than the cervical or thoracic vertebrae. The pedicles are wider and broader, and they are usually able to accept bone screws. The facet joints are oriented sagittally with the inferior facet of the segment above medial to the superior facet of the segment below. The transverse processes project straight lateral from the superior facets and are quite large. The posterior elements (lamina and spinous processes) are also larger in the lumbar spine.

The **sacrum and coccyx** are normally fused and attach the axial skeleton to the pelvis by the sacrotuberous and sacrospinous ligaments and sacroiliac joint.

Ligamentous Anatomy

The ligaments of the spinal column support the osseous structures. We distinguish between those supporting the anterior and middle columns and those stabilizing the posterior column. The stabilizers of the anterior and middle column are the **anterior longitudinal ligament** and the **posterior longitudinal ligament,** which extend the entire length of the spine and insert on the vertebral bodies. They are the major stabilizers of the vertebral bodies and discs in flexion and extension. The anterior longitudinal ligament is closely attached to the intervertebral disc and has a ribbon-like structure. The posterior longitudinal ligament is widest in the upper cervical spine and narrows as it proceeds caudally. It thins over the vertebral bodies and thickens over the intervertebral discs.

The ligamentous structures stabilizing the posterior column include the **supraspinous ligament, the interspinous ligament, the facet joint capsule,** and **the ligamentum flavum.** The ligamentum flavum runs from the superior margin of the caudad lamina to the ventral surface of the cephalad lamina. There are right and left ligaments separated by a small fissure which merges with the interspinous ligaments posteriorly and medially, and the fibrous facet capsules laterally. The posterior ligamentous structures are stabilizers during flexion.

The ligamentous structures of the upper cervical spine are unique. The odontoid process is held snugly against the posterior wall of the anterior arch of the atlas by the **transverse ligament.** Additional stability is afforded by the **apical ligament** and the paired **alar ligaments** that run superiorly from the odontoid process to the anterior rim of the foramen magnum. This allows rotation of C1 on C2, but prevents posterior translation of the dens within the ring of the atlas, which would place the spinal cord at risk.

The **intervertebral discs** are complex structures made up of an outer annulus fibrosis and an inner nucleus pulposus. The **annulus fibrosis** is a laminated structure consisting of collagen fibers which are oriented 30° from horizontal. The inner layers are attached to the cartilaginous endplates, whereas the outer fibers are firmly secured to the osseous vertebral bodies. The annulus surrounds and contains the **nucleus pulposus,** a matrix of protein, glycosaminoglycans, and water. Injury to the intervertebral disc may not be obvious on conventional radiography, but it must be considered when evaluating overall spinal stability and potential neurologic compromise. MRI allows direct visualization of the intervertebral disc.

BIOMECHANICS

In the sagittal projection, the spine is made up of three smooth curves: cervical lordosis, thoracic kyphosis, and lumbar lordosis, with a smooth transition between these curves. The center of gravity passes anterior to the midthoracic spine and just posterior to the midlumbar spine before intersecting the top portion of the sacrum. This implies that most of the spinal column experiences compressive forces anteriorly through the vertebral bodies, and tensile forces through the posterior elements and ligaments.

The distribution of materials and their properties match the function of the spine. The vertebral bodies are well equipped for handling compressive loads. The majority of the vertebral bodies are made of trabecular bone, which is the primary weight-bearing component of the vertebral bodies in compression. Removing the cortex of the vertebral body reduces its strength by only 10 percent. The marrow contents of the vertebral body act as a hydraulic system when compressed. This viscoelastic property allows the vertebral body to absorb more energy.

Posteriorly, the major stabilizers of the spine are the ligamentous structures of the posterior column. These structures are predominantly made of collagen and are very strong when loaded in tension.

The intervertebral discs are important to the structural stability of the spine. The inner layers of the annulus and the nucleus transmit loads from vertebra to vertebra. With significant force application, the annular fibers fail, allowing the potential for segmental instability and traumatic disc herniations.

The rib cage stabilizes the thoracic spine. This increased thoracic spine stability creates stress risers at the junction of the more mobile cervical spine above and lumbar spine below.

The criteria for determining traumatic **spinal instability** are controversial. The three-column concept of spinal anatomy provides a framework in which to consider specific anatomical areas of injury. Thus, when only one column is injured, the spine is usually stable. When two or three columns are injured, it is usually unstable (i.e., unable to adequately function as a support column and to protect the neural elements). This definition is applicable both acutely and chronically. Thus, in many situations, the question of spinal stability is unclear and rests on the interpretation of pertinent radiographs, the neurologic exam, and sound clinical judgment.

Neurologic Injuries

Based on the anatomic location of the spinal injury, there are three categories of neurologic injury: spinal cord, conus medullaris, and cauda equina lesions. Injuries to the cervical and thoracic spine may directly affect the spinal cord or nerve roots (Table 14–2). The distal spinal cord is termed the conus medullaris and usually lies at the thoracolumbar

TABLE 14–2 Upper Extremity Neurologic Exam

Root	Motor	Sensory	Reflex
C4	Diaphragm	Top of shoulder	
C5	Elbow flexion (biceps)	Lateral arm	Biceps
C6	Wrist extensors (ECRL/ECRB)	Lateral forearm thumb/index finger	Briachioradialis
C7	Elbow extension (triceps)	Middle finger	Triceps
C8	Finger flexors (FDP)	Medial forearm ring/little finger	
T1	Finger abduction (interossei)	Posterior shoulder	

junction at the pedicle level of L1. The sacral nuclei which control bowel and bladder function are located in the conus. The cauda equina consists of all lumbar and sacral roots below the conus (usually L2 and below). Injuries to the cauda equina are peripheral nerve root injuries; they have a better prognosis for return of function than spinal cord or conus injuries.

Spinal cord injuries in the cervical or thoracic spine are designated as complete or incomplete. **Complete** lesions are characterized by total loss of motor, sensory, and reflex function below the level of injury. These injuries result in quadriplegia in the upper cervical spine and paraplegia in the thoracic spine. Complete spinal cord injuries of the cervical spine are described by the lowest level of cervical root function. This has implications for functional independence of the patient. A C3 quadriplegic is ventilator-dependent without any upper or lower extremity function. Patients with C6 or below quadriplegia function independently.

Complete spinal cord injuries in the thoracic spine produce paraplegia. The location of the lesion is irrelevant to the functional outcome for the patient because the segmental thoracic nerve roots only supply sensation to the thorax and innervation to the intercostal muscles. However, a proximal thoracic paraplegic versus a distal thoracic paraplegic has an increased risk of respiratory problems because of increased intercostal paralysis.

Incomplete spinal cord injuries are categorized into four types based on the cross-section location of the injury within the spinal cord: anterior cord, posterior cord, central cord, and Brown-Séquard syndromes. In the **anterior cord syndrome,** the injury is to the anterior spinal cord which contains the corticospinal motor tracts. This results in motor paralysis with preservation of deep pressure sensation and proprioception due to the intact posterior columns. The **posterior cord syndrome** is rare and results from damage to the posterior columns. This results in loss of proprioception and deep pressure sensation, but the maintenance of motor function due to the intact anterior motor columns. **Central cord syndrome** results from damage to the central gray matter and centrally oriented white matter tracts. In the cervical spine, the centrally oriented white matter tracts provide motor innervation to the upper extremities. As a result, the upper extremities will be more involved than the lower. In the thoracic region, a central cord injury affects the proximal musculature of the lower extremities more than the distal. In the **Brown-Séquard syndrome,** half the cord is damaged in the coronal projection. Thus, there is ipsilateral motor paralysis and loss of position sense, and contralateral loss of pain and temperature sensation. This is because the motor tracts and posterior columns decussate in the brainstem while the sensory tracts decussate one to two levels above where they enter the spinal cord. Frequently, there is overlap between these syndromes.

The second group of neurologic injuries involves the **conus medullaris.** These injuries occur with trauma to the thoracolumbar junction and frequently involve elements of the lower spinal cord and cauda equina. Injuries at this level are very difficult to accurately diagnose in the acute setting, especially in the face of spinal shock. Because the conus medullaris usually ends at the level of the L1 pedicle, spinal injuries at this level may damage the upper motor neurons of the sacral cord or the lower motor neurons to the sacral or lumbar roots which have already exited the spinal cord. Thus, it is not unusual to regain motor strength in the lower extremities which are innervated by lumbar nerves, but continue to have absent bowel and bladder function due to a conus injury damaging sacral nerve root innervation to the bowel and bladder.

Cauda equina injuries occur with fractures or dislocations of the L2 level and below. The neurologic deficit may range from a single nerve root injury to a **cauda equina syndrome** in which there is marked weakness of the lower extremities and involvement of the nerve roots supplying the bowel and bladder.

The decrease in spinal canal cross-sectional area following fracture or dislocation does not always correlate with the severity of neurologic injury or the prognosis for recovery. This is because the size of the canal, and the presence of bone or disc material within it, only reflects the final resting place of these fragments, not the magnitude of energy absorbed, the maximum displacement, or the trajectory of the displaced fragments. However, residual spinal canal compromise of greater than 50 percent or absolute spinal canal dimensions less than 10 to 13 mm indicate acute or impending neurologic dysfunction.

Decompression of the spinal canal in complete spinal cord injuries does little or nothing to improve neurologic outcome. Surgical decompression is recommended for incomplete spinal cord, conus, or cauda equina lesion. Significant improvement in neurologic outcome is possible, especially with cauda equina (lower motor neuron) lesions.

The incidence of penetrating spinal trauma from **gunshot wounds** is increasing. Rarely is the spinal column rendered unstable from a gunshot wound; however, neurologic injury is frequent. Cervical and thoracic level injuries often produce quadriplegia or paraplegia, respectively. Similarly, injury to the cauda equina occurs with lumbar gunshot wounds. Most of the neural damage is secondary to the kinetic energy transference to the neural tissues. Surgical removal of bullet is rarely indicated except in incomplete spinal cord or cauda equina lesion with a space occupying fragment of bone or bullet identified. Because of the heat generated, these bullet wounds have a low infection rate, except if they traversed the colon prior to entering the spinal column. This is one indication for elective removal of the bullet if lodged in the spinal column or canal.

Diagnosis and Initial Management

The diagnosis and initial management of patients with spinal fractures and dislocations depends to a great degree on the area of the spine involved. Nevertheless, there are commonalities.

Patients with spinal injuries may have additional life-threatening injuries; therefore, initial priorities are to secure an airway, ventilation, and hemodynamic stabilization.

Precautions for the stabilization of the entire spinal column begin at the accident site. Patients with a history of trauma to the head, neck, or back, or conscious patients who report any neurologic symptoms are immobilized in a cervical collar with complete head and neck immobilization on a spine board until an appropriate evaluation is performed. A history of the mechanism of injury, as well as a detailed report of any neck or back pain and motor or sensory changes in the extremities, are essential. Unconscious patients with major trauma are a more difficult challenge and suspicion must remain high until a thorough examination for potential spinal injury is performed.

A thorough neurologic exam is performed as soon as possible. Neurologic exams include complete assessment of motor, sensory, and reflex function for both upper and lower extremities. Perianal sensation and a rectal exam are critical to determine the function of the sacral roots and sacral cord. Sacral sensory sparring or any trace of distal motor function implies possible return of function. Also, spinal shock for the first 24 to 48 h may give the appearance of a complete spinal cord injury in patients who will later be found to have sensory and motor function. The resolution of spinal shock is indicated by the return of the **bulbocavernosus reflex.** This is tested while performing a digital rectal exam. Pulling on the foley catheter will result in contraction of the anal sphincter when the bulbocavernosus reflex is present. When the bulbocavernosus reflex returns in the face of a complete spinal cord injury, the chances are that the neurologic deficit is permanent.

Radiographic Examination

Screening radiographs include an anteroposterior as well as a lateral. On the lateral radiograph, one should examine the height of all the vertebral bodies as well as the intervening disc spaces. These heights should be fairly uniform and symmetric. When the vertebral body height is decreased, an angulatory deformity (i.e., kyphosis) is produced on the lateral radiograph. The anterior and posterior vertebral body lines should align throughout the whole spine. With injury to the middle column (posterior vertebral body), retropulsion of bone into the spinal canal may be evident on the lateral view. The lateral radiograph also will show the posterior elements, including the facets, lamina, and spinous processes. Widened interspinous process distance is indicative of distraction injury to the posterior column.

The anteroposterior radiograph of the spine is examined. Each vertebral body should sit directly on top of the one below with a symmetric and evenly placed disc space between them. The right and left borders of the vertebral bodies should be well aligned. The two round pedicle shadows of each vertebral body should be present and symmetric. Widening of the interpedicular distance at one level may be indicative of a middle column burst-type injury. Careful examination delineates the posterior elements of the spine. The posterior elements of a segment are somewhat distal to the corresponding vertebral body. The spinous process shadow is usually visible allowing for comparison of the interspinous process distance at each level. Finally, the transverse processes at each level are examined for fracture, as well as the ribs in the thoracic spine, the sacrum, SI joints, and iliac wings of the pelvis.

It is very important in patients with spinal trauma to not miss additional spinal injuries. Up to 10 percent of patients with spinal trauma at one site will have another injury to their spinal column at an adjoining or distant site. This is especially important in cervical or thoracic spine-injured patients who may have spinal cord injuries resulting in sensory loss to more distal areas of their thoracic and lumbar spine, making it more difficult to diagnose injuries there.

Initial Management

All patients are kept supine on a well-cushioned mattress and log-rolled every 2 h to decrease pressure on sensitive areas. Antiembolism stockings are used for deep vein thrombosis prophylaxis. Cardiac status and oxygen saturation are monitored continuously. A nasogastric tube is placed for the accompanying gastrointestinal ileus. A foley catheter provides for accurate determination of urine output and simplifies nursing care. Intravenous fluids maintain an adequate fluid volume. Complete blood counts are obtained at presentation and then several times in the early postinjury period. Intravenous pain medications are dictated by the age, medical status, and amount of pain. Physical therapy for range of motion exercises of uninjured extremities is begun early in the hospital course.

The initial care for a cervical spine injury patient is somewhat different. Patients with a cervical spine injury causing spinal malalignment,

regardless of the neurologic status, are placed in **skeletal tongs traction.**
We use graphite Gardner-Wells tongs that are MRI compatible. They
are placed one finger breadth above the earlobe in line with the external
auditory canal. The skull bolts are finger tightened until the pressure
valve is released in the center of the bolt indicating adequate force.
Tongs are applied in the emergency room when spinal malalignment
is identified. Approximately 5 lb per level of injury is slowly added to
the traction apparatus under close neurologic and radiographic surveil-
lance. Thus, a patient with a C4 to C5 facet dislocation may require
25 lb or more for reduction of the malalignment. It is not uncommon
to require anywhere from 50 to 100 lb of traction weight for lower
cervical spine dislocations to accomplish reduction in large adults.
Once reduction is achieved, 10 to 15 lb is sufficient to maintain
reduction. A lateral cervical spine radiograph ensures maintenance
of proper cervical spine alignment and should be checked frequently,
especially after returning from tests that require mobilization of the
patient.

The pharmacologic treatment of acute spinal cord injury is administration of steroids in an attempt to diminish edema around the neural
elements following injury. Indications for steroids are all cervical spine-
injured patients with any neurologic deficit, thoracic spine injuries with
incomplete paraplegia, incomplete cauda equina lesions with neurologic
deterioration, and the inability to promptly take the patient to surgery.
Steroids are administered to complete cervical spine-injured patients.
They are not administered to complete thoracic spine-injured patients.
This is because of the significant benefit of saving or gaining a functional
root level in a complete cervical spine-injured patient. Thirty mg/kg
of methylprednisolone is administered as a loading dose intravenously
over 30 min. A continuous intravenous drip of methylprednisolone at
a dose of 5.4 mg/kg per h is continued for 24 h and then discontinued.
Any neurologic deterioration while on methylprednisolone merits re-
consideration of its use. The risk of this high-dose steroid regimen
is gastrointestinal hemorrhage; therefore, all patients are protected
with H_2 antagonists, such as Cimetidine or Ranitidine for a minimum
of 72 h.

Spine injuries are divided into four groups based on the involved
segment: upper cervical, subaxial cervical, thoracic and lumbar, and
sacral.

UPPER CERVICAL SPINE INJURIES (OCCIPUT TO C2)

Classification

There are eight types of upper cervical spine injuries encountered.
The four most frequently encountered are: atlas fractures, atlantoaxial
subluxations, odontoid fractures, and traumatic spondylolisthesis of the

axis (C2 hangman's fractures). The four less common injuries are: occipital condyle fractures, atlantooccipital dislocation, atlantoaxial rotary subluxation, and C2 lateral mass fractures.

Atlas fractures result from impaction of the occipital condyles on the arch of C1. This causes single or multiple fractures of the ring of C1 which usually splay apart and thus increase the space for the spinal cord; therefore, neurologic injury is rare. There are four types of atlas fractures. The first two are stable injuries: isolated anterior or posterior arch fractures. Anterior arch fractures are usually avulsion injuries from the anterior portion of the ring. Posterior arch fractures result from hyperextension with compression of the posterior arch of C1 between the occiput and C2. The third type of atlas fracture is a lateral mass fracture. The fracture lines run anterior and posterior to the articular surface of the C1 lateral mass with asymmetric displacement of the lateral mass from the remainder of the vertebrae. This is best seen on an open-mouth odontoid view of the C1 to C2 complex. The fourth type, burst fractures of the atlas (or Jefferson's fracture), classically has four fractures in the ring of C1—two in the anterior portion and two in the posterior ring. Potential instability of these fractures is best identified by examining the overhang of the C1 lateral masses on the C2 articular facets as noted on the open-mouth odontoid view. Total lateral displacement on both sides of more than 6.9 mm indicates rupture of the transverse ligament with resultant atlantoaxial instability.

Atlantoaxial subluxation is secondary to rupture of the primary stabilizer of the atlantoaxial articulation, the transverse ligament. This produces atlantoaxial instability which may place the spinal cord at risk. Thus, potential complications from this injury include neurologic injury resulting from the odontoid compressing the upper cervical cord against the posterior arch of C1.

Identification of **odontoid process fractures** requires a high index of suspicion. Odontoid process fractures must be ruled out in all patients with neck pain following a motor vehicle accident, and elderly patients involved in trivial trauma to the head and neck region. If there is significant anterior, or more commonly posterior, displacement of the odontoid process, spinal cord injury may result. The incidence of neurologic injury is approximately 10 percent. Odontoid fractures are further classified into three types based on the anatomic level at which they occur (Fig. 14–2). **Type I** fractures represent an avulsion fracture from the tip of the odontoid process where the alar ligament inserts.

Type II fractures are the most common type of odontoid fracture and occur in the midportion of the dens proximal to the body of the axis. The limited blood supply and small cross-sectional cancellous surface area lead to a high incidence of nonunion. Other risk factors for nonunion are angulation, anterior or posterior displacement of more than 4 mm, and patient age greater than 40 years.

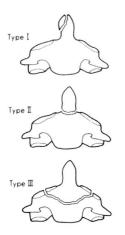

ODONTOID PROCESS FRACTURES

FIG. 14–2   The three types of odontoid fractures.

Type III injuries are those in which the fracture line extends into the vertebral body of C2. Because of the larger cross-sectional area and the presence of cancellous bone with a rich blood supply, these type III fractures consistently unite, providing they are adequately aligned (Fig. 14–3).

Traumatic spondylolisthesis of the axis, or hangman's fracture, is a bipedicular fracture with disruption of the disc and ligaments between C2 and C3 resulting most commonly from hyperextension and distraction. This fracture is named for the injury resulting from judicial hanging with rope in the submental position.

Hangman's fractures are further classified based on the amount of displacement and angulation of the C2 body in relation to the posterior elements (Figs. 14–4 through 14–7). **Type I** injury is a fracture of the neural arch without angulation, and with as much as 3 mm of anterior displacement of C2 on C3.

Type II fractures have anterior displacement greater than 3 mm or angulation of C2 on C3. These fractures usually result from hyperextension and axial load followed by severe flexion that stretches the posterior annulus and disc and produces the anterior translation and angulation. **Type IIA** injuries are a flexion-distraction variant of type II fractures. They demonstrate severe angulation of C2 on C3 with minimal displacement, apparently hinging on the anterior longitudinal ligament. It is important to recognize this type of hangman's fracture because the application of traction may distract the C2 to C3 disc space and further displace the fracture.

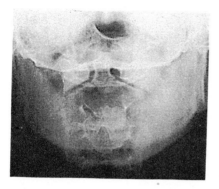

FIG. 14–3 An open-mouth view indicating a type III odontoid fracture.

Type III injuries are bipedicle fractures associated with unilateral or bilateral facet dislocations. These are serious, unstable injuries and have a high rate of neurologic sequelae.

Fractures of the **occipital condyles** result from combined axial loading and lateral bending. There are two types: avulsion fractures or comminuted compression fractures.

Atlantooccipital dislocations are rare injuries resulting from total disruption of all ligamentous structures between the occiput and the atlas. The mechanism of injury is usually extension or flexion. Death is

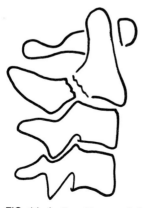

FIG. 14–4 Type I hangman's fracture.

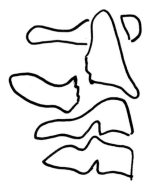

FIG. 14–5   Type II hangman's fracture.

usually immediate due to severe brain stem involvement with complete respiratory arrest.

Atlantoaxial rotary subluxation occurs most often secondary to vehicular accidents. The main difficulty is lack of early recognition.

Lateral mass fractures of the axis are the result of combined axial loading and lateral bending forces.

Associated Injuries

Associated injuries include spinal cord or cervical nerve root compression; head injuries; and other spine fractures, particularly of the cervical spine. Fractures of the occipital condyles are associated with severe

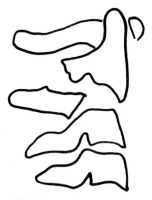

FIG. 14–6   Type IIA hangman's fracture.

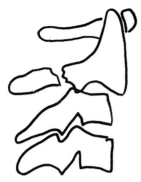

FIG. 14–7 Type III hangman's fracture.

head trauma and are accompanied by cranial nerve palsies. Fifty percent of patients with a fracture of the posterior arch of the atlas have another cervical spine injury, the most common being a traumatic spondylolisthesis of the axis or a displaced odontoid fracture. A high index of suspicion and careful physical and radiographic examination are the best method of finding associated injuries.

Diagnosis and Initial Management

Physical Examination

The patient has pain localized to the neck, and there may be a feeling of instability or fixed deformity. The initial asssesment is performed as described.

Radiographic Examination

Initially, a cross-table lateral is obtained in all patients with suspected cervical spine injuries. This radiograph includes all seven cervical vertebrae, as well as the C7 to T1 junction. When this is not possible due to interposition of the shoulders in patients with short necks, the patients' arms are pulled down to lower the shoulders, or, alternatively, one arm is extended above the head while keeping the other arm at the side while shooting (swimmer's view) (Fig. 14–8).

Additional required views include an AP view and odontoid, or openmouth, view, which details the C1 to C2 articulation in the coronal plane (Fig. 14–3). Right or left obliques and voluntary flexion-extension views are obtained as indicated.

Four lines are essential to examine on the lateral radiograph: the anterior vertebral body line, the posterior vertebral body line, the spinal laminar line, and the line connecting the tips of the spinous processes. All of these landmarks should align in a smooth arc from C1 to T1

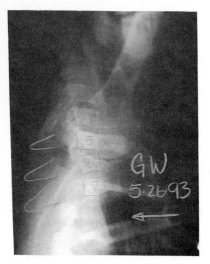

FIG. 14-8   Swimmer's view of cervical spine.

(Fig. 14–9). Any malalignment indicates potential vertebral subluxation or dislocation occurring with a spinal injury.

The soft tissue shadows in lateral cervical spine radiographs represent the retropharyngeal and retrotracheal shadows. These soft tissue shadows are expanded by the accompanying hematoma produced following cervical spine injury and may be the only indication of subtle injuries. The soft tissue shadow should be no more than 6 mm from the anterior aspect of C2, and no more than 2 cm at the anterior edge of C6 (i.e., 6 at 2 and 2 at 6).

Fractures of the occipital condyles are difficult to visualize on plain radiographs and require axial CT studies for delineation.

Atlantoocipital dissociation is identified on the lateral radiograph of the cervical spine or lateral view of the skull, which profiles the atlantoocipital junction quite well. There is dissociation between the base of the occiput and the C1 arch and severe soft tissue swelling.

Fractures of the atlas are diagnosed on a lateral cervical spine radiograph and/or an open-mouth odontoid view. The lateral cervical spine radiograph demonstrates fracture lines within the posterior arch of C1. The open-mouth view indicates splaying of the lateral masses of C1 on the articular surfaces of the axis. An axial CT scan is helpful in evaluation.

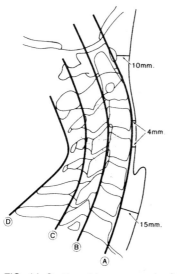

FIG. 14–9   Normal bony arcs and soft tissue shadows seen on the lateral of the cervicle spine. (*a*) anterior vertebral body line, (*b*) posterior vertebral body line, (*c*) laminar line, and (*d*) spinous process line.

Atlantoaxial subluxation due to disruption of the transverse ligament is best demonstrated on lateral flexion-extension views and is indicated by an increase in the atlantodental interval (ADI), which is normally less than 3.5 mm. This is measured from the posterior aspect of the anterior arch of C1 to the anterior aspect of the odontoid process (Figs. 14–10 and 14–11.) However, spinal extensor muscle spasm accompanying an acute injury may prevent adequate voluntary flexion-extension radiographs. Once recognized, an axial CT scan is obtained to ascertain if instability is purely ligamentous or due to a bony avulsion.

Radiographs following atlantoaxial rotary subluxation are often reported as normal because it is difficult to obtain radiographs parallel to the plane of both C1 and C2 due to the accompanying torticollis. Open-mouth radiographs often help recognize this injury by demonstrating a "wink sign." This occurs because of the unilateral overlap of the lateral mass of C1 on C2. A CT scan is helpful in describing the direction and rotation of C1 on C2.

Odontoid fractures are seen on lateral cervical spine radiographs or an open-mouth view. Occasionally, three-dimensional CT reconstruction or conventional tomography may be necessary to identify and fully

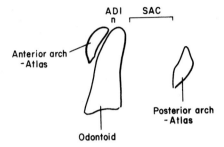

FIG. 14—10 Normal relation of the atlas and dens seen on the lateral.

evaluate these fractures. Axial CT scans may miss the fracture line as it is in the plane of the axial image.

Hangman's fractures are seen on the lateral radiograph. Lateral mass fractures with minimal comminution may require CT scanning for identification.

Initial Management

Occipital condyle fractures are managed initially in a cervicle orthosis. Fractures of the occipital condyles are generally stable injuries which can be treated with orthotic immobilization with a two-poster orthosis or a rigid Philadelphia collar. Most of these fractures heal uneventfully, although occasionally posttraumatic arthritis occurs requiring posterior atlantooccipital fusion.

Traction is contraindicated following atlantooccipital dislocation. Even 5 lb may overdistract and stretch the brain stem with catastrophic results. Initial treatment is application of a halo vest to maintain stability

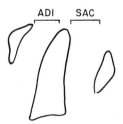

FIG. 14—11 Atlantoaxial subluxation as indicated by an increase in the ADI.

of the spine, while attention is placed on the patient's respiratory and neurologic status. Once the patient is stabilized, a posterior occiput to upper cervical spine fusion is performed with continued immobilization in a halo vest for approximately 3 months.

Initial management of types I, II, and III fractures of the atlas is a cervical orthosis. Jefferson's fractures are placed in traction.

Atlantoaxial subluxation and atlantoaxial rotary subluxation are managed initially with a cervical orthosis.

Type I odontoid fractures are managed with a cervical orthosis. Type II and III fractures are initially managed with cervical tongs traction to reduce and/or maintain sagittal alignment.

Type I and II hangman's fractures are managed with a cervical orthosis. The initial management of type III fractures is application of traction in order to reduce the facet dislocation. Reduction by closed means may not be possible because of the dissociation between the vertebral body and the posterior elements.

Definitive Management

Definitive management of fractures of the atlas is based on the type of fracture. Types I and II may be managed in a cervical orthosis in a compliant patient, whereas type III injuries are managed with a halo vest. Type IV, or Jefferson's, fractures with a competent transverse ligament (less than 6.9 mm displacement of the lateral masses) are stable and are also managed in a halo vest. Jefferson's fractures with an incompetent transverse ligament (more than 6.9 mm displacement) are unstable and managed with extended cervical traction to reduce the splaying until the bony fragments are sticky. This is necessary because the halo vest is unable to provide the axial distraction necessary to maintain fracture reduction. After preliminary healing, application of a halo vest for the remainder of the 3- to 4-month period allows complete healing. When a C1 fracture is presumed healed, voluntary lateral flexion-extension radiographs of the cervical spine are obtained to ensure there is no significant atlantoaxial subluxation. If there is more than 5 mm of atlantoaxial subluxation in an adult, posterior C1 to C2 fusion is performed.

Atlantoaxial subluxation due to bony avulsion of the transverse ligament is managed with a halo vest for 3 months. Purely ligamentous injuries are managed with a C1 to C2 posterior fusion.

Atlantoaxial rotary subluxation recognized within several weeks of injury is reduced with cervical traction. This may require up to 30 to 40 lb of traction to reduce the rotary dislocation. Often a "pop" is heard and felt at reduction. A halo vest is applied. Even with prolonged halo vest treatment, long-term stability may not be achieved because the C1 to C2 facet joint is a saddle-type joint and depends on ligamentous restraint for stability. Atlantoaxial arthrodesis is the treatment of choice for chronic instability and pain, or for patients with an associated neurologic deficit. For chronic injuries, closed reduction via cervical traction is not possible; they are managed with open reduction and C1 to C2 arthrodesis.

Type I odontoid fractures are stable injuries which are managed with an orthosis for symptomatic comfort. Type I avulsion injuries are often seen in association with atlantooccipital dislocations; therefore, evaluation must be performed for this more serious injury. There are four types of definitive treatment for type II odontoid fractures: halo vest management of minimally displaced or angulated fractures followed by posterior C1 to C2 arthrodesis if healing does not occur within 4 months; primary posterior C1 to C2 arthrodesis as long as the posterior arch of C1 is intact; posterior C1 to C2 facet screw fixation and fusion; and anterior screw fixation of the dens under biplanar fluoroscopy. The theoretical advantage of anterior screw fixation is that it does not require a C1 to C2 fusion and thus preserves motion of the upper cervical spine. Provided type III odontoid fractures are adequately reduced, halo vest immobilization for 3 months is the treatment of choice. When reduction is lost after halo vest placement, cervical traction for 3 to 4 weeks to allow early fracture healing before continuing with the halo vest is required.

Type I hangman's fractures are stable injuries and are managed in a cervical orthosis for 3 months in a compliant patient. Type II fractures displaced less than 5 mm and minimally angulated are managed with a halo vest if reduction can be maintained. Fractures displaced more than 5 mm are managed in cervical tongs traction with slight extension for approximately 3 to 6 weeks prior to application of the halo vest. Traction is contraindicated for Type IIA fractures. These fractures are managed with early halo application under fluoroscopic guidance, and compression across the fracture site for maintenance of reduction. Type III fractures are reduced open when closed reduction is not possible, and posterior spinal fusion of C2 to C3 is performed. Postoperatively, halo vest immobilization is maintained 3 months for these injuries.

Lateral mass fractures of the atlas are stable injuries which only require orthotic immobilization. Occasionally, with late symptomatic facet degeneration, some of these may require posterior fusion for pain relief.

Complications

The complication of high cervical fractures is bony or ligamentous instability. Management is posterior fusion of the unstable segments. Also, not identifying an upper cervical spine injury is not too infrequent an occurrence, especially in multiply traumatized patients. Neurologic injury is rare due to the large amount of space available for the spinal cord in the upper cervical spine.

SUBAXIAL CERVICAL SPINE INJURIES

Although bony injuries are often the obvious manifestation of cervical spine trauma, it is essential to accurately identify ligamentous components of injury to the subaxial cervical motion segments. It is often this ligamentous failure which allows cervical motion segment translation that may account for severe neurologic damage. It is also well accepted that ligaments heal with scar tissue that is weaker than the preinjured ligamentous structure and may result in chronic instability.

An important difference between upper and subaxial cervical spine injuries is the increased risk of cervical cord injuries in the lower cervical spine. This is a reflection of two factors: the overall diminished size of the spinal canal in the lower cervical spine, and the increasing prevalence of injuries which narrow rather than expand the canal. Thus, the immediate and long-term goals for injuries in the lower cervical spine are to obtain and maintain spinal column alignment to optimize the environment for the spinal cord and existing nerve roots.

Classification

There are five types of **subaxial cervical spine** injuries: isolated posterior element fractures, minor avulsion and compression fractures, vertebral body-burst fractures, teardrop fractures, and facet injuries causing spinal malalignment.

Isolated posterior element fractures of the lamina, articular process, or spinous process may occur by a compression extension sequence with impaction of the posterior elements upon one another. Additional lesions include unilateral or bilateral laminar fractures and, often, contiguous posterior element fractures secondary to the impaction of the adjacent posterior elements.

Minor avulsion and compression fractures of the subaxial cervical spine include anterior compression or avulsion injuries of the vertebral body and combined anterior and posterior bony injuries with minimal displacement and angulation.

Vertebral body-burst fractures are usually the result of axial-loading injury with varying amounts of flexion possible, as seen in diving accidents. They involve the anterior column as well as the middle column, with the potential for bony retropulsion into the spinal canal.

Teardrop fractures of the subaxial cervical spine are a particular group of fractures with a high association of severe spinal cord injury and spinal instability. These injuries occur when the neck is in a flexed position with axial compression as the main loading force. The inferior tip of the proximal vertebral body is driven down into the caudad body by compression and flexion. This produces the typical teardrop fragment on the anteroinferior aspect of the affected body. The true significance of this injury lies in the three-column instability pattern produced. The typical fracture line proceeds from superior to inferior and exits through the disc space, which is severely damaged. Posterior element ligament and bony damage is characteristic of the teardrop injury. This produces a grossly unstable injury of all three spinal columns in which the entire vertebral body is retropulsed into the spinal canal causing either partial or complete spinal cord injury.

Facet injuries are divided into fractures and ligamentous injuries. Both may allow segmental translation with subluxation or dislocation of the vertebral segments. The primary mechanism of injury is a posterior distraction force applied to the already flexed spine. This produces a spectrum of injury which ranges from an interspinous ligament sprain to complete posterior ligamentous and facet joint failure producing facet subluxation or facet dislocation. These injuries are further divided into unilateral or bilateral facet injury. Thus, facet injuries are described as **unilateral or bilateral facet fractures with or without subluxation, unilateral facet dislocations, perched facets, or bilateral facet fractures.** Unilateral facet fractures or dislocations display a variety of neurologic injuries ranging from a normal exam to single root deficits or spinal cord syndromes. The increasing spectrum of distraction and flexion injuries produces the perched facet injury. This occurs with bilateral facet injuries causing perching of the inferior facet on the superior facet with segmental kyphosis between the two affected vertebral body segments. Neurologic deficits are variable but most commonly include isolated root deficits. The most severe facet injury is bilateral facet dislocation. This is a purely ligamentous injury with disruption of the entire posterior ligamentous complex, including the interspinous ligament; ligamentum flavum; both facet capsules; and, in severe cases, disruption of the posterior longitudinal ligament and intervertebral disc. This injury produces the highest incidence of neurologic deficit of any facet injury due to the loss of space available for the spinal cord as a result of vertebral translation. The incidence of bilateral facet fractures associated with dislocations is extremely small. Both of these injuries predispose to rotational as well as translational instability.

Diagnosis and Initial Management

Physical Examination

The primary sign of a subaxial cervical spine injury may be the associated neurologic deficit. Other than neck pain and a sense of instability, there may be no symptoms indicating a cervical spine fracture without neurologic deficit. Patients with unilateral facet dislocation have a mild rotational deformity of their neck—the head is tilted and rotated to the contralateral side of the facet dislocation.

Radiographic Examination

A common, isolated posterior element fracture, the unilateral vertebral arch fracture, often is not evident on the initial lateral cervical spine radiograph. Oblique views or nonstandard views, such as a 20° oblique or pillar view, may be necessary to establish the diagnosis. When both an ipsilateral pedicle and laminar fracture occur, the articular process may rotate into the frontal plane and be viewed as a "transverse facet" on the anteroposterior radiographic view.

Vertebral body-burst fractures involve the anterior and middle columns of the cervical spine. The lateral radiograph indicates compression of the anterior and middle columns with retropulsion of the middle column posteriorly into the spinal canal. Burst fractures always require an axial CT or MRI exam to document the amount of middle column retropulsion. As anterior compression approaches 50 percent, middle column injuries or concomitant posterior ligamentous injuries must be considered. It is difficult to identify posterior ligamentous injuries in a patient with a burst fracture because voluntary flexion-extension views are unobtainable. Warnings include a widened interspinous process distance; fractured posterior elements, including facet fractures; or sagittal MRI evidence of ligamentous damage.

Teardrop fractures are first suspected on the lateral cervical spine radiograph, which will show retrodisplacement of the cephalad vertebral body on the caudad and, possibly, the anteroinferior teardrop fragment. Posterior element fractures may also be noted on the lateral or the anteroposterior radiograph. CT scans or MRI scans through the involved segment also demonstrate the fractures as well as the diminished spinal canal diameter due to the significant retrolisthesis.

Facet dislocations are identified on the lateral radiograph. Unilateral dislocations are characterized by approximately 25 percent anterior olisthesis of the cephalad vertebra on the caudad vertebra; bilateral dislocations have 50 percent anterior olisthesis (Fig. 14–12). An axial CT scan further defines the injury. Perched facets are diagnosed on the lateral radiograph by the increased distance between the spinous processes. There is also an obvious segmental kyphosis seen between the involved vertebral bodies, as well as anterior translation of the cephalad vertebral body on the caudad body.

Initial Management

Initial management of isolated fractures of the posterior elements and minor avulsion and compression fractures is a cervical orthosis.

Initial management of burst fractures with greater than 25 percent loss in height, retropulsion, or neurologic deficit is cervical tongs traction to stabilize the spinal segment and attempt an indirect reduction of retropulsed fragments via ligamentotaxis, thereby decompressing the neural canal.

Initial management of teardrop fractures is application of cervical tongs traction to increase the spinal canal diameter by indirect reduction via ligamentotaxis.

Initial management of unilateral or bilateral facet injuries causing

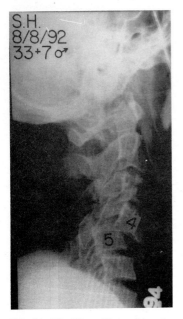

FIG. 14–12   Bilateral facet dislocation of C4 on C5.

any spinal subluxation or dislocations, perched facets, and bilateral facet dislocations is cervical tongs traction for reduction (Fig. 14–13). The one caveat is that there is a small but significant incidence of disc herniations accompanying bilateral facet dislocations. In these patients, there is the potential that a closed reduction maneuver will retropulse the injured disc into the spinal canal and cause further neurologic compromise. The disc herniation is best identified by MRI exam, but is suspected when the disc space at the dislocated level is markedly decreased in height on the lateral radiograph. Therefore, in patients with a normal neurologic exam, reduction is performed in an incremental fashion with careful attention paid to the neurologic exam and radiographic reduction sequence.

In an awake patient with a complete neurologic injury, reduction is attempted prior to obtaining an MRI exam. In an awake patient with an incomplete neurologic deficit, reduction is attempted as long as the

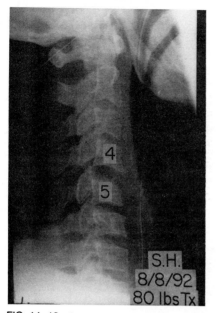

FIG. 14-13   Same patient as in Fig. 14-12 following closed reduction.

neurologic exam does not deteriorate. If at any time the neurologic exam deteriorates, the reduction maneuver is halted and the patient is immediately taken for an MRI exam or cervical myelography if MRI is not available. Treatment of a traumatic disc herniation associated with a facet dislocation is anterior discectomy and fusion preceding a single level posterior instrumentation and fusion. Unilateral facet dislocation is often difficult, if not impossible, to reduce with pure longitudinal cervical traction. These require a manual reduction maneuver after application of the appropriate amount of cervical traction weight. Manually turning the rotated head and chin toward the ipsilateral side of injury often produces a palpable clunk and feeling of reduction for the patient. This obviously must be done with careful neurologic monitoring and radiographic control. This reduction maneuver unlocks the dislocated facet and places it back into the normal position, that is, the superior facet sits anterior to the inferior facet.

Associated Injuries

Associated injuries are identical to those of the upper cervicle spine.

Definitive Management

Definitive treatment options for subaxial cervical spine injuries include:
(1) orthotic immobilization with SOMI (sternal-occipital-mandibular-immobilizer) (Fig. 14–14); (2) halo vest immobilization (Fig. 14–15);
(3) posterior fusion and stabilization utilizing wires, cables, clamps and/or screws, and plates; (4) anterior approaches for decompression and strut graft fusion with or without plate and screw stabilization; and (5) a combination of these four treatment modalities. The two primary considerations for choosing a particular treatment plan include the presence of neural compression and actual or anticipated spinal instability.

Traditionally, posterior stainless steel wire constructs have provided adequate stabilization for fusion in the subaxial cervical spine by utilizing spinous processes and/or facet wiring techniques. Sublaminar wire

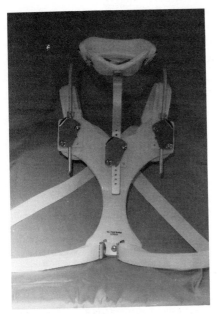

FIG. 14–14   SOMI orthosis.

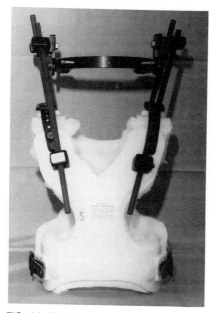

FIG. 14–15   Halo vest.

techniques are not recommended in the subaxial cervical spine following trauma due to risk of iatrogenic neurologic injury. However, with the presence of posterior bony element injury, these wiring techniques may be impossible or must be extended to normal levels above and/or below the injury. Recently, lateral mass-plating techniques have been developed in an attempt to provide stabilization to areas with spinous process and lamina injuries, but intact lateral masses. This technique requires screw placement into the lateral masses, which has some risk of neurologic and vascular complications associated with it; long-term results are not yet available for this technique (Fig. 14–16).

The halo vest is often a useful modality in the management of subaxial cervical spine bony injuries. As a general rule, the more osseous injuries involved, the more useful the halo vest. Ligamentous injuries will heal with scar tissue in a halo that will not maintain long-term spinal stability. For single or multilevel bony injuries, the halo vest is often the optimal treatment device. However, there are many potential complications in utilizing a halo vest, most commonly pin tract infections causing pin

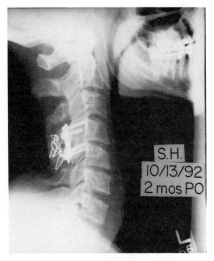

FIG. 14–16   Same patient as in Fig. 14–12 following posterior plating and fusion.

loosening. Thus, these patients must be followed closely when being treated as an outpatient.

The majority of isolated posterior element fractures are stable without major neurologic deficit (except for isolated cervical root deficits) and are managed in a SOMI. Occasionally, with multiple injuries spanning several segments, a halo vest provides better control of alignment.

Minor avulsion and compression fractures are managed in a cervical orthosis.

The definitive management of cervical burst fractures is dependent on the loss of height of the vertebral body, retropulsion, neurologic status, kyphosis, and the presence of posterior element injury. Fractures with less than 25 percent loss of height, minimal retropulsion, and kyphosis in a neurologically intact patient are managed in a halo vest for approximately 3 months. With increasing middle column retropulsion, there is an increased likelihood of spinal cord injury. These patients are candidates for anterior decompression via corpectomy and strut graft stabilization. If the posterior ligaments are intact, stability is maintained with an anterior strut graft and halo vest for approximately 3 months. An alternative to provide additional stability is an anterior cervical plate attached to the segments above and below the fractured vertebral body, internally stabilizing the strut graft. In patients with vertebral body-burst fractures and posterior ligamentous disruption, anterior strut grafting with anterior plate fixation cannot resist flexion forces, posterior stabilization is also necessary.

Definitive management of teardrop fractures is based on the extent of bony, ligamentous, and neurologic damage. When there is significant spinal canal compression, anterior corpectomy of the retropulsed vertebral body is performed with autogenous iliac crest strut grafting. Application of an anterior cervical plate is an option to further stabilize these segments. Because of the posterior column instability, either halo vest placement (for posterior bony injuries) or posterior instrumentation and fusion is performed.

Unilateral facet fractures without subluxation are managed in a SOMI orthosis or halo vest for 3 months or until bony healing is noted. The residual rotatory instability of a facet fracture with subluxation may be uncontrolled in a halo vest; therefore, these may heal in a malunited rotated position, which may exacerbate a nerve root deficit. For those injuries in which reduction cannot be maintained with a halo vest, management is anterior cervical discectomy and fusion with anterior cervical plating, as well as a halo vest to provide reduction and stability for posterior column healing.

When closed reduction of a facet dislocation is successful, the patient's neurologic status as well as overall medical condition is monitored. When the patient is considered neurologically and medically stable, single-level posterior instrumentation with fusion is performed. Posterior wiring techniques are the traditional method of internal stabilization. Posterolateral mass plating techniques are also being utilized for internal stabilization of these injuries (Fig. 14–16). With both of these techniques, patients are kept out of a halo, which aids in both pulmonary and psychologic recovery. Bilateral facet fractures are approached anteriorly because the posterior column involvement precludes posterior instrumentation. Anterior cervical discectomy and fusion with or without anterior cervical plating is performed at the involved level. Postoperative treatment with a halo vest is necessary to immobilize the posterior element fractures.

Complications

Complications of burst fractures include lack of appreciation of posterior ligamentous injuries and progressive kyphosis with potential neurologic sequelae. With greater than 50 percent loss of height in the neurologically intact patient, voluntary flexion-extension radiographs after healing of the compression fracture are necessary to rule out posterior ligamentous injury which will result in chronic instability. Complications in the use of anterior strut grafts include anterior dislodgment with esophageal compression, posterior dislodgment with potential spinal cord compression, and breakage or nonunion of the strut graft.

Complications of teardrop fractures revolve around the difficulty in stabilizing unrecognized posterior ligamentous injuries. Management with anterior corpectomy and strut graft in the face of posterior column injury has resulted in graft dislodgment, late kyphotic deformities, and the need for reoperation even with postoperative halo vest treatment. Anterior and posterior surgical approaches with internal stabilization via plates anteriorly and posteriorly appear to maximally stabilize these injuries.

Complications of cervical facet injuries are the development of acute or chronic instability. This is frequently due to inadequately treating ligamentous injuries in a halo which will not produce long-term stability, failure to recognize a concomitant disc herniation in the presence of a facet subluxation or dislocation during the closed reduction maneuver, and failure to anticipate rotational instability and using interspinous wiring techniques which do not control rotational instabilities. Acute and chronic cervical instability has been quantified to be present with >3.5 mm of segmental translation or >11° of segmental angulation present. Patients who satisfy these criteria, even if asymptomatic, should be considered for posterior instrumentation and fusion.

THORACIC AND LUMBAR SPINAL INJURIES

Spinal fractures of the thoracic, thoracolumbar, and lumbar spine are classified into four general categories: compression fractures, burst fractures, flexion-distraction injuries (chance fractures), and fracture-dislocations.

The most common and benign of thoracic and lumbar fractures are simple **compression fractures.** These typically are wedge-shaped fractures of the vertebral body involving only the anterior column. They occur after trivial trauma in elderly patients with osteoporosis, or following more significant trauma in younger patients. They are located in any part of the thoracic or lumbar spine, most frequently in the midthoracic to the midlumbar spine (Fig. 14–17).

Burst fractures involve the anterior and middle columns with or without injury to the posterior column. The mechanism of injury is high-energy axial loading with slight flexion. The vertebral body literally explodes or ''bursts,'' often resulting in posterior vertebral body wall retropulsion into the spinal canal (Fig. 14–18).

Flexion-distraction injuries (chance fractures) are three-column injuries with the fracture propagating through the posterior elements, pedicle, and exiting through the vertebral body. These can also be completely ligamentous injuries entering through the posterior ligaments and exiting through the disc space or combined bony and ligamentous injuries. Chance fractures often occur during a head-on automobile collision in which the patient is wearing a lap belt. The mechanism of injury is acute flexion of the torso on the lap belt. During impact, the

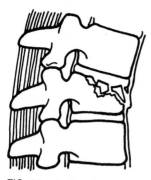

FIG. 14–17   Compression fracture of the lumbar spine.

upper part of the body is accelerated anteriorly over the seat belt producing a distraction force posteriorly around a fixed fulcrum just anterior to the abdomen (Fig. 14–19).

   Fracture-dislocations are the result of significant energy applied to the spine with a variety of forces including flexion, distraction, extension, rotation, shear, and axial-loading components producing spinal malalignment. These injuries always involve all three columns of the spine and are extremely unstable. They have a high propensity for profound neurologic injury (Fig. 14–20).

Diagnosis and Initial Management

History and Physical Examination

The neurologic examination is critical in patients with thoracic and lumbar spinal injuries, and particularly so in burst fractures. Clinically,

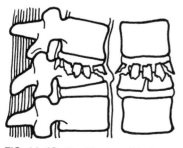

FIG. 14–18   Burst fracture of the lumbar spine.

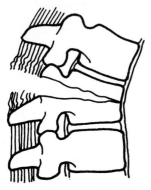

FIG. 14–19   Flexion-distraction, or chance, fracture of the lumbar spine.

patients may have tenderness to palpation over the affected posterior elements if these are injured also.

The diagnosis of flexion-distraction spinal injuries includes a high index of suspicion from the mechanism of injury as noted previously. Often, these patients present to the emergency room with a seat belt type of abrasion over their anterior abdominal wall. A tender, palpable gap may be present when examining the back indicative of the distracted spinous processes. The incidence of neurologic complications in flexion-distraction injuries is low in patients without an associated dislocation. Patients with fracture-dislocations often have multisystem injuries due to the violent nature of the trauma. Gross spinal malalingment may be

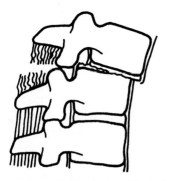

FIG. 14–20   Dislocation of the lumbar spine.

obvious when examining the back, which may have a palpable step-off in the posterior spinal contour.

Radiographic Examination

The diagnosis of a compression fracture is normally made on routine lateral radiographs of the affected region of the spine. Typically, loss of anterior body height versus posterior height is noted, depending on the amount of compression seen. For more subtle injuries, technetium bone scanning with or without a CT scan may be necessary to identify the injury. Axial CT scanning can reliably document an intact posterior vertebral body wall, confirming an intact middle column, and thus verifying an anterior compression injury.

The diagnosis of burst fracture is either made on plane radiographs or CT scan. Radiographic signs of a burst fracture include a widened interpedicular distance at the fractured level on the anteroposterior projection, and vertebral body compression with segmental kyphosis and retropulsion of the posterior cortex of the vertebral body on the lateral projection. The plane radiographs are also examined for subluxation or dislocation in the coronal or sagittal planes, as well as evidence of posterior column injury. The axial CT scan demonstrates a break in the posterior cortical wall with varying degrees of spinal canal compression from retropulsed bone (Fig. 14–21).

Plain radiographs are essential in the diagnosis of flexion-distraction injuries. The lateral radiograph indicates widening of the posterior column either within or between the bony elements and localized kyphosis. There are also varying degrees of distraction of the middle column, and thus either a fracture propagating through the pedicles or a widening of the posterior disc space. The anteroposterior radiograph indicates a widened interspinous distance indicative of ligamentous posterior column injury, fracture through the spinous process lamina, or splayed posterior elements. If translational forces are present and sustained, ligamentous flexion-distraction injuries may progress to unilateral or bilateral facet subluxation or dislocation. Unilateral dislocation is characterized by anterior displacement of the superior vertebra on the inferior by 25 percent on the lateral radiograph. When displacement is 50 percent or greater, a bilateral facet dislocation is likely.

Plain radiographs indicate fracture dislocations of the thoracic and lumbar spine in either the coronal or sagittal planes or both (Fig. 14–22). Occasionally, thoracic subluxations are quite subtle and may involve only a slight lateral translation of one vertebral body on another, or slight olisthesis in the sagittal plane. When subluxation proceeds to frank dislocation, the spinal malalignment is obvious on the lateral radiograph. CT scanning is mandatory for these fractures to assess unrecognized posterior element fractures which may affect operative management. Axial CT scanning often demonstrates two vertebral bodies in the same transaxial slice, indicating dislocation of a vertebral

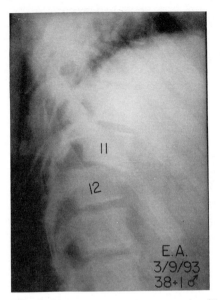

FIG. 14–21   CT scan indicating compromise of the spinal canal following a burst fracture.

segment. The empty facet sign is present when there is complete facet dislocation. Unlike burst fractures, the middle column is often intact when the primary mechanism of injury is a shearing force. In this instance, the vertebral canal compromise is secondary to the extreme vertebral malalignment rather than retropulsed bone.

Initial Management

The initial treatment of a patient with a spinal thoracic or lumbar fractureincludes supine bed rest with log-rolling to minimize pressure-dependent areas. A thorough system review for associated injuries is performed. It is essential to perform serial neurologic exams on patients who are awaiting definitive treatment of their fractures. Deterioration in the neurologic exam is an indication for emergent surgery.

Associated Injuries

There is a high incidence of multisystem trauma, such as liver or spleen lacerations, aortic arch tears, and intraabdominal trauma associated with high-energy thoracolumbar fractures. Twenty-five percent of patients

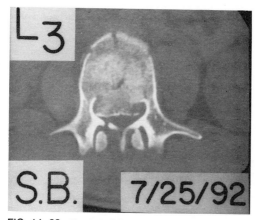

FIG. 14–22   Fracture-dislocation of T11 on T12.

with flexion-distraction injuries have associated intraabdominal injuries. Conversely, 25 percent of patients with intraabdominal injuries from wearing a lap belt have a flexion-distraction spine injury. Patients with thoracic spinal injuries also may have concomitant rib fractures with hemothorax or pneumothorax.

Definitive Management

Definitive management of thoracic and lumbar compression fractures depends on the age of the patient, location of the injury, amount of compression deformity, and any evidence of posterior column distraction injury. Elderly patients with multiple osteoporotic compression fractures of the spine often are treated symptomatically without any immobilization. Concern for possible pathologic involvement with tumor or infection must be maintained in the elderly patient population. Compression fractures with less than 50 percent loss of height are usually stable injuries which can be treated with a spinal orthosis for pain control during healing in younger patients. For lesions in the thoracolumbar junction and lumbar spine, a hyperextension orthosis attempts to limit the kyphosis which occurs after these injuries. However, even with a well-molded hyperextension cast or orthosis, some settling does occur during the healing process in the majority of these patients, but usually it is of little significance as long as the middle and posterior columns are intact.

For patients with greater than 50 percent compression deformity, it is essential to rule out middle column involvement and posterior column distraction. Radiographs demonstrate a widened intraspinous process distance or posterior element fracture, and the sagittal MRI may document a posterior ligamentous injury as well. These injuries may require surgery with posterior compression instrumentation and fusion with or without an anterior corpectomy, and anterior fusion to prevent a progressive kyphosis and neurologic sequelae.

Definitive management of thoracic and lumbar burst fractures depends on neurologic status, patient age, fracture location, spinal canal compromise, posterior element involvement, coronal or sagittal subluxation, amount of segmental sagittal kyphosis present, concomitant multisystem injuries, and body habitus. Methods of management are nonoperative bracing or casting, or operative stabilization via anterior, posterior, or combined surgical approaches.

Burst fractures are managed **nonoperatively** when the patient is neurologically intact, there is minimal segmental kyphosis and bony retropulsion (less than 50 percent canal compromise), no coronal or sagittal subluxation, and no posterior column involvement. A molded, two-piece hyperextension spinal orthosis is applied. Younger patients with kyphosis and a thin body habitus are managed with a hyperextension risser cast in an attempt to limit the postinjury settling of the fracture. When L4 or L5 are fractured, a single thigh is incorporated into the cast or brace to increase control of the lower lumbar spine sagittal alignment. The nonoperative treatment of lumbar burst fractures in neurologically intact patients with greater than 50 percent canal compromise is controversial. The majority of these patients with this clinical scenario heal their burst fractures uneventfully without neurologic sequelae. The spinal canal remodels over time to increase the space available for the neural elements. However, settling of the burst fracture usually results in an increase in segmental kyphosis.

Indications for **operative** management of a burst fracture in a **neurologically intact** or minimally involved patient are three-column injuries, subluxation in the coronal or sagittal plane, significant segmental sagittal kyphosis at the fracture site, spinal canal compromise greater than 60 percent, and concomitant injuries or body habitus which will not allow orthotic or cast treatment. Fractures of the thoracolumbar junction or upper lumbar spine are approached posteriorly, reduced, bone grafted, and stabilized. The preservation of sagittal alignment and maintenance of motion segments is important and is accomplished by utilizing posterior pedicle screw fixation systems when the pedicles are of sufficient size. In cases in which there is inadequate anterior and middle column support, anterior corpectomy and strut grafting is performed as a second stage procedure. Significant burst fractures of the thoracic spine in the neurologically intact patient are usually managed with combined anterior corpectomy and fusion, followed by posterior compression instrumentation and fusion to minimize the risk of further bony retropulsion and neurologic injury.

Operative management of burst fractures associated with **significant neurologic deficit** is individualized. The primary concern is spinal canal decompression. The anterior approach to the spine is the most thorough method of clearing the spinal canal of retropulsed bone and disc material, and it is the treatment of choice for this group of patients. The surgical approach is dictated by the level of pathology: a thoracotomy for T1 to T10 fractures; a thoracoabdominal approach usually through the tenth rib for T11, T12, and L1 fractures; and a retroperitoneal flank approach below the diaphram for L2 to L5 fractures. The intervertebral discs above and below the fracture are excised and a subtotal corpectomy of the injured vertebra is performed leaving the anterior and deep cortex intact.

Following spinal canal decompression, a strut graft is placed from the inferior end-plate of the cephalad vertebra to the superior end-plate of the caudad vertebra. Success or failure of the surgery rests mainly on the stability and healing of the graft more than on any instrumentation placed. Anterior instrumentation devices secure the strut graft and the spine is also instrumented and fused posteriorly in a second stage with rods and hooks over the same levels as the anterior construct for further stabilization.

The spine is approached posteriorly first for burst fractures with significant posterior column disruption or subluxation. The posterior instrumentation is utilized for reduction and restoration of sagittal plane alignment. At the same sitting, an anterior corpectomy and strut graft fusion is performed.

Definitive management of flexion-distraction injuries depends on the anatomic structures involved and the amount of displacement. Lesions occurring entirely through bone are managed in a hyperextension cast. This is particularly successful when the fracture line has propagated through the pedicles bilaterally. Injuries in which the fracture involves the pars interarticularis and pure soft tissue are managed operatively. This is because the pars has very little cancellous bone, which means fracture healing is less reliable and ligamentous healing does not result in adequate stability. It is important to identify traumatic disc disruptions and herniations prior to the surgical reduction of displaced posterior elements, as posterior compression forces may displace herniated disc material into the spinal canal causing neurologic injury. A short segment fixation with pedicle screw intrumentation and fusion is performed via a posterior approach. A thoracolumbar orthosis is worn 4 months postoperatively.

Definitive management of fracture dislocations is posterior operative reduction, stabilization, and fusion. Thoracic injuries are instrumented three to four segments above and below the fracture dislocation utilizing hook and rod constructs. Thoracolumbar and lumbar injuries are instrumented with pedicle screw and rod constructs, limiting the number of distally instrumented and fused motion segments, if possible. Postoperative bracing is usually provided to enhance the fusion rate and protect the instrumentation until fusion occurs.

The timing of operative reduction and stabilization is determined by the neurologic status and overall medical condition. The primary indication for emergent operative reduction is a neurologically incomplete patient with a progressing neurologic deficit. Patients with complete spinal cord injuries are stabilized as soon as possible to decrease the duration of enforced bedrest. A patient with an incomplete neurologic injury which is improving is observed until improvement plateaus. The spine is then reduced and stabilized.

Complications

The most significant complication of compression fractures is progressive kyphosis resulting from: settling of the vertebral body, unrecognized posterior column ligamentous injuries, and the presence of multiple contiguous compression fractures and pathologic fractures. Neurologic abnormalities are not seen with typical compression fractures, which involve only the anterior column.

Complications of nonoperative management of burst fractures are residual segmental kyphosis, progressive kyphosis secondary to unrecognized posterior column injury, and vertebral collapse due to settling. All these have a potential for increasing neurologic deficits. Complications of operative management of burst fractures are failure of instrumentation due to inadequate anterior column reconstruction, vascular or neurologic injury during the surgical approach, and dislodgment of strut grafts. Pseudarthrosis is rare either with operative or nonoperative treatment.

Complications of flexion-distraction injuries are inadequate posterior column reduction with casting for bony injuries, unrecognized ligamentous components of the injury, and rare traumatic disc herniations. The latter may retropulse into the spinal canal during operative reduction by posterior compression forces.

Complications of fracture-dislocations of the spine are an increase in spinal deformity due to inadequate treatment in a spinal orthosis, or a charcot spinal arthropathy below a complete spinal cord injury.

SACRAL FRACTURES

Classification

Sacral fractures are classified anatomically into zone I, II, and III. **Zone I fractures** are lateral to the neural foramen. Neurologic deficits result from superiorly displaced sacral fracture fragments compressing the L5 nerve root against the undersurface of the L5 transverse process. Zone I injuries also include various ligamentous avulsion injuries around the periphery of the sacrum.

Zone II fractures are longitudinal fractures through the sacral foramen. These are associated with a 28 percent incidence of neurologic deficits. The neurologic injury is usually characterized by S1 compression associated with sciatica. L5 is involved when fracture fragments are displaced superiorly, and other sacral nerve roots can be involved if the fracture extends through these levels causing displacement. Because these fractures are unilateral, incontinence is rare, but sensory changes over the involved dermatomes is common.

Zone III fractures involve the central canal and have a high (57 percent) incidence of neurologic deficits with loss of sphincter control, saddle anesthesia, and acute cauda equina symptoms. Transverse fractures occur as isolated injuries as the result of a flexion force imparted to the lower part of the sacrum and the coccyx. Below S4, there is little chance of a significant neurologic deficit because the sacral nerve roots have exited proximal to this.

Diagnosis and Initial Management

History and Physical Examination

Sacral fractures occur most frequently in high-energy trauma. Physical findings are back and buttock pain, ecchymosis over the sacrum, and sacral pain on rectal exam. Specific low lumbar and sacral root neurologic deficits should prompt consideration of sacral fractures. The fifth lumbar root is often involved when it is trapped between the transverse process of L5 and the superiorly migrating fragment of the sacral ala. Evaluation of the Achilles and bulbocavernosus reflex is mandatory when assessing sacral root function. Sacral fractures may result in anesthesia over the sacral dermatomes, impotence, and a flaccid bowel and bladder. Incontinence rarely occurs with unilateral root injury between S2 and S5. Decreased sensation is a more usual consequence. When in doubt about the integrity of the structures innervated by the sacral segments, urodynamics is helpful in the assessment of motor function of the bladder.

Radiographic Examination

Radiographic documentation of sacral fractures is difficult because of the complex shape of the sacrum and pelvis. Fifty percent of sacral fractures without neurologic deficit are missed on initial exam. The initial radiographc examination includes lateral and anteroposterior, or Fergusson, projections. The Fergusson projection centers the proximally directed beam on the sacrum. Radiographic findings associated with sacral fractures are low lumbar transverse process fractures, asymmetrical sacral foramen, and irregular trabeculation of the lateral masses of the proximal sacral segments. CT scans are the most accurate method of evaluating sacral fractures. Suspected fractures are identified on bone scan when the sacral segments are too osteopenic to produce reliable radiographic images.

Initial Management

The focus of initial management of sacral fractures is pain relief. The patient is kept at bed rest and log-rolled from side to side until the pain subsides to the point where mobilization can be initiated, usually 7 to 10 days.

Associated Injuries

Multisystem injuries and neurologic injuries are associated with fractures of the sacrum.

Definitive Management

Isolated sacral fractures without anterior pelvic ring fractures or neurologic deficits are stable and do not require treatment beyond relief of symptoms. After the initial period of bed rest, the patient is mobilized with nonweight-bearing on the affected side for 4 to 8 weeks, and then weight-bearing as tolerated. Sacral fractures which present as elements of a pelvic injury are managed to reestablish the pelvic ring.

Complications

Complications of sacral fractures are chronic pain secondary to sacroiliac arthritis or change of alignment of the sacrum, and loss of voluntary control of bowel and bladder. Sacroiliac arthritis is managed with arthrodesis.

Neurologic deficits associated with zone II injuries are managed with observation because many of these injuries are neuropraxias which will resolve spontaneously. Symptoms which persist beyond 6 to 8 weeks may benefit from foraminal decompression. Deficits associated with zone III injuries should undergo aggressive radiologic examination to identify the cause of the neurologic injury because early posterior decompression may result in return of bowel and bladder control and reversal of foot drop. Late decompression is often complicated by epidural fibrosis and minimal return of function.

SELECTED READINGS

Allen GL, Ferguson RL, Lehmann TR, O'Brien RP: A mechanistic classification of closed, indirect fractures and dislocations of the lower cervical spine. *Spine* 7:1–27, 1982.

Bohlmann HH: Acute fractures and dislocations of the cervical spine, an analysis of 300 hospitalized patients and review of the literature. *J Bone Joint Surg* 61A:1141, 1979.

Bohlmann HH: Treatment of fractures and dislocations of the thoracic and lumbar spine-current concepts review. *J Bone Joint Surg* 67A:165–169, 1985.

Clark CR, White AA III: Fractures of the dens. A multi center study. *J Bone Joint Surg* 67A:1340, 1985.

Denis F: The 3-column spine and its significance in the classification of acute thoracolumbar spinal injuries. *Spine* 8:817–831, 1983.

Haher TR, Selnly WF, O'Brien MO: Diagnosis and management of thoracic and lumbar spinal fractures. *In* Bridwell KH and Dewald RL (eds). *Textbook of spinal surgery,* 1st ed. Philadelphia, Lippincott, 1991.

McAfee PC, Bohlman HH, Yuan HA: Anterior decompression of traumatic thoracolumbar fractures with incomplete neurological deficit using a retroperitoneal approach. *J Bone Joint Surg* 47A:89–103, 1985.

Sabiston CP, Wing PC: Sacral fractures: Classification and neurologic implications. *J Trauma* 26:1113–1115, 1986.

Vaccaro AR, An HS, Lin S, Sun S, Balderston RA, Cotler JM: Noncontiguous injuries of the spine. *J Spinal Disord* 5:320–329, 1992.

White AA, Southwick WO, Panjabi MM: Clinical instability in the lower cervical spine, a review of past and current concepts. *Spine* 1:15–27, 1976.

Fractures and Dislocations
of the Pelvic Ring
and Acetabulum

D. Kevin Scheid

This chapter reviews fractures and dislocations of the pelvis and acetabulum and dislocations of the hip.

ANATOMY OF THE PELVIC RING

The bony pelvic ring consists of two innominate bones (hemipelvis) and the sacrum held together by an intricate ligamentous network. Each innominate bone consists of three parts: ilium, ischium, and pubis, which fuse at the acetabulum upon skeletal maturity. The **anterior column,** or iliopubic column, includes the anterior wall of the acetabulum, the anterior ilium, and the superior pubic ramus. The **posterior column,** or ilioischial column, includes the posterior wall of the acetabulum, and extends from the posterior-inferior ilium at the greater sciatic notch to the ischial tuberosity (Fig. 15–1). Specific landmarks on the anterior column helpful during surgery include the anterosuperior iliac spine, anteroinferior iliac spine, iliopubic line, iliopubic eminence, and pubic tubercle. Landmarks on the posterior column include the greater sciatic notch, lesser sciatic notch, ischial spine, and ischial tuberosity.

Each innominate bone articulates with the sacrum posteriorly at the sacroiliac joints. The joints are covered with hyaline cartilage on the sacral side and fibrocartilage on the iliac side. All sacroiliac joint stability is derived from **interosseous, posterior sacroiliac, and anterior sacroiliac ligament complexes** (Fig. 15–2). The anterior pelvic ring is joined at the cartilage-covered pubic symphysis and held by an enveloping fibroligamentous complex. Two additional (sacroischial) ligaments, the sacrospinous and sacrotuberous, confer additional stability to the pelvic ring. Together, these ligament complexes resist vertical and rotational forces on each hemipelvis. The pelvic brim divides the upper (false pelvis) and lower (true pelvis).

Vascular, neurologic, and genitourinary structures lie within and along the inner pelvis making them susceptible to injury during pelvic disruption. The **common iliac artery** gives rise to the **internal iliac and external iliac arteries. The superior and inferior gluteal, vesical, and lumbosacral arteries** all arise from the internal iliac artery. The **sacral venous plexus** is particularly susceptible to injury and is difficult to control or embolize.

The **lumbosacral plexus,** which includes the fourth and fifth lumbar and sacral nerve roots, lies along the anterior sacrum. The sciatic, gluteal, and splanchnic nerves arise from this plexus. The obturator

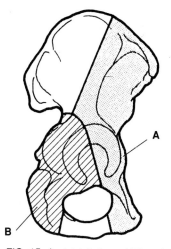

FIG. 15–1   (a) Anterior and (b) posterior columns of the pelvis.

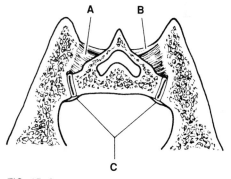

FIG. 15–2   Transverse section through sacroiliac joints: (a) interosseous ligaments, (b) posterior sacroiliac ligaments, and (c) anterior sacroiliac ligaments.

nerve runs along and below the pelvic brim to exit the obturator foramen.

The bladder, urethra, vagina, and rectum are all susceptible to puncture and/or tear by bony spicules and shear forces.

FRACTURES AND DISLOCATIONS OF THE PELVIS

Classification

Pelvic fractures are classified according to the mechanism of injury as: lateral compression, anteroposterior compression, vertical shear, and complex.

There are three types of **lateral compression** injuries. Type I injuries are stable and have anterior rami fractures and a minor sacral body or ala crush (Fig. 15–3). Type II injuries usually internally rotate the hemipelvis to such a degree that either the posterior sacroiliac ligaments rupture or the posterior ilium or sacrum fractures (Fig. 15–4). Type II injuries result in a hemipelvis which is unstable to internal rotational forces, but is vertically stable due to the intact sacroischial and anterior sacroiliac ligaments. Type III injuries are a continuation of type II injuries with an external rotation or anteroposterior compression injury to the contralateral hemipelvis (Fig. 15–5). The hemipelvis is vertically stable.

There are three types of **anteroposterior compression** injuries. Type I injuries are a disruption of the pubic symphysis or fracture of the anterior rami with strain of the anterior sacroiliac ligaments. Because the posterior ligaments are not disrupted, this injury is stable rotationally and vertically (Fig. 15–6). Type II injuries externally rotate the hemipelvis to such a degree that the anterior sacroiliac ligaments rupture along with the sacroischial ligaments. This injury leaves the hemipelvis unstable to external rotation, but vertically stable due to an intact posterior sacroiliac ligament complex (Fig. 15–7). Type III injuries are the continuation of type II and are a disruption of the entire posterior sacroiliac ligament complex, allowing both rotational and vertical instability (Figs. 15–8 and 15–9).

Vertical shear injuries are both rotationally and vertically unstable due to complete posterior ligamentous disruption or an unstable posterior ring fracture in combination with anterior diastasis or fracture (Fig. 15–10).

Complex injuries include bilateral injuries and associated ring injuries with ipsilateral acetabular fractures.

Diagnosis and Initial Management

History and Physical Examination

There is always a history of significant trauma. A rapid initial physical exam includes inspection for pelvic, abdominal, and perineal bruising; rectal or vaginal tears indicating an open fracture; blood at the urethral

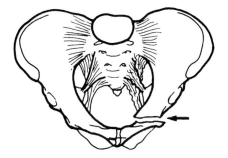

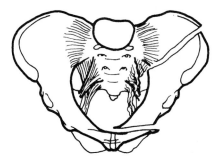

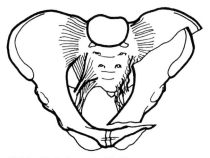

FIGS. 15–3 through 15–5   Type I, II, and III lateral compression fractures of the pelvis.

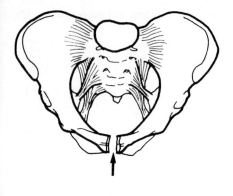

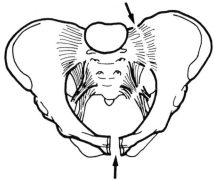

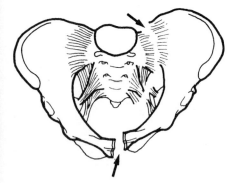

FIGS. 15–6 through 15–8 Type I, II, and III anteroposterior compression fractures of the pelvis.

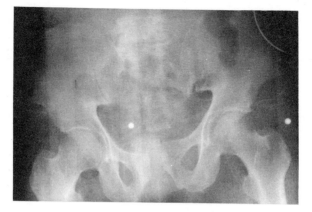

FIG. 15–9   Radiograph of a type III anteroposterior compression fracture. The hemipelvis is rotated and vertically displaced.

meatus indicating possible urethral tear; pelvic asymmetry; iliac crest mobility; lower extremity malrotation; leg length discrepancy; and a focused neurologic and vascular exam of the lower extremities.

Radiographic Examination

An anteroposterior pelvis film confirms the diagnosis. Inlet and outlet views and CAT scans define the posterior injury and, thus, pelvic ring stability. Instability is documented fluoroscopically by exam under anesthesia, if equivocal.

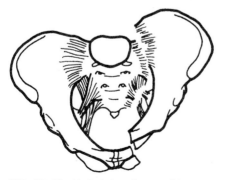

FIG. 15–10   Vertical shear fracture of the pelvis.

Initial Management

Hemodynamically stable patients are closely monitored. When there is significant vertical displacement, 20 to 30 lb of femoral traction is applied. When there is no vertical displacement, the patient is log-rolled every hour. Hemodynamic instability is a life-threatening emergency. Hemodynamically unstable patients are put in a MAST suit (antishock trousers) to increase peripheral vascular resistance and decrease motion of the fracture by direct pressure. Use of the MAST suit for other than initial transport and stabilization is not indicated because of complications secondary to prolonged inflation. Immediate intervention for the bleeding pelvis following removal of the MAST suit is rapid reduction and external fixation to tamponade bleeding vessels. Anterior ring stabilization alone will suffice to tamponade retroperitoneal hemorrhage, even if there is vertical instability; however, skeletal traction is added to reduce vertical migration of the hemipelvis. If bleeding continues as indicated by continued hemodynamic instability, selective arterial embolization is attempted. Indications for emergent open control of hemorrhage are rare: open fracture and inability to control hemorrhage, major vessel disruption uncontrollable by embolization, and lifesaving hemipelvectomy.

Associated Injuries

Pelvic fractures frequently are associated with vascular and genitourinary system injuries. Anteroposterior compression injuries have a greater incidence of associated injuries than lateral compression injuries. **Vascular injuries** are life-threatening and must be aggressively managed. Rapid evaluation is required to rule out thoracic, intraperitoneal, or external bleeding, and to direct management of the patient in extremis toward the retroperitoneum and the pelvic fracture. The hypovolemic patient with an unstable pelvic ring fracture is assumed to have significant retroperitoneal hemorrhage due to injury of the sacral venous plexus, bleeding fractured bone, and major or minor arterial injuries.

Genitourinary injury is suspected with any pelvic fracture. Blood at the urethral meatus, fractures of the ischial and pubic rami, and a floating prostate on rectal examination indicate urethral injury. A retrograde urethrogram determines the presence of a urethral tear prior to catheterization of the bladder. A cystogram determines whether the bladder is intact.

Definitive Management

The goal of management is stabilization of the unstable pelvis. This is most frequently accomplished by application of an anteroexternal fixater.

In **rotationally unstable** fractures, anterior ring stability only is required to convert an unstable pelvic ring to a stable structure. Type II and III lateral compression fractures require anterior stabilization for reduction of internal rotation deformity. Type II anteroposterior compression injuries with greater than 2.5 cm of symphysis dissociation or gross radiographic and clinical instability warrant stabilization of the anterior pelvic ring. In equivocal cases, examination with image under general anesthesia will assess the degree of rotational instability.

In **vertically unstable** fractures (i.e., type III anteroposterior compression, vertical shear, and some complex fractures), anterior and posterior stabilization is required.

Anterior stabilization is accomplished in most cases with an external fixater. Relative indications for internal fixation of the symphysis pubis or pubic rami fractures include exposure of the area for laparotomy or bladder repair; an acetabular fracture stabilized with an anterior column plate that can be continued across the pubic symphysis; and when external fixater pins would violate an acetabular surgical incision, increasing the chance of postoperative infection. The **technique of external fixation** follows many of the guidelines set forth for external fixater use in long bones. Two to three pins at least 5 mm in diameter are placed in each hemipelvis. Increased pin spacing improves stability. External fixater systems which do not require parallel pin placement allow individual angling of pins for optimum positioning. The shape of the iliac wing makes it a challenge to insert the pins between the two cortical tables. Pins are placed via an incision over the iliac crest. The starting point for the first pin is 2 cm posterior to the anterosuperior iliac spine. The second pin is inserted in the broad iliac tubercle 6 to 10 cm posterior to the first pin. A drill hole is made in the cortex of the crest only, and pins are inserted by hand using a T-handled chuck, while palpating inner and outer iliac tables. Directing each pin toward the rectum offers an initial threedimensional mental landmark for pin placement within the cortical tables. Maximum pin depth with the tip of the pins ending in the ilium, just above the acetabulum, affords the greatest stability and longevity of the pin. Rotating the fluoroscope in various directions allows tangential views of each pin verifying placement between the cortical tables. A simple quadrilateral frame is attached to the pins, the pelvis is reduced by manipulation under fluoroscopy, and the frame is tightened to hold the reduction.

The **technique of open reduction and internal fixation** of the anterior pelvic ring is via a horizontal Pfannenstiel or vertical laparotomy incision. Two anterior plates oriented 90° to each other afford considerable increased stability over single plate fixation. A foley catheter in the bladder not only decompresses the bladder, but affords an easily palpable landmark for bladder location.

There is no anteroexternal fixater construct or internal fixation that gives enough stability to maintain reduction of a vertically unstable fracture. Therefore, when there is vertical instability, the posterior ring must be stabilized. Various **techniques of posterior fixation** have evolved and their use depends on the location of the posterior injury and the surgeon's experience. **Posterior iliac fractures** are stabilized using standard plating techniques. Lag screws compress the fracture, and a neutralization plate is applied. The approach is anterior via an iliac crest incision exposing the inner table, or posterior with the patient in a lateral decubitus or prone position. Exposure of the more lateral iliac fracture is easier through an inner pelvic approach. Posterior iliac fractures are more easily exposed through a posterior approach, especially in the obese patient.

Sacroiliac joint stabilization is via an anterior inner pelvic approach, a posterior approach, or percutaneously. Nonanatomic reduction results in posttraumatic osteoarthritis.

The majority of patients presenting for posterior fixation have had an external fixater placed on admission or during the recessitation. This may make an anterior sacroiliac approach difficult, especially if the pins communicate with the surgical wound. The external fixater is removed to allow mobility of the hemipelvis for anatomic reduction.

Anterior fixation with two- or three-hole plates has been used successfully for many years. Two-hole plates offer increased stability and are preferable, especially when there is room for only one screw on the sacral side due to the proximity of the L5 nerve root and sacral foramina.

The disadvantage of the **posterior approach** is the incidence of wound breakdown. In cases in which nerve decompression or acute sacroiliac fusion is needed, exposure is via a posterior incision parallel with the sacroiliac joint. If transiliac plating is used, two incisions are needed.

The advantage of **percutaneous iliosacral lag screws** is the direct fixation of the ilium to the sacrum. The disadvantages are potential iatrogenic neurologic injury from screw penetration into the sacral foramina or spinal canal, and violation of the sacroiliac joint itself with the screws. Two large diameter cannulated screws are inserted from the posterolateral ilium into the Sl body or sacral ala. Washers or small plates are used to prevent migration of the screw head through the ilium as the screw is tightened. The technique requires clear visualization using image intensification. Patient position must allow enough undertable clearance to obtain appropriate inlet, outlet, and lateral views using the fluoroscope. When there is inadequate visualization of the sacral foramina on the outlet view, due to obesity or bowel gas, alternative methods of fixation are used, or the procedure is delayed until the bowel is well prepped. On the inlet view, the pin is angled slightly posterior to prevent anterior penetration of the concave sacral ala and an L5 nerve root injury. The tip of the guidepin is placed in the anterior one-third of the S1 body to maintain the maximum distance away from the sacral spinal canal. On the outlet view, the guidepin should be either horizontal or angled slightly cephalad ending in the upper one-half of the Sl body. A final check with a true lateral view will ensure guidepin tip placement.

Sacral fractures are stabilized in situ using the percutaneous iliosacral screw technique described for sacroiliac joints. Problems unique to sacral fractures are loss of foraminal landmarks secondary to fracture pattern, and crushing of interposed nerves between bone fragments while the screws are being tightened. When anatomic reduction of the sacral fracture is not achieved by closed methods, a combination open and percutaneous approach is used. The patient is positioned prone, and the sacrum exposed through a posterior longitudinal incision. The fracture is reduced and nerves decompressed. With the help of fluoroscopy, percutaneous iliosacral screws are placed through the buttock. If direct visualization of the sacroiliac joint is needed, the same combined approach can be used. This obviates the need for stripping the gluteal muscles off the posterior ilium, decreasing the incidence of wound breakdown.

Complications

Complications include posttraumatic arthritis of the sacroiliac joint, symptomatic malunion resulting in leg length discrepancy, malrotation, and neurologic symptoms due to inflammation and entrapment of lumbar and sacral nerve roots. **Arthritis** of the sacroiliac joint is managed conservatively initially, and with arthrodesis if necessary. Symptomatic **malunion** is managed with a shoe lift and gait modification. Occasionally, a correctional osteotomy is indicated. **Neuritis** is managed with nonsteroidal anti-inflammatories, and nerve decompression only if extremely symptomatic.

ACETABULAR FRACTURES

Classification

The anatomic classification of acetabular fractures was published by Judet in the 1960s and later refined by Letournel. Acetabular fractures are classified into five **simple** and five **associated** fractures.

Simple Fractures

Posterior wall fractures represent posterior dislocation of the femoral head. They involve a varying amount of the posterior rim of the acetabulum. Sciatic nerve injury and marginal impaction of the remaining intact posterior wall are common (Fig. 15–11). The mistake frequently made is classifying a large posterior wall fracture as a posterior column fracture.

Posterior column fractures by definition require disruption of the ilioischial line on the anteroposterior pelvis view. They include the

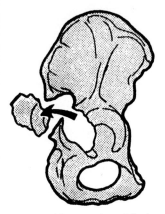

FIG. 15–11   Posterior wall fracture.

ischial portion of the bone, and involve a disruption of the obturator foramen (Fig. 15–12).

Anterior wall fractures are rare. They involve varying portions of the anterior rim or half of the acetabulum. The fracture does not involve the inferior pubic ramus (Fig. 15–13).

Anterior column fractures are characterized by disruption of the iliopectineal line. Low-column fractures involve the inferior acetabulum

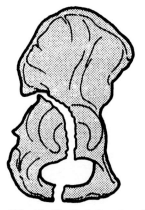

FIG. 15–12   Posterior column fracture.

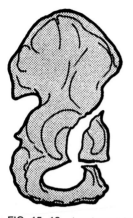

FIG. 15–13   Anterior wall fracture.

and have disruption of the inferior pubic ramus. Superior fractures involve varying parts of the anterior one-half of the ilium (Fig. 15–14).

   Transverse fractures divide the hemipelvis into superior and inferior halves. The line can traverse the articular surface at any level, and the obturator foramen is intact (Figs. 15–15 and 15–16).

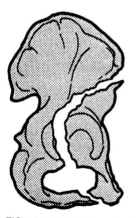

FIG. 15–14   Anterior column fracture.

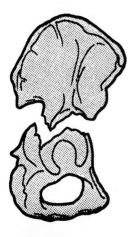

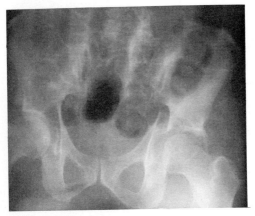

FIGS. 15–15 and 15–16   Transverse fracture.

Associated Fractures

Posterior column-posterior wall fractures represent a dislocation of the hip with an associated posterior column fracture. There is a break in the obturator foramen (Fig. 15–17).

T-shape fractures are transverse with an associated vertical fracture

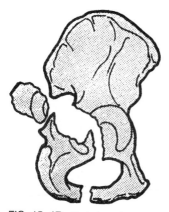

FIG. 15–17   Posterior column-posterior wall fracture.

into the obturator foramen and out through the inferior ramus (Fig. 15–18).

Anterior wall or column fracture with posterior hemitransverse, as the name implies, combines an anterior wall or column fracture with the posterior one-half of a transverse fracture (Fig. 15–19).

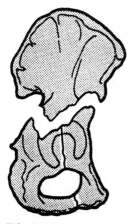

FIG. 15–18   T-shaped fracture.

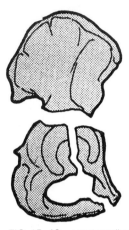

FIG. 15–19   Anterior wall or column fracture with a posterior hemitransverse fracture.

Both-column fractures are diagnosed more often than they occur. A true both-column fracture has no articular surface attached to the intact portion of the ilium, which remains attached to the sacrum (Fig. 15–20).

Transverse with posterior wall fractures do not have a break in the obturator foramen (Fig. 15–21).

Diagnosis and Initial Management

History and Physical Examination

There is always a history of significant injury. The patient has pain localized to the hip. The leg may be rotated and shortened. Motion of the hip elicits severe pain.

Radiographic Examination

Radiographic evaluation is important for preoperative planning. Virtually all fractures can be classified with an anteroposterior pelvis film and two oblique views. Although both-column outlines can be seen on the anteroposterior view (Fig. 15–22), the two oblique, or Judet, views at 45° best display the individual columns. The **iliac oblique** view is taken with the fractured side tilted down, or away, from the x-ray tube. This view profiles the ilium and best displays the posterior column of the affected side (Fig. 15–23). The **obturator oblique** view taken with the fractured side tilted up toward the tube best displays the outline of

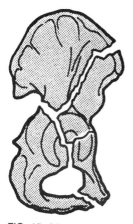

FIG. 15–20   Both-column fracture.

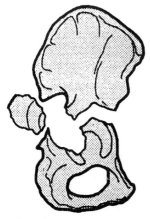

FIG. 15–21   Transverse with posterior wall fracture.

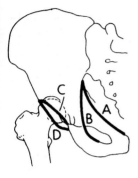

AP

A Iliopectineal line
B Ilioischial line
C Anterior rim
D Posterior rim

FIG. 15–22   Anteroposterior view of the hemipelvis.

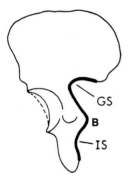

ILIAC-OBLIQUE

P   Outline post column
GS Greater sciatic notch
IS Ischial spine

FIG. 15–23   Iliac oblique projection.

the anterior column (Fig. 15–24). CT scans add additional information not easily found on plain films, for example, undisplaced ilium fragments or impacted segmental fragments of the acetabulum. Downfalls of axial CT scanning include the inability to determine dome step-off and difficulty in classification without comparison to plain films. Three-dimensional CT scans are accurate representations of the fracture, but usually add little additional information.

Associated Injuries

Associated injuries of the femoral head, pelvis, genitourinary system, and sciatic nerve occur frequently. Unfortunately, the best acetabular reconstruction may have a poor result due to **damaged articular surface of the femoral head.** Some of this damage occurs postinjury as the subluxed head articulates with fractured bony edges. For this reason, the patient is placed in skeletal traction until it is determined that the fracture is undisplaced and that there are no intraarticular fragments. A concomitant **pelvic ring** injury complicates the preoperative planning. **Genitourinary** injuries are less frequent than with pelvic ring disruptions. **Sciatic nerve** contusion with selective injury to the peroneal section of the nerve is not uncommon in posterior column and wall fractures. Local soft tissues are frequently compromised and are care-

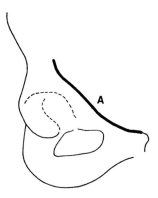

OBTURATOR-OBLIQUE

A Pelvic brim of anterior
    column

FIG. 15–24   Obturator oblique projection.

fully inspected prior to determining the timing of surgery and the approach.

Initial Management

Similar to pelvic ring injuries, acetabular fractures frequently occur with injuries to other organ systems. During recussitation, an anteroposterior pelvis film will reveal most acetabular pathology. When hemodynamic stability is achieved, Judet views and a CT scan are obtained to determine whether traction is necessary. Distal femoral skeletal traction is applied in the emergency room or on the floor. Twenty to thirty pounds of skeletal traction will suffice to partially reduce the femoral head and disimpact the joint.

A dislocated femoral head is reduced as though there were no acetabular fracture. If necessary, skeletal traction is applied while the reduction is held manually. Open reduction is necessary for the rare irreducible dislocation.

Definitive Management

Goals of surgery include reduction of the articular surface, removal of debris from the joint, and stable fixation which will allow nonweight-bearing ambulation and range of motion. The primary relative indication for nonoperative management is a congruous joint that is stable without traction. Posterior wall fractures that involve up to one-half of the posterior articular surface may be stable. If posterior stability is documented, nonoperative management is considered. Very low, transverse T-shaped and anterior column fractures can be managed nonoperatively if the weight-bearing portion of the joint is stable and congruous.

Surgical approaches are divided into two categories: limited and extensile. The term "limited" implies visualization of one column. The term "extensile" implies exposure of part or all of both columns through one incision. Occasionally, two limited incisions are used to achieve the exposure of both columns. The approach used depends on the type of fracture and the surgeon's experience.

The **limited** approaches are the Kocher-Langenbeck and ilioinguinal approaches. The **Kocher-Langenbeck** approach exposes the posterior column and posterior one-half of the superior dome. Fractures that can be exposed through this approach include posterior wall, posterior column, and associated posterior column-posterior wall. Transverse and transverse with posterior wall fractures can be reduced and stabilized via this approach if the anterior fracture does not require fixation, or if it can be stabilized with a percutaneous lag screw.

The **ilioinguinal** approach affords exposure of the anterior column from inside the pelvis. Exposure from the anterior sacroiliac joint around the inner pelvic brim and down to the pubic symphysis is possible. This exposure is demanding but extremely valuable for certain fractures.

Fractures routinely exposed through this approach include anterior wall and anterior column fractures. Like the Kocher-Langenbeck approach, other fractures can be stabilized through this approach including transverse; anterior column with posterior hemitransverse; and, occasionally, both-column fractures. When the ilioinguinal approach is used for a transverse or associated fracture, the posterior fracture must either not require fixation or be secured with a blind posterior column lag screw.

The two **extensile** approaches are the triradiate and the extended iliofemoral. The advantage of these approaches is that they expose both columns and the articular surface. The disadvantage is the increased soft tissue dissection and resultant propensity for heterotopic bone formation.

The **triradiate** approach combines the posterior Kocher-Langenbeck approach with an anterior limb designed to give exposure of the inferior one-half of the ilium and the proximal one-half of the anterior column.

The **extended iliofemoral** approach gives similar exposure of the two columns as the triradiate approach, but greater exposure of the proximal one-half of the ilium.

The indication for an extensile approach is a fracture which cannot be satisfactorily reduced and stabilized via a limited approach.

Complications

Complications of acetabular fractures are similar to those of hip dislocation and are covered in the ''Dislocations of the Hip'' section.

DISLOCATIONS OF THE HIP

Classification

Dislocations of the hip are classified according to the location of the femoral head as being posterior, anterior, or obturator. **Posterior** dislocations are by far the most common type of dislocation. The mechanism of injury is an axial load applied to the flexed adducted hip, such as would occur when the knee strikes a dashboard. **Anterior and obturator** dislocations are caused by hyperabduction of the hip. The greater trochanter impinges on the acetabular rim and levers the head out of the acetabulum. Extension and external rotation force the hip anteriorly, resulting in an anterior dislocation. Flexion and internal rotation force the hip inferiorly, resulting in an obturator dislocation.

Associated Injuries

Multisystem injuries; sciatic nerve injury; and fracture of the femur, knee, acetabulum, femoral head, and neck are associated with hip dislocations. Multisystem injuries reflect the high-energy trauma required to dislocate a hip. The presence of injuries to other systems is determined by adhering to the assessment guidelines outlined in Chapter 1. Sciatic nerve injury follows posterior dislocation of the hip and is the result of the femoral head impacting and stretching the nerve. The injury is almost always a neurapraxia and manifested by partial loss of function, most frequently peroneal nerve function. The most accurate method of determining whether the femoral head and acetabulum are fractured is a CT scan. Fractures about the knee are ruled out by a focused examination and radiographs.

Diagnosis and Initial Management

History and Physical Examination

The patient has severe pain. When the hip is dislocated posteriorly, there is a history of significant trauma. The leg is shortened. The hip is flexed approximately 30° and internally rotated. Anterior dislocations are often the result of less significant trauma and are characterized by external rotation and varying degrees of abduction. Obturator dislocations are caused by significant trauma and are characterized by at least 45° of fixed abduction of the hip.

Radiographic Examination

The diagnosis is confirmed by an anteroposterior radiograph of the pelvis. Spot anteroposterior and lateral radiographs of the hip are also obtained to evaluate the femoral head and acetabulum. Radiographs of the femoral neck, femoral diaphysis, and knee are examined to rule out fracture. Following reduction, new films are obtained to asses whether the reduction is concentric. In equivocal cases, a CT scan is obtained.

Initial Management

Initial management is reduction. The patient is sedated. Posterior dislocations are reduced by flexing the patient's knee, applying traction in line with the femur, and adducting the hip. Anterior and obturator dislocations are reduced by pulling in line with the femur, while an assistant pulls the thigh laterally. For anterior dislocations, the hip is also internally rotated. Straight traction is safe in the reduction of hip dislocations. Internal and external rotation must be performed very gently because of the risk of fracturing the femoral neck. If reduction is not possible with intravenous sedation, the patient is anesthetized in the operating room, and reduction with the aid of fluoroscopy is performed. Interposition of the capsule and external rotators in the acetabulum may prevent closed reduction, necessitating open reduction.

Definitive Management

Definitive management is skeletal traction until pain and muscle spasm have resolved (usually 7 to 14 days). Nonweight-bearing is maintained an additional 6 weeks. Surgical intervention is necessary for irreducible dislocations and to debride the joint when the reduction is not concentric.

The joint is approached posteriorly. If the dislocation is posterior, very little dissection is necessary once the gluteus maximus has been split. The acetabulum is cleared of debris and the femoral head is reduced. Postoperative management is as described in the "Initial Management" section.

Complications

Complications of acetabular fractures and hip dislocation are posttraumatic arthritis, hetcrotopic ossification, avascular necrosis, and instability. **Arthritis** is characterized clinically by pain with motion and radiographically by loss of joint space and formation of osteophytes. Management is conservative with nonsteroidal anti-inflammatories. If conservative management fails, older patients are managed with an arthroplasty. Patients under 50 years of age are managed with arthrodesis. **Heterotopic ossification** is more common following an extensile surgical approach and when there is concomitant head injury. Indocin decreases the severity of heterotopic ossification and is administered to patients who are not threatened by a prolonged bleeding time. Once heterotopic ossification has been diagnosed, passive range of motion exercises are stopped for a minimum of 8 weeks, or until the bony mass shows radiographic signs of maturing. The position of the hip is determined. If it is not in a position of function (i.e., 0° of abduction, 10 to 20° of flexion, and neutral rotation), the patient is placed in skeletal traction to improve the alignment, as there is a high probability of ankylosis. The bony mass may be excised after it matures. Maturity is indicated by normal serum alkaline phosphatase levels and a cold bone scan. **Avascular necrosis** of the femoral head is rare following acetabular fracture or hip dislocation. Its diagnosis and management are covered in Chapter 16. **Chronic instability** is extremely rare following dislocation without fracture. It has been successfully managed with imbrication of the posterior capsule of the hip joint. Chronic instability following acetabular fracture is managed with reduction, stabilization, and bone grafting of the nonunion if there are no signs of posttraumatic arthritis. If there is arthritis, an arthroplasty or arthrodesis is performed.

SELECTED READINGS

Fractures and Dislocations of the Pelvis

Bucholz RW: The pathological anatomy of malgaigne fracture-dislocations of the pelvis. *J Bone Joint Surg* 63A:400–404, 1981.

Hanson PB, Milne JC, Chapman MW: Open fractures of the pelvis: Review of 43 cases. *J Bone Joint Surg* 73B:325–329, 1991.

Moreno C, Moore EE, Rosenberger A, Cleveland, HC: Hemorrhage associated with major pelvic fracture: A multispecialty challenge. *J Trauma* 26:987–993, 1986.

Acetabular Fractures

Judet R, Judet J, Letournel E: Fractures of the acetabulum: Classification and surgical approaches for open reduction: Preliminary report. *J Bone Joint Surg* 46A:1615, 1964.

Letournel E: *Fractures of the Acetabulum.* New York, Springer-Verlag, 1981.

Matta J, Anderson L, Epstein H, Hendricks P: Fractures of the acetabulum: A retrospective analysis. *Clin Orthop* 205:230–240, 1986.

Dislocations of the Hip

Epstein HC: *Traumatic Dislocations of the Hip.* Baltimore, Williams & Wilkins, 1980.

16 | Intracapsular Fractures of the Proximal Femur

Clayton R. Perry

Intracapsular fractures of the proximal femur are low-energy fractures of the femoral neck, high-energy fractures of the femoral neck, and fractures of the femoral head.

ANATOMY

The three important anatomic considerations of femoral head and neck fractures are the intracapsular location of the fracture, the degree of osteopenia, and the vascular supply of the femoral head.

The intracapsular location means that the fracture site is bathed in synovial fluid that lyses the fracture hematoma, decreasing healing potential. The neck is covered with synovium and the head with articular cartilage. Therefore, healing is endosteal; periosteal healing does not occur. Finally, intracapsular hematoma increases intracapsular pressure, resulting in avascular necrosis.

Osteopenia leads to loss of fixation and, therefore, is a relative indication for hemiarthroplasty. The Singh index correlates the degree of osteopenia with the trabecular systems remaining (Fig. 16–1). There are six grades of osteopenia. Grade VI indicates normal bone with all trabecular systems present. Grade I indicates extreme osteopenia with all trabecular systems absent, except the principle compressive trabeculae, of which only a few remain.

Disruption of the **vascular supply to the femoral head** results in avascular necrosis. The three groups of vessels that supply the femoral head are ascending cervical or retinacular vessels, intramedullary vessels, and the artery of the ligamentum teres (Fig. 16–2). Of these three, the retinacular vessels are the most important. They arise from the extracapsular arterial ring formed by the medial and lateral circumflex arteries, and run along the femoral neck beneath the synovium, piercing the femoral neck just distal to the margin of the articular cartilage. A second arterial ring which is intraarticular and subsynovial is formed by terminal branches of the retinacular vessels at the margin of the articular cartilage of the femoral head. This ring also gives off branches which supply the femoral head.

Descending intramedullary metaphyseal arteries anastomose with ascending branches from the nutrient artery system of the femoral shaft. The intramedullary vessels are disrupted in all displaced femoral neck fractures.

The artery of the ligamentum teres takes origin from the obturator artery. It supplies the area around the fovea, but is not adequate to

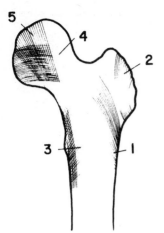

FIG. 16–1 The Singh index. Numbers 1, 2, and 3 indicate secondary trabecular systems which disappear in the early stages of osteoporosis (grades V and VI). Number 4 indicates the principle tensile trabeculae. This system is reduced in grades III and IV and absent in grade II osteoporosis. Number 5 indicates the principle compressive traveculae. This system is the last to disappear.

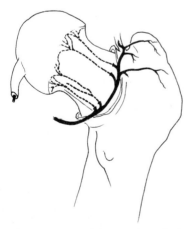

FIG. 16–2 Retinacular arteries and artery of the ligamentum teres.

supply the entire femoral head. Fractures of the femoral head occurring distal to the fovea have a high incidence of avascular necrosis of the fragment because the vascular supply from the artery of the ligamentum teres is disrupted.

LOW-ENERGY FEMORAL NECK FRACTURES

Classification

Low-energy femoral neck fractures are classified according to a system described by Garden (Fig. 16–3). Stage I is an incomplete fracture frequently in slight valgus. Stage II is a complete but undisplaced fracture. Stage III is a complete fracture partially displaced, but with an intact posterior retinacular attachment (ligament of Whitebrecht). Stage IV fractures are completely displaced with tearing of all retinacular vessels.

Diagnosis and Initial Management

History and Physical Examination

There is hip, groin, or thigh pain. If the fracture is not displaced, pain is the only physical finding. If the fracture is displaced, the leg is externally rotated; however, unlike intertrochanteric fractures, there is minimal shortening.

Radiographic Examination

Anteroposterior and lateral radiographs of the hip and an anteroposterior radiograph of the pelvis confirm the diagnosis and estimate the degree of osteopenia.

Initial Management

Prior to surgery the injured extremity is prevented from rotating externally with Buck's traction and pillows. Patients with undisplaced fractures (i.e., Garden I and II) are moved carefully to prevent displacement.

Associated Injuries

These low-energy fractures are usually not associated with other injuries; however, many patients with femoral neck fractures have medical problems. Cardiovascular and pulmonary systems are addressed specifically. Infections of the genitourinary system are common, and, if present, treatment is initiated.

Definitive Management

The definitive management is either pinning or hemiarthroplasty. The procedure is based on Garden's classification system, the age of the patient, and the degree of osteopenia. Osteoarthritis is an indication for

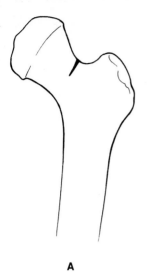

A

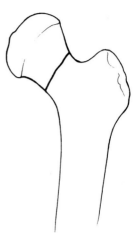

B

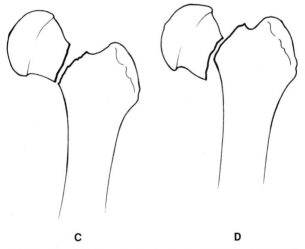

C

D

FIG. 16–3   The Garden classification system: (*a*) stage I, (*b*) stage II, (*c*) stage III, and (*d*) stage IV.

arthroplasty, but is uncommon in patients with low-energy femoral neck fractures.

Surgical Technique

Stage I and II fractures are stabilized with screws or pins. Reduction is not necessary for these undisplaced fractures. Two to four screws are inserted percutaneously. They must be parallel with each other and the long axis of the neck so that with weight-bearing the fracture will collapse along the axis of the screws. The most dense bone in the femoral head is subchondral; therefore, the screws must penetrate to within 0.5 cm of the subchondral bone. The threads should not cross the fracture or they will prevent collapse.

Garden III fractures have an intact vascular supply, and potentially the femoral head can be salvaged. If the patient is younger than 75 years of age or extremely ill and cannot undergo a significant operation, the fracture is reduced and fixed. If the patient is more than 75 years old, not a high-demand user, and can withstand a significant operative procedure, a hemiarthroplasty is performed. The fracture is reduced by separating the fragments by externally rotating the leg. Traction is then applied to bring the fracture out to length and the leg is internally rotated, reducing the fracture and preventing apex anterior angulation. An absolutely anatomic reduction is mandatory. There is a high incidence of avascular necrosis with fractures stabilized in more than 20° of valgus (an anteroposterior alignment index of 180°), and a high incidence of nonunion in fractures stabilized in varus or with more than 20° of apex anterior angulation (lateral alignment index of 160°) (Fig. 16–4). If reduction within these limits is not possible, a hemiarthroplasty is performed. Inability to achieve reduction is most frequently due to incorrect staging of the fracture (i.e., the fracture is stage IV).

Garden IV fractures are managed with a hemiarthroplasty (Figs. 16–5 and 16–6). The decision to use cement is made at the time of surgery. We use an anterolateral approach which is a modification of the approach described by Hardinge. The anterolateral approach minimizes wound problems associated with posterior approaches and gives better exposure than a straight anterior approach.

Postoperatively, weight-bearing as tolerated is allowed. Anterior precautions, including an abduction pillow between the legs while the patient is sleeping, are enforced for 3 weeks.

Complications

Low-energy femoral neck fractures are frequently the beginning of the end for debilitated patients. The incidence of mortality at 1 year approaches 30 percent. The incidence of postoperative infection is high, presumably because of decreased resistance, other foci of infection (e.g., the urinary tract and decubiti), and incontinence leading to contam-

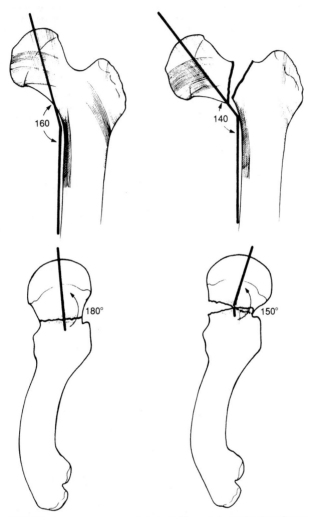

FIG. 16–4 The anteroposterior index is the angle formed by the primary compressive trabeculae and the medial cortex of the femoral diaphysis. The lateral index is the angle formed by the primary compressive trabeculae and the axis of the neck.

ination of the incision. Infection can be managed by two-stage revision or by chronic suppression with oral antibiotics. Avascular necrosis and nonunion are best managed by hemiarthroplasty.

HIGH-ENERGY FEMORAL NECK FRACTURES

Classification

High-energy femoral neck fractures have a worse prognosis and occur in younger patients than low-energy fractures.

We classify high-energy fractures into four groups: Type I—undisplaced, type II—simple displaced fractures, type III—comminuted displaced fractures, and type IV—fractures with associated fracture of the acetabulum or femur (Fig. 16–7). In addition to the displacement and the presence of associated injuries, verticality of the fracture line is assessed according to the classification system described by Pauwels (Fig. 16–8). More vertical fractures (i.e., Pauwels' type III) have a higher incidence of nonunion secondary to increased shear and decreased compression across the fracture.

Diagnosis and Initial Management

History and Physical Examination

Pain and external rotation are usually present; associated injuries may mask these findings.

Radiographic Examination

An anteroposterior and lateral radiograph of the hip and an anteroposterior radiograph of the pelvis confirm the diagnosis.

Initial Management

During the initial evaluation, skeletal or Buck's traction is applied.

Associated Injuries

There is a high incidence of other associated system injuries (e.g., chest contusion) and of associated injuries to the musculoskeletal system (e.g., pelvic fractures or ipsilateral knee injuries).

Definitive Management

Patients with high-energy fractures are most commonly young. Salvage of the femoral head is of paramount importance and hemiarthroplasty is acceptable only as a last resort.

Type I (undisplaced) fractures are stabilized with percutaneous screws.

Type II (simple displaced) fractures are reduced closed. If there is any doubt as to the adequacy of reduction, the femoral neck is reduced

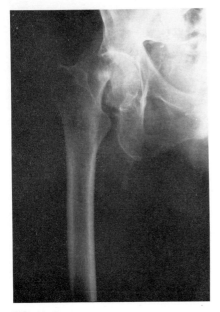

FIG. 16–5   Garden IV fracture.

under direct vision via the Watson-Jones approach. This approach utilizes the interval between the tensor fascia lata and the gluteus medius, and can be extended distally and laterally for the placement of a lag screw and side-plate.

Type III (comminuted) fractures are exposed through a posterolateral approach with the patient in the lateral decubitus position on a fracture table. The neck is reduced and stabilized with a lag screw and side-plate. Cancellous bone graft from the distal femur or iliac crest is used to augment the fixation.

In Type IV (associated with fracture of the acetabulum or femur) fractures, stabilization of the fractured femoral neck is the primary goal. If there is a posterior fracture of the acetabulum or hip dislocation, the femoral neck is approached posterolaterally. Management of femoral neck fractures associated with a diaphyseal femoral fracture is dependent on the type of femoral neck fracture. In undisplaced neck fractures, a reconstruction locked nail is used for both fractures. Displaced fractures are managed with the patient supine on the fracture table. An open

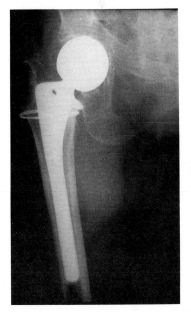

FIG. 16–6 Hemiarthroplasty for Garden IV fracture.

reduction of the femoral neck is performed, and fixation is with screws. The femoral shaft fracture is stabilized with a plate or retrograde nail.

Complications

The complications unique to high-energy intracapsular femoral neck fractures are nonunion and avascular necrosis. Risk factors for these complications include the degree of initial displacement, time to reduction and stabilization, bone density, and quality of reduction and stabilization. Theoretically, core decompression is of value in the management of **avascular necrosis** if done prior to arthritic changes. When symptomatic segmental collapse occurs, there are two options: osteotomy or fusion. Osteotomies are designed to move the involved portion of the femoral head from under the weight-bearing surface of the acetabulum and to replace it with healthy bone. Osteotomies are either rotational about the long axis of the femur or varus/valgus. If an osteotomy is not possible (i.e., the avascular portion is too large), a hip fusion is performed. In patients with **nonunion,** an intertrochanteric osteotomy

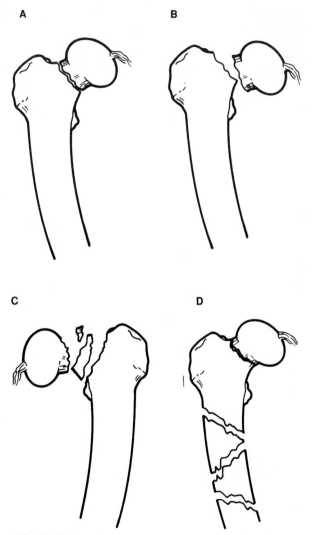

FIG. 16–7 The classification of high-energy femoral neck fractures: (a) type I, (b) type II, (c) type III, and (d) type IV.

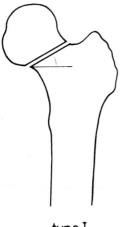

type I
<30°

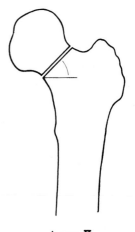

type II
>30° <50°

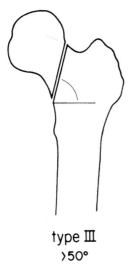

type III
>50°

FIG. 16–8   Pauwels' classification system of femoral neck fractures.

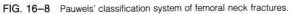

designed to make the plane of the nonunion more horizontal, thereby decreasing shear stresses across the nonunion, is performed. In addition, the nonunion is bone grafted.

FRACTURES OF THE FEMORAL HEAD

Classification

The third type of intracapsular fracture of the femur is fracture of the femoral head. Although femoral head fractures are invariably associated with a dislocation of the hip joint, we include them in this chapter because their anatomy, pathology, and management are very similar to that of high-energy femoral neck fractures.

Femoral head fractures are classified into four types. In type I fractures, the fracture is below the fovea. In type II fractures, the fracture line extends above the fovea. Type III and IV fractures are type I or II injuries associated with a fracture of the femoral neck or acetabular rim, respectively (Fig. 16–9).

Diagnosis and Initial Management

History and Physical Examination

The physical findings are those of a posterior dislocation of the hip. The hip is flexed and adducted, and the extremity is shortened.

Radiographic Examination

Anteroposterior and lateral radiographs of the hip indicate a dislocation of the hip with a retained fragment of the femoral head in the acetabulum (Fig. 16–10). CT scans and tomography confirm the diagnosis.

Initial Management

Initial management is reduction of the dislocation. Type I, II, and IV fractures are reduced closed without any specific precautions. In general, the easier the reduction, the less stable it is. Type III fractures are reduced while being monitored with fluoroscopy. If the femoral neck fracture is being displaced, the closed reduction is abandoned and open reduction performed emergently. Unstable reductions are maintained with skeletal traction and abduction of the hip.

Associated Injuries

Sciatic nerve injury is associated with these dislocations. Frequently, there are associated multisystem injuries.

Definitive Management

Definitive management is surgical. The goals of surgery are to obtain a stable concentric reduction of the hip joint, and either to reduce

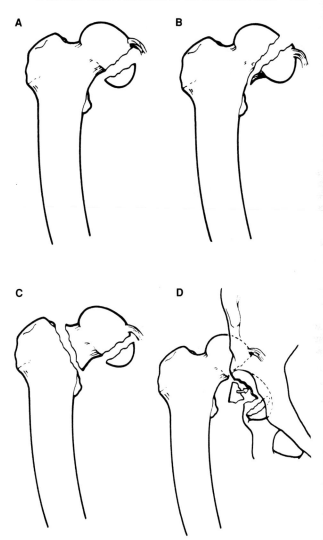

FIG. 16–9   Classification of femoral head fractures: (*a*) type I, (*b*) type II, (*c*) type III, and (*d*) type IV.

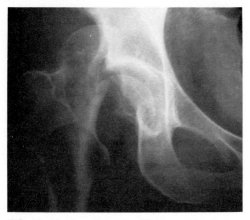

FIG. 16–10   Type II fracture of the femoral head.

anatomically and fix the femoral head fracture or to excise nonessential fragments. Type I and II injuries are exposed via a posterolateral (Kocher-Langenbeck) approach to the hip. The external rotators and capsule are invariably torn posteriorly; therefore, as the fibers of the gluteus maximus are split, the hip joint is exposed. The hip is dislocated posteriorly, and internal rotation of the femur affords limited exposure of the medial fragment and the hip joint. The medial fragment has synovial attachments called the "retinacular leash."

Type II fractures have, in addition, the ligamentum teres attached to the medial fragment. The dislocation is reduced, and the head fracture is stabilized with screws placed in the lateral aspect of the head and neck and directed medially toward the fragment.

Type III injuries have an associated femoral neck fracture. The Kocher-Langenbeck approach is used to expose both fractures. The head fracture is reduced and stabilized first. The neck fracture is reduced and stabilized with screws under fluoroscopic control. Older patients are managed with a hemiarthroplasty.

Type IV injuries have an associated acetabular fracture, usually a posterior lip fracture. When it does not require stabilization, the head fracture is approached as if it were a type I or II injury. If the acetabulum requires stabilization, the Kocher-Langenbeck approach is used to expose the hip joint. The hip is dislocated, and the joint and fractures are debrided of bone fragments and hematoma. The hip is reduced, the femoral head fracture is stabilized with screws, and the acetabulum is stabilized according to its fracture pattern.

Postoperatively, the extremity is placed in balanced suspension with the hip abducted 30°. At 4 weeks, the patient is allowed to ambulate nonweight-bearing on the affected side. At 12 weeks, full weight-bearing is allowed.

Complications

Long-term complications include postraumatic arthritis and avascular necrosis. Nonunion has not been reported. Arthritis and symptomatic avascular necrosis are managed with hip fusion in younger patients or with hip replacement in older patients.

SELECTED READINGS

Low-Energy Femoral Neck Fractures

Garden RS: Low-angle fixation in fractures of the femoral neck. *J Bone Joint Surg* 43B:647–661, 1961.
Niemann KMW, Mankin HJ: Fractures about the hip in a institutionalized patient population. *J Bone Joint Surg* 50A:1327–1340, 1968.

High-Energy Femoral Neck Fractures

Swiontkowski MF, Winquist RA, Hansen ST: Fractures of the femoral neck in patients between the ages of twelve and forty-nine years. *J Bone Joint Surg* 66A:837–846, 1984.
Protzman RF, Burkhalter WE: Femoral neck fractures in young adults. *J Bone Joint Surg* 58A:689–695, 1976.

Fractures of the Femoral Head

Pipkin G: Treatment of grade IV fracture-dislocation of the hip. A review. *J Bone Joint Surg* 39A:1027–1042, 1957.
Butler JE: Pipkin type II fractures of the femoral head. *J Bone Joint Surg* 63A:1292–1296, 1981.

General

Hardinge K: The direct lateral approach to the hip. *J Bone Joint Surg* 64B:17–19, 1983.
Singh M, Nagrath AR, Maini PS: Changes in trabecular pattern of the upper end of the femur as an index of osteoporosis. *J Bone Joint Surg* 52A:457–467, 1970.

17 Intertrochanteric Fractures

Enes Kanlic   Clayton R. Perry

This chapter reviews intertrochanteric fractures and isolated fractures of the greater and lesser trochanters. Intertrochanteric fractures are extracapsular fractures of the proximal femur. The major fracture lines are located between the base of the femoral neck and the lesser trochanter.

ANATOMY

The proximal extent of the intertrochanteric region of the **femur** is the intertrochanteric line anteriorly and the intertrochanteric crest posteriorly. The distal extent of the intertrochanteric region is the lesser trochanter. The osseous tissue in this region is cancellous bone surrounded by a thin shell of cortical bone. The cancellous bone forms the secondary compressive, secondary tensile, and greater trochanteric trabeculae (see the "Anatomy" section in Chapter 16). The calcar is a thick plate of bone underlying the lesser trochanter. As the calcar extends proximally, it fuses with the cortex of the posterior medial femoral neck. The linea aspera, a thickened ridge of cortical bone on the posterior aspect of the femur, extends from the greater trochanter distally down the diaphysis.

Numerous **muscles** insert on, or take origin from, the intertrochanteric region. The gluteus medius and minimus, the piriformis, and short external rotators insert on the greater trochanter. The iliopsoas inserts on the lesser trochanter. Because of the muscular insertions and origins, the intertrochanteric region has an extremely rich vascular supply. Post-traumatic avascular necrosis of the femoral head does not occur following an intertrochanteric fracture in contrast to intracapsular fractures of the proximal femur. In addition, the muscular attachments tend to prevent displacement of the fragments following fracture. The rich vascular supply and the broad surfaces of cancellous bone lead to rapid healing if the fracture is reduced and stabilized appropriately.

Classification

We classify intertrochanteric fractures according to the degree of osteopenia and the configuration of the fracture.

The Singh index is used to estimate the **degree of osteopenia.** Osteopenia plays an important role in the configuration of the fracture, its healing potential, and its management.

The **fracture configuration** is classified into one of four groups: type I—undisplaced, type II—stable displaced, type III—unstable displaced, and type IV—reverse obliquity (Fig. 17–1). **Undisplaced fractures**

236

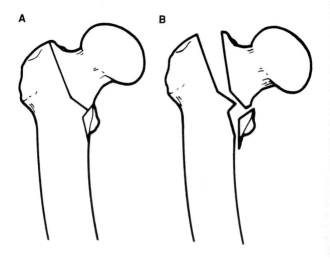

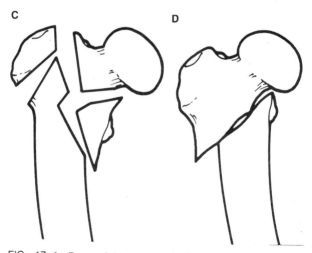

FIG. 17–1 Types of intertrochanteric fractures: (a) undisplaced, (b) stable displaced, (c) unstable displaced, and (d) reverse obliquity.

(type I) are usually simple fractures along a line between the greater and lesser trochanters.

Stable displaced fractures (type II) are those fractures which are stable when reduced. The sine qua non of stability is bone-to-bone contact across the fracture along the medial cortex of the femur. Fracture of the lesser trochanter does not always indicate an unstable fracture (i.e., there may be enough intact medial cortex for adequate bone-to-bone contact).

Unstable displaced fractures (type III) are those fractures that have posteromedial comminution that is so extensive it prevents bone-to-bone contact across the fracture. This comminution is usually a single large fragment which includes the lesser trochanter. Frequently, there is an associated fracture of the greater trochanter.

Reverse obliquity fractures (type IV) are those fractures in which the fracture line runs parallel to the long axis of the femoral neck (i.e., from lateral inferior to medial superior). This fracture pattern is unstable because the gluteus medius and minimus and piriformis externally rotate and abduct the proximal fragment while the adductors displace the distal fragment medially.

Diagnosis and Initial Management

History and Physical Examination

There is pain and inability to bear weight. There is usually a history of a minor fall. The injured leg is completely externally rotated, the lateral part of the foot often touching the surface of the bed. In addition to external rotation, there is shortening. Occasionally there is ecchymosis of the proximal thigh. Patients with femoral neck fractures usually do not have these physical findings, as extreme external rotation is prevented by a partially intact hip capsule, and fracture hematoma is contained by the capsule, thus minimizing ecchymosis.

Radiographic Examination

The clinical diagnosis is confirmed by the radiographic examination. A radiograph of the pelvis in the anteroposterior projection is of most use. The contralateral hip should be internally rotated 20° to profile the femoral neck to determine the Singh index. In addition to the anteroposterior pelvic radiograph, anteroposterior and lateral radiographs centered on the injured hip help to determine the fracture configuration. The lateral projection is obtained with the patient in the Danelius-Miller position (supine with the uninjured hip flexed). The film is placed lateral to the injured hip and the x-ray beam is directed through the hip. Other radiographic examinations (e.g., tomograms and CAT scans) are rarely useful in the evaluation.

Initial Management

The two goals of initial management are to make the patient as comfortable as possible and to prepare the patient for surgery as expeditiously as possible. Early stabilization of the fracture allows mobilization of the patient and minimizes the incidence of problems associated with prolonged recumbency (e.g., pneumonia and decubiti).

The patient is made as comfortable as possible by positioning the injured extremity. This is accomplished by applying skin traction with the knee flexed 10 to 20° over a pillow. External rotation is prevented by placing pillows laterally at the knee and foot. Because many patients with intertrochanteric fractures have fragile skin, the skin traction must be applied carefully to avoid skin breakdown. The malleoli and other bony prominences are carefully padded and no more than 5 to 10 lb of weight is used. Skeletal traction is applied through a distal femoral traction pin if there is skin breakdown or if surgery will be delayed more than 2 days.

Associated Injuries

The most frequent associated injuries are due to the patient's osteopenia and are to other areas of the body. They are sustained at the same time as the intertrochanteric fracture. The patient must be carefully examined for any signs of wrist fracture or head injury. Radiographs of the femur and knee, in addition to those of the pelvis, are obtained.

Prior to surgery, the patient's medical status is optimized. These patients are frequently dehydrated. Dehydration coupled with the blood loss associated with fracture results in severe volume restriction, which must be corrected. In addition, patients who have sustained an intertrochanteric fracture are likely to have other medical problems. Their cardiac, pulmonary, genitourinary, and neurologic systems are carefully assessed.

Definitive Management

The definitive management of intertrochanteric fractures is operative reduction and stabilization. The most important factors affecting the eventual outcome are the age and general health of the patient, the degree of osteopenia, the configuration of the fracture, the quality of reduction, and the stability of fixation. Of these factors, the surgeon controls two: the quality of reduction and the stability of fixation.

The goal of **reduction** is to obtain bone-to-bone contact along the medial cortex; realign the fracture fragments; and, in particular, avoid varus angulation. The anesthetized patient is placed on the fracture table. The reduction and stabilization are monitored with fluoroscopy. Reduction is accomplished by gently externally rotating the extremity to "unlock" the fragments and then applying axial traction. After the fracture is out to length, the extremity is internally rotated to align the fragments. The exact amount of internal rotation is determined by fluoroscopy (usually about 30°). The reduction is assessed fluoroscopically in the anteroposterior and lateral planes. In the anteroposterior plane, the fracture should be out to length and the neck shaft angle at least 130°. If there is shortening or varus angulation, the reduction maneuver of external rotation, more traction, and internal rotation is repeated. Slight abduction of the extremity may help reduce the fracture. Two bits of information are obtained from the lateral fluoroscopic projection: the direction of the axis of the femoral neck, and the relative position of the shaft of the femur to the femoral neck. Knowing the direction of the axis of the femoral neck helps in the accurate placement of the implant. The relative position of the femoral shaft to the femoral neck is important in that if they are not aligned, further reduction is necessary after the fracture is exposed (i.e., the femoral shaft has to be lifted anteriorly).

There are two basic types of implants that are used to **stabilize** intertrochanteric fractures: sliding screw-plate assemblies and intramedullary devices.

The **sliding screw-plate** allows controlled collapse and impaction of the fracture fragments, thus making an osteotomy unnecessary and minimizing shortening (Fig. 17–2). Several important points of this technique are: the screw is located inferiorly in the femoral head, and it should extend to within 0.5 cm of the subchondral bone to prevent cut-out; the barrel of the side-plate should not extend across the fracture or it will prevent postoperative impaction across the fracture; two-thirds of the barrel should be occupied by the lag screw to prevent disengagement or binding of the lag screw in the barrel; and the traction should be released intraoperatively to assess the amount of shortening that will occur.

Intramedullary devices are used most frequently to stabilize type III (unstable displaced) and type IV (reverse obliquity) fractures. The intramedullary location prevents medial displacement of the distal fragment and is a mechanical advantage over the sliding screw-plate. Flexible retrograde intramedullary nails (e.g., Ender's nails) are inserted by a closed technique; therefore, there is minimal blood loss. This technique has the disadvantage of insertion site symptoms if the nails back out. Important points regarding this technique are: the medullary canal must be "stacked" or filled with nails to prevent them from backing out; at least two nails must be inserted to within 1 cm of the subchondral bone to adequately stabilize the fracture; and the nails must have an anteversion bend to prevent an external rotation deformity.

The technique or method of stabilization depends on the configuration of the fracture. Type I (undisplaced) and type II (stable displaced) fractures are stabilized with a sliding screw-plate device. If the fracture

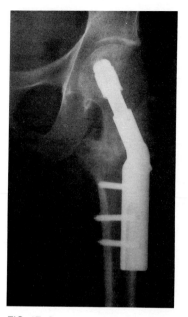

FIG. 17-2   A stable displaced intertrochanteric fracture stabilized with a sliding screw-plate device. An expanding dome has been substituted in place of the lag screw.

is type III (unstable displaced), there are two options: (1) to restore bone-to-bone contact along the medial cortex, or (2) to impact the fragments into a more stable configuration. Bone-to-bone contact can be restored if there is a single large fragment posteromedially which can be reduced and held in place with lag screws or cerclage wires. The advantage of this option is that leg length is maintained. The disadvantage is that it is very difficult to stabilize the posteromedial fragment, and if its fixation fails, uncontrolled shortening of the fracture with loss of fixation will occur. Impaction of the fragments into a more stable configuration is done by displacing the distal fragment medially and placing the medial cortex of the proximal fragment into the medullary canal of the distal fragment. The fracture is deliberately aligned in valgus, and a "high angle" (e.g., 145°) screw-plate assembly is used to stabilize it. The advantage of this option is that fixation is extremely stable and loss of reduction is rare. The disadvantage is that the extremity is shortened 2 to 4 cm. Type IV (reverse obliquity) fractures cannot be stabilized with a screw-plate assembly because they will shorten and displace (Fig. 17–3). Either a 95° screw-plate device or an intramedullary device (Figs. 17–4 and 17–5) is used to stabilize reverse obliquity fractures.

If there is severe osteopenia (i.e., Singh grade I or II), fixation is augmented with polymethylmethacrylate (PMMA). Care is taken to avoid placing cement between bone fragments, which inhibits bone healing.

Complications

Complications following intertrochanteric fracture include loss of reduction with cut-out of the fixation, and infection. Other complications, such as nonunion and avascular necrosis, are extremely rare.

Loss of reduction with cut-out of the fixation is the most frequently encountered complication. It is more common in patients with severe osteopenia (i.e., Singh index of I or II) who have sustained unstable

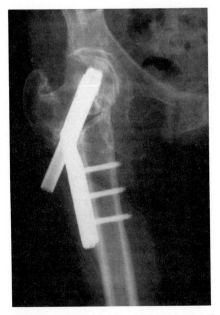

FIG. 17–3   A reverse obliquity intertrochanteric fracture has been stabilized with a sliding screw-plate device. Uncontrolled shortening has occurred.

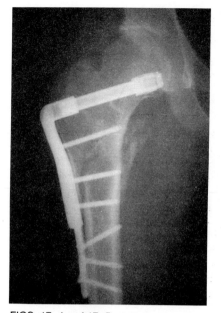

FIGS. 17–4 and 17–5 Anteroposterior radiographs of two hips illustrating the alternative methods of stabilization of reverse obliquity fractures: a 95° screw side-plate device or flexible intramedullary nails.

displaced or reverse obliquity fractures. It is best managed operatively by removing the fixation device, revising the reduction to a more stable configuration, and reinserting the fixation device. PMMA is used to increase the stability of fixation. If the articular surfaces of the femoral head and acetabulum have been damaged, an arthroplasty with a calcar replacement prosthesis is performed.

Infection is more common following open reduction and internal fixation of intertrochanteric fractures than other closed fractures because the patients are debilitated. Implants that provide stability are left in place until healing of the fracture has occurred. Antibiotics, based on the sensitivities of the pathogenic organisms, are administered as long as necessary to control the infection. Once the fracture has healed, the implants are removed, the area is debrided of avascular tissue, and antibiotics are administered for 6 weeks.

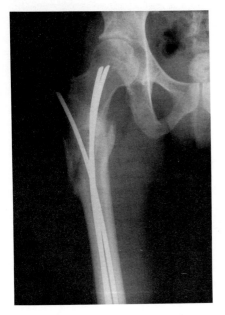

FIG. 17–5

ISOLATED FRACTURES OF THE GREATER AND LESSER TROCHANTERS

Isolated fractures of the greater trochanter are the result of a direct blow or an avulsion. When they are minimally displaced they will heal. If they are displaced, nonunions frequently develop but they are usually asymptomatic. Fractures of the lesser trochanter are rare injuries. They are the result of an avulsion of the iliopsoas tendon and are treated conservatively. The primary importance of isolated fractures of the trochanters is that they may signal an undisplaced intertrochanteric fracture. Radiographs should be carefully examined to rule out this possibility.

SELECTED READINGS

Laros GS, Moore JF: Complications of fixation in intertrochanteric fractures. *Clin Orthop* 92: 147, 1973

Miller WC: Survival and ambulation following hip fracture. *J Bone Joint Surg* 60A:930–933, 1978

Kenzora EJ, McCarthy ER, Lowell JD, Sledge BC: Hip fracture mortality. *Clin Orthop* 186:45–56, 1984

Boyd HB, Griffen LL: Classification and treatment of trochanteric fracture. *Arch Surg* 58:853–866, 1949

Kenneth A. Davenport

The femoral diaphysis is the tubular section extending from the intertro-chanteric region to the supracondylar region.

ANATOMY

The important anatomical features of the femoral diaphysis are its shape, vascular supply, surrounding muscles, and neighboring neurovascular structures.

The femur has an **anterior bow** which varies widely from patient to patient, but averages 12 to 15°. Posteriorly, the cortex thickens into a ridge called the **linea aspera** which is the origin of the medial and lateral intermuscular septa.

The **blood supply** is via endosteal and periosteal vessels. Endosteal vessels are from one or two nutrient arteries which enter the proximal third of the femur via foramina in the linea aspera. These nutrient arteries originate from the profunda femoris artery and supply the inner two-thirds of the diaphyseal cortex. Periosteal vessels supply the outer one-third and originate from arteries supplying the surrounding muscles. Following fracture, the periosteal vessels become the dominant vascular supply.

The muscles of the thigh form three **compartments** separated by intermuscular septa. The anterior compartment contains the knee extensors. The posterior contains the knee flexors. The medial contains the hip adductors.

Unopposed action of muscles results in predictable displacement dependent on the level of the fracture. In fractures proximal to the isthmus of the medullary canal, the proximal fragment is abducted (gluteus), flexed, and internally rotated (iliopsoas). Fractures distal to the isthmus are in varus (adductors) and angulated posteriorly (knee extensors and gastrocnemius).

Neurovascular structures of the thigh are the sciatic nerve, the femoral nerve, the superficial femoral artery, and the deep femoral artery. The sciatic nerve is cushioned from the femur by muscles; therefore, it is seldom injured in association with fractures of the femur. The femoral nerve enervates the quadriceps femoris. The superficial femoral artery enters the posterior compartment of the thigh from the medial compartment via the adductor hiatus, or Hunter's canal, located just proximal to the distal metaphyseal flare of the femur. The artery is tethered by the intermuscular septum, and a fracture at this level is likely to result in its injury. The deep femoral artery gives off approximately four perforating branches prior to ending proximal to the knee. The perforators enter the anterior compartment from the posterior compartment through the lateral intermuscular septum. Their clinical significance is that when they are cut, they retract beneath the lateral intermuscular septum and are a source of uncontrolled bleeding.

Classification

Fractures of the femoral diaphysis are classified according to location and stability. The location is defined as being proximal, middle, or distal third. Fractures of the proximal third are subtrochanteric fractures, and fractures of the distal third merge with supracondylar fractures.

The key to classifying fractures of the femoral diaphysis is the concept of **stability** (Fig. 18–1). Stability is defined in terms of the percentage of the circumference of the cortex that is intact and the obliquity of the fracture. Fractures with at least 50 percent of the cortex intact and an obliquity of less than 30° are stable. When reduced, stable fractures have intrinsic axial and rotational stability; unstable fractures will shorten or rotate. Type I fractures are simple transverse or oblique fractures with no comminution. Type II fractures are comminuted, but more than 50 percent of their cortex is intact. Type III fractures have more than 50 percent of their cortex comminuted, but there is some cortical contact between the proximal and distal fragments. Type IV fractures have segmental comminution. Type V fractures have a long oblique pattern.

Diagnosis and Initial Management

History and Physical Examination

A history of injury, pain, swelling, and obvious deformity are present.

Radiographic Examination

Anteroposterior and lateral radiographs are obtained and examined to rule out undisplaced comminution. Radiographs of the knee and pelvis rule out associated injuries.

Initial Management

Initial management makes the patient as comfortable as possible and optimizes his condition for surgery. If surgery is to be performed within 12 h of admission, 5 to 10 lb of skin traction is applied with the thigh resting on a pillow. If surgery is delayed, 10 to 20 lb of skeletal traction is applied via a tibial pin to minimize the chance of contaminating the distal femur. Ligamentous injury of the knee is ruled out prior to applying traction through a tibial pin. Initially, the hip and knee are flexed 30°, and the calf is supported in a sling. Radiographs are obtained

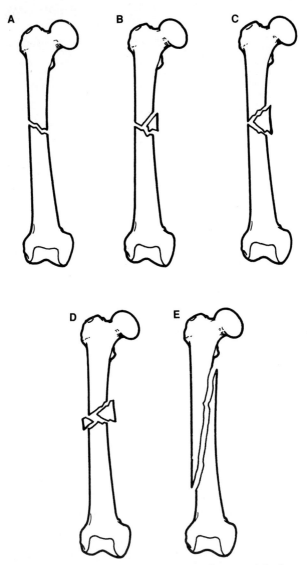

FIG. 18–1 The classification of diaphyseal fractures of the femur: (a) type I, (b) type II, (c) type III, (d) type IV, and (e) type V.

in traction and traction is adjusted accordingly. Ideally, the fracture is aligned and distracted 0.5 cm.

Associated Injuries

Neurovascular injuries and compartment syndrome of the thigh and buttock are ruled out by a focused examination of the injured extremity.

Skeletal injuries associated with fractures of the femoral diaphysis are fracture of the **femoral neck, hip dislocation, pelvic ring** injury, and **ligamentous injury of the knee.** The presence of a femoral neck fracture, hip dislocation, or pelvic ring injury is determined by radiographs of the hip and pelvis. Anteroposterior and lateral radiographs of the knee are obtained, and the knee is carefully examined for an effusion and pain with palpation of the patellar ligament and medial- and lateral-collateral ligaments. When it is not possible to rule out ligamentous injury, the patient is reexamined following fracture fixation.

Definitive Management

Fractures of the femoral diaphysis are managed with open reduction and plating, reduction and application of an external fixater, or closed reduction and intramedullary nailing.

Relative indications for **plating** are inability (usually due to other injuries) to place the patient on the fracture table, a grade III open fracture, fractures around other implants (e.g., the femoral stem of a total hip arthroplasty), an associated fracture of the femoral neck or intercondylar fracture of the distal femur, and obliteration of the medullary canal (usually due to a previous fracture). The disadvantages of plating fractures of the femoral diaphysis are a higher risk of infection and the prolonged postoperative nonweight-bearing. Surgical exposure is via a lateral approach through the interval between vastus lateralis and the lateral intermuscular septum. The vastus lateralis is elevated subperiosteally from the femur. Fracture fragments are identified and anatomically reduced. A broad dynamic compression plate on the lateral side of the femur is used to stabilize the fracture. A minimum of eight cortices are proximal and distal to the fracture. Medial cortical defects are grafted with autogenous cancellous bone to stimulate healing and decrease the incidence of plate failure. Postoperatively, motion of the hip and knee is encouraged. Strict nonweight-bearing is maintained until trabeculae cross the fracture, usually at 10 to 12 weeks after fixation.

The primary indication for **external fixation** is a grade III open fracture. The advantages of external fixation are that it is quick; it stabilizes the fracture, but does not place a foreign body in a contaminated wound; and it allows access to the wound. The disadvantages are that stability is not absolute; the pins placed through the lateral muscles of the thigh "tack" these muscles to the femur, resulting in loss of knee motion; and there is a high incidence of nonunion.

The fracture is reduced through the open wound after debridement and irrigation. A lateral frame is applied with two to four half-pins proximal and distal to the fracture. If possible, the pins are located outside of the zone of injury. The fascia lata and underlying muscles around each pin are incised proximally and distally to minimize irritation and loss of knee motion. The postoperative management is tailored to the patient. Generally, toe touch weight-bearing is maintained until the fracture has healed. Knee and hip motion are encouraged. After the soft tissue has healed, the incidence of nonunion is minimized by grafting the fracture with autogenous cancellous bone, or by removing the fixater and stabilizing the fracture with an intramedullary nail. An intramedullary nail is inserted only if there have been no signs of infection of the fracture or pin sites.

The majority of fractures of the femoral diaphysis are managed with **intramedullary nailing.** The advantages are a low incidence of infection, a high incidence of healing, and the ability to bear weight postoperatively.

Nails are either inserted through the proximal femur and driven distally (i.e., antegrade nailing), or through the distal femur and driven proximally (i.e., retrograde nailing). **Antegrade nails** are rigid and the femur is always reamed prior to their insertion. **Retrograde nails** are rigid or flexible and the femur is not necessarily reamed prior to their insertion. Type I and type II fractures of the femoral diaphysis are managed with either type of intramedullary nail. Type III, IV, and V fractures of the femoral diaphysis are managed with antegrade statically locked nails.

Antegrade intramedullary nailing (Figs. 18–2 and 18–3) is performed with the patient supine on the fracture table. The fluoroscopy machine is brought in from the medial side of the thigh. The fracture is reduced. The nail is inserted through the piriformis fossae at the superior aspect of the base of the femoral neck. The cortex is perforated with a drill, and a guide wire is inserted into the proximal fragment and driven across the reduced fracture. The femur is sequentially reamed. The appropriate size nail is driven across the fracture. In type I and II fractures, the nail is locked dynamically. If the fracture is in the distal third of the femur, the nail is locked distally. If the fracture is in the proximal two-thirds of the femur, the nail is locked proximally. In type III, IV, and V fractures, the nail is locked statically. Postoperatively, patients with stable fractures are allowed to weight-bear as tolerated. Patients with statically locked nails weight-bear 50 percent on the injured side. If radiographic healing progresses over the first 3 to 4 months, weight-bearing is advanced as tolerated. If radiographic signs of healing are delayed, full weight-bearing is delayed; then at 4 to 6 months the fracture is grafted with autogenous cancellous bone.

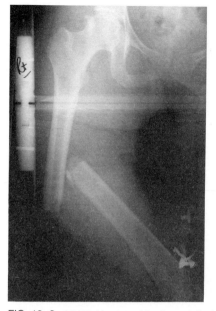

FIG. 18–2 Midthird fracture of the femoral diaphysis. This is a type II fracture because there is comminution involving less than 50 percent of the circumference. In addition, the fracture is open with a grade II soft tissue injury.

Alternatively, the nail is dynamized by removing either proximal or distal locking screws. If the nail is dynamized, the patient is followed carefully for signs of shortening or rotation. If these occur, the nail is relocked statically.

Retrograde nailing of the femoral diaphysis is performed with the patient supine on the fracture table. The fluoroscopy machine is brought in from the lateral side of the thigh. The fracture is reduced. The medial and lateral metaphyseal cortices are perforated with a one-fourth-in. drill bit, and the hole is enlarged with an awl. The appropriate length nail is selected, and nails are driven from the medial and lateral portals simultaneously across the fracture. The lateral nail is driven into the greater trochanter. The medial nail is driven into the base of the femoral neck. The nails are locked dynamically by driving screws through the eyes into underlying bone. Postoperatively, knee flexion is encouraged when incisional pain allows and weight-bearing is tolerated.

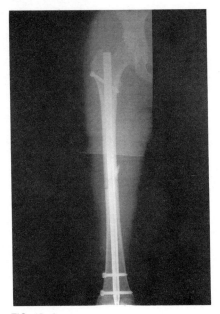

FIG. 18–3   Stabilization with a reamed antegrade statically locked nail.

Complications

The complications of fractures of the femoral diaphysis include malunion, nonunion, and infection.

Rotational and angular **malunion** is managed by osteotomy, realignment, and stabilization of the femur. A statically locked nail or plate
is used for stabilization. Fractures which have healed with significant
shortening are a difficult problem. Significant shortening is defined as
greater than 3 cm, or as resulting in gait disturbance or back pain not
relieved by a shoe lift. Management options include lengthening the
involved femur, lengthening the ipsilateral tibia, or shortening the contralateral femur. Lengthening the involved femur is the most attractive
option because it corrects the deformity. Lengthening is achieved by
applying an external fixater, osteotomizing the femur, and lengthening
the femur in 1 mm increments per day. This procedure requires excep-
tional patient compliance. Lengthening the tibia is a simpler procedure,
but the patient's knees are at different heights. Shortening of the contra-

lateral femur is done closed; it has the lowest morbidity, but results in overall loss of height.

Nonunion is managed by stabilizing the fragments and autogenous bone grafting, or by dynamic compression applied with an external fixater. Intramedullary nails are usually the best method of stabilization, but plates are occasionally indicated (e.g., if there is a fragment of a broken nail in the canal which cannot be retrieved). If dynamic compression is used, a fixater is used to compress the ends of the nonunion together, usually at the rate of 0.25 mm per day. This technique can be combined with lengthening techniques to manage nonunions associated with a segmental defect or shortening.

Infection is managed with debridement, stabilization, and administration of antibiotics. When there is an associated nonunion, delayed grafting with autogenous cancellous bone or dynamic compression with an external fixater is performed.

SELECTED READINGS

Brumback RJ, Reilly JP, Poka A, Lakatos RP, Bathon GH, Bugess AR: Intramedullary nailing of femoral shaft fractures. Part I: Decision-making errors with interlocking fixation. *J Bone Joint Surg* 70A:1441–1452, 1988.

Kempf I, Grosse A, Beck G: Closed locked intramedullary nailing. Its application to comminuted fractures of the femur. *J Bone Joint Surg* 67A:709–719, 1985.

Pankovich AM, Goldflies ML, Pearson RL: Closed ender nailing of femoral-shaft fractures. *J Bone Joint Surg* 61A:222–32, 1979.

Winquist RA, Hansen ST Jr: Comminuted fractures of the femoral shaft treated by intramedullary nailing. *Orthop Cl Na* 11:633–648, 1980.

Injuries About the Knee

Robert C. Schenck, Jr.   Clayton R. Perry

This chapter reviews fractures of the distal femur (supracondylar, intra-condylar, and medial and lateral condyles); fractures of the proximal tibia (the tibial spines, and medial and lateral condyles); injuries of the extensor mechanism (the tibial tubercle, ruptures of the patellar or quadriceps tendon, and fractures of the patella); and dislocations of the knee.

ANATOMY

The knee is a compound joint consisting of a sellar joint between the condyles of the femur and the patella, and two condylar joints between the condyles of the femur and the tibial plateaus.

The **distal femur** consists of condyles and epicondyles. Medial and lateral condyles form the articular surface. They are narrower anteriorly, and the medial condyle projects further distally than the lateral condyle, which results in the distal articular surface forming an angle of 7° with the diaphysis. The lateral condyle projects further anteriorly (preventing lateral patellar subluxation) and posteriorly than the medial. The distal and posterior surfaces of both condyles are convex and articulate with the corresponding tibial plateau. The anterior surface of the distal femur is the coalescence of medial and lateral condyles. Its concave surface corresponds to the articular surface of the patella.

The **proximal tibia** expands to form the medial and lateral condyles, or plateaus, and tibial tuberosity. The articular surface of the tibia is the cartilage-covered medial and lateral plateaus which match the corresponding articular surfaces of the femur. Congruency is further increased by the medial and lateral menisci. The two plateaus are separated by the anterior and posterior tibial spines (i.e., the intercondy-lar eminence). The anterior tibial spine is the insertion of the anterior cruciate ligament, and the attachment of the anterior and posterior horns of the lateral meniscus and anterior horn of the medial meniscus. The posterior tibial spine is the attachment of the posterior horn of the medial meniscus. The posterior intercondylar areas are the insertion of the posterior cruciate ligament. The fibular facet on the lateral condyle faces laterally, distally, and posteriorly.

The **tibial tuberosity** is the anterior projection of the tibia into which the patellar ligament inserts. It is 2 cm distal to the articular surface of the tibia. Its upper surface is directly behind the patellar ligament and is an insertion site for intramedullary nailing.

The **patella** is the largest sesamoid bone of the body. It increases the lever arm of the quadriceps and protects the anterior articular surface of the distal femur. It is located 2 cm proximal to the articular surface of the tibia when the knee is extended. A more proximal location is referred to as "patella alta," and a more distal location as "patella baja." With the exception of the apex, or lower pole, the posterior surface of the patella is covered with articular cartilage. The lower pole serves as the origin of the patellar ligament. The articular surface of the patella is convex and is divided into smaller medial and larger lateral sections by a vertical ridge. The medial and lateral halves are further divided into two or three pairs of facets by faint horizontal ridges in the articular surface. The lateral facets are more distinct than the medial, and the upper lateral facet is slightly concave. In addition, there is a single facet on the extreme medial border of the patella which runs the length of the patella and articulates with the medial femoral condyle when the knee is flexed.

FRACTURES OF THE DISTAL FEMUR

Fractures of the distal femur involve the distal metaphysis and articular surface of the femur.

Classification

Distal femoral fractures are classified according to whether there is intraarticular extension and whether one or both condyles are fractured into three types: type I—extraarticular fractures, type II—intraarticular fractures in which both condyles are involved, and type III—fractures of a single condyle.

Extraarticular fractures (type I), also known as supracondylar fractures, are divided into simple fractures and those with supracondylar comminution (Figs. 19–1 and 19–2).

Intraarticular fractures (type II), or intracondylar fractures, are divided into four subtypes based on the presence of intraarticular displacement and metaphyseal comminution. The subtypes are simple metaphyseal fractures with undisplaced intraarticular component, simple metaphyseal fractures with displaced intraarticular component, comminuted metaphyseal fractures with undisplaced intraarticular component, and comminuted metaphyseal fractures with displaced intraarticular component (Figs. 19–3 through 19–8).

Fractures of a single condyle (type III) are further divided into four subtypes based on the plane of the fracture and the condyle involved. The subtypes are fractures in the coronal plane of the medial or lateral condyles, and fractures in the sagittal plane of the medial or lateral condyles (Figs. 19–9 and 19–10).

Associated Injuries

Injuries associated with supracondylar fractures of the femur are fractures and dislocations of the proximal femur and pelvis, ligamentous

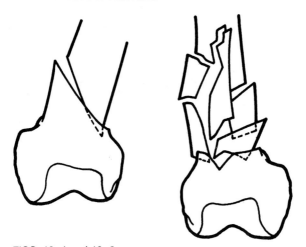

FIGS. 19–1 and 19–2   Type I supracondylar fractures.

disruption of the knee, injury of the popliteal artery, and injury of the peroneal and tibial nerves. These injuries are more likely to occur in association with high-energy fractures.

Associated **fractures and dislocations of the proximal femur and pelvis** are most likely to occur in an automobile accident as part of the "dashboard injury" complex. They are ruled out by physical examination and review of radiographs of the proximal femur and entire pelvis.

The most frequently disrupted **ligament** is the patellar ligament. Disruption of the collaterals and cruciates also occurs. Accurate physical examination of the ligaments is usually not possible prior to fracture fixation. Radiographic signs of ligamentous injury are loss of parallelism between the articular surfaces of the femoral condyles and tibial plateaus, and bony avulsion of the cruciates (Figs. 19–7 and 19–8). Following stabilization of the fracture, all ligaments are examined and repaired if injured.

Early identification of an associated **popliteal artery** injury is key. The cardinal finding is decreased dorsalis pedis and posterior tibial pulses. This may be due to torsion or traction of the vessels. If aligning the fracture does not result in the return of pulses within 5 min, the assumption is that there is a popliteal artery injury and an angiogram is obtained. Once the location of the vascular injury is determined, surgery to stabilize the fracture and restore circulation is performed emergently. Occasionally, the popliteal artery injury is an intimal tear, and pulses which are initially present will suddenly disappear with

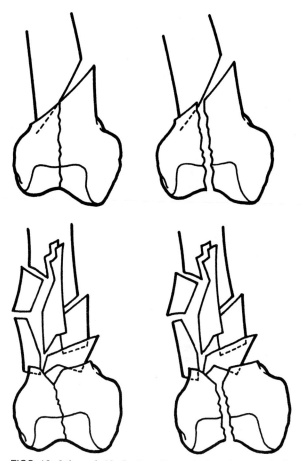

FIGS. 19–3 through 19–6 Type II intraarticular or intracondylar fractures.

artery thromboses. For this reason, vascular checks are performed every 2 h for the first 36 h after injury.

Injuries of the **peroneal and tibial nerves** are identified by assessing sensation and the ability to plantarflex and dorsiflex the ankle. They are managed with range of motion exercises of the ankle and foot, and splinting in a functional position.

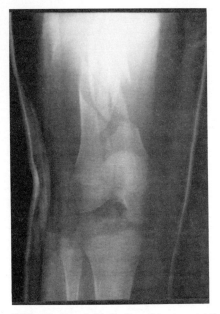

FIGS. 19–7 and 19–8   Type II fracture stabilized with a retrograde nail after the condyles had been lagged together. The tibial spines are avulsed, indicating a cruciate injury.

Diagnosis and Initial Management

History and Physical Examination

There is pain and a history of injury. Obvious instability and deformity is present with type I and II fractures, but may not be present with fractures of a single condyle.

Radiographic Examination

Radiographs in the anteroposterior and lateral projections are sufficient to evaluate the injury. The tunnel view of the distal femur in which the anteroposterior radiograph is obtained with the knee flexed to 30° is helpful, but painful for the patient. Radiographs of the pelvis, hip, femur, and tibia are examined for associated injuries.

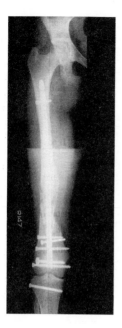

Initial Management

The key factor in the initial management is evaluation of the vascular status of the leg. If a vascular injury has not occurred, the leg is immobilized in a toe-to-groin splint and iced. If splinting does not adequately immobilize the fracture, skeletal traction is used. A proximal tibial pin is inserted, the knee is placed on pillows, the calf is supported in a sling, and 10 to 20 lb of traction is applied. Posttraction radiographs are obtained to assess alignment and to determine whether the knee joint is being distracted due to ligamentous disruption.

Definitive Management

The definitive management of supracondylar fractures is surgery. The surgical approach, stabilization device, and whether bone graft is used is based on the type of fracture.

We stabilize fractures without intraarticular extension with an ante-grade or retrograde intramedullary nail. **Antegrade locked nailing** of a supracondylar fracture is performed as described in Chapter 18. To

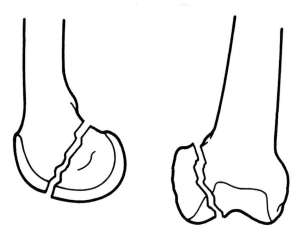

FIGS. 19–9 and 19–10   Fractures of a single condyle in the coronal and sagittal planes.

decrease the incidence of nail breakage through a distal locking hole, there should be at least 5 cm of intact bone proximal to the distal screw holes; therefore, this method can be used only for very proximal supracondylar fractures.

The fracture can be stabilized with a **rigid retrograde nail** inserted through the intercondylar notch. The objections to this technique are the intraarticular insertion portal, possible synovial metalosis, and the potential difficulty of removing the nail (Figs. 19–7 and 19–8).

Intracondylar fractures (type II) are managed with a plate and screws. Intramedullary nails are not an option because of the intraarticular component. Intercondylar fractures with a simple metaphyseal component and undisplaced condyles are stabilized with a 95° side-plate and lag screw. To minimize the potential that the undisplaced condyles will displace during lag screw insertion, they are stabilized with two large cancellous screws prior to reaming for the lag screw. Fractures with metaphyseal comminution and an undisplaced intracondylar component are managed similarly; however, the medial side of the metaphysis is grafted with autogenous cancellous bone. Anatomic reduction of comminuted metaphyseal fragments is not mandatory as long as the relationship of the condyles to the distal diaphysis is restored.

The management of intracondylar fractures with a simple metaphyseal component and displaced condyles is more complex. The condyles must be reduced and, therefore, it is necessary to use a surgical approach which exposes the distal articular surface. A straight anterior incision is made. The quadriceps tendon is split in line with its fibers; this incision is continued distally as a lateral parapatellar incision. If necessary, the tibial tuberosity is predrilled, osteotomized, and reflected proximally for better exposure. The condyles are reduced and held in place with Kirschner wires and screws. The fixation of the intercondylar fracture is planned so that it does not interfere with placement of the device used to fix the condyles to the femur (e.g., a side-plate and lag screw). Fractures with metaphyseal comminution and a displaced intracondylar component are managed similarly; however, the medial side of the metaphysis is grafted with autogenous cancellous bone. In fractures with segmental comminution, the medial side of the metaphysis is plated through the same incision. The medial plate functions as a buttress and is fastened to the bone with unicortical screws.

Supracondylar and intracondylar fractures which are complicated by osteopenia are stabilized as described, but polymethylmethacrylate (PMMA) is used to provide more stable fixation. After the fragments have been reduced, the PMMA, while in its doughy state, is inserted into the medullary cavity across the fracture. This is done through a cortical window at the level of the fracture. After the PMMA has hardened, the fracture is stabilized with plates and screws. If PMMA is used, it is mandatory to graft the medial side with autogenous bone.

Fractures of the medial or lateral condyles in the sagittal plane are exposed via a medial or lateral parapatellar surgical approach. The condyle is reduced and held in place with lag screws or a buttress plate. Fractures in the coronal plane involve the posterior portion of the condyle. They are exposed via a midmedial or midlateral incision. The surface of the fragment is covered with articular cartilage and is stabilized with countersunk screws.

Following stabilization of supracondylar, intracondylar, and single condyle fractures, early motion is encouraged as soon as incisional pain becomes tolerable. The duration of nonweight-bearing is dependent on the stability of the fracture, the stability of fixation, and the rate of healing.

Complications

Complications are nonunion, malunion, and posttraumatic arthritis. **Nonunion** is managed with autogenous bone graft and rigid stabilization. A stiff knee worsens the prognosis. In cases in which the knee is stiff or in which stabilization of the distal fragment is impossible because of its small size or osteopenia, arthrodesis is performed. If there is no prior history of infection, an intramedullary rod is used. If there is a history of infection, an external fixater is used.

Varus and valgus **malunions** are invariably symptomatic and eventually result in arthritis. Extension and flexion malunions are better tolerated. Symptomatic malunion is managed with corrective osteotomy of the femur.

Posttraumatic arthritis is managed with nonsteroidal anti-inflammatories and local injection of steroids. Arthroscopic debridement gives short-term relief of symptoms. The last resort is arthroplasty or arthrodesis. Arthroplasty is reserved for low-demand elderly patients.

FRACTURES OF THE TIBIAL PLATEAU

Fractures of the tibial plateau involve the proximal articular surface of the tibia.

Classification

Tibial plateau fractures are classified into seven types: type I—split fracture of the lateral plateau, type II—depressed fracture of the lateral plateau, type III—split-depressed fracture of the lateral plateau, type IV—low-energy fracture of the medial plateau, type V—high-energy fracture of the medial plateau, type VI—bicondylar plateau fracture, and type VII—any of the first six types of fractures associated with a metaphyseal fracture (Figs. 19–11 through 19–17).

Split fractures of the lateral plateau occur in young patients with dense bone. The mechanism of injury is high-energy (e.g., a blow to the lateral side of the knee). The fracture, which is best seen on the anteroposterior projection, is vertical and seldom displaced more than 3 mm. The lateral meniscus may be torn peripherally and dislocated into the fracture site (Fig. 19–11).

Depressed fractures occur in osteopenic bone. The mechanism of injury is a low-energy valgus stress—the lateral femoral condyle sinks into and depresses the lateral plateau. The lateral plateau including the metaphyseal cortex is tilted laterally (Fig. 19–12).

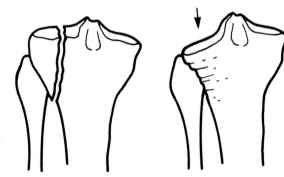

FIGS. 19–11 through 19–17 Types of tibial plateau fractures.

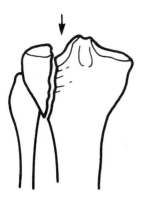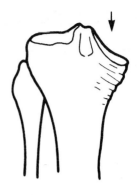

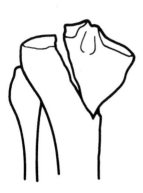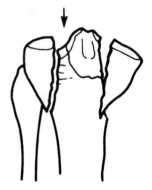

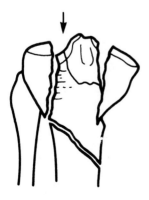

Split-depressed fractures are the most common type of tibial plateau fractures. The mechanism of injury is a valgus stress which impacts the lateral femoral condyle against the plateau, fracturing the lateral portion of the plateau from the proximal tibia. As the femoral condyle continues to impact the remaining portion of the lateral plateau, it drives a segment of articular surface into the metaphysis. This depressed segment is always on the medial side of the fracture, not on the split fragment. Whether the depressed segment is anterior or posterior depends on the degree of flexion at the time of injury (extension is associated with anterior depression; flexion with posterior depression) (Figs. 19–13, 19–18, and 19–19).

Low-energy medial plateau fractures are similar to depressed fractures of the lateral plateau, but are the result of a varus force across the knee. The entire medial plateau is tilted medially (Fig. 19–14).

High-energy medial plateau fractures are fracture dislocations frequently associated with neurovascular injuries. They are caused by an axial and valgus force across the knee resulting in the lateral femoral

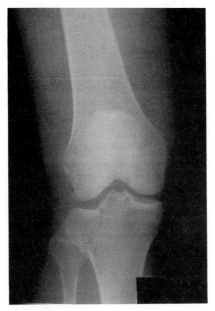

FIGS. 19–18 and 19–19 Split-depressed tibial plateau fracture reduced and stabilized with a plate.

condyle impacting the tibial spines along a vector directed medially and distally. The medial tibial condyle, along with the tibial spines, is fractured and driven along this vector. The lateral-collateral ligament is ruptured; the cruciates and medial-collateral ligaments are intact (Fig. 19–15).

Bicondylar plateau fractures involve both condyles and are the result of complex high-energy trauma. Associated neurovascular and ligamentous injuries and compartment syndrome are common (Fig. 19–16).

Plateau fractures associated with a fracture of the proximal metaphysis are similar to bicondylar fractures in that they are the result of high-energy trauma and frequently have associated neurovascular injuries. There is a high incidence of nonunion and postoperative infection due to the magnitude of the injury and the extensive surgical exposure necessary to reduce and stabilize the fracture (Fig. 19–17).

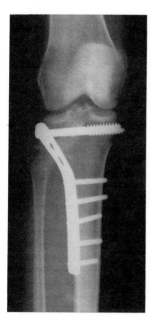

Associated Injuries

Injuries which are frequently associated with fractures of the tibial plateaus are ruptures of the collateral ligaments, occlusion of the popliteal artery or trifurcation, compartment syndrome, and injury of the posterior tibial or common peroneal nerve.

Fracture of the medial or lateral plateau may be associated with a rupture of the contralateral **collateral ligament.** Apparent ligamentous laxity may be a misinterpretation of motion occurring through the fracture site. To definitively determine if there is a ligamentous injury, the knee is stressed under fluoroscopy.

Injuries of the **popliteal artery or trifurcation** are most likely to occur with high-energy medial-tibial plateau and bicondylar fractures. If distal pulses are absent, an arteriogram is obtained.

Compartment syndrome is indicated by the presence of the classic signs of increased intracompartmental pressure: pain at rest, pain with passive stretch of muscles, tense compartments, and numbness in the first web space.

Injuries of the **posterior tibial and peroneal nerves** are identified by assessing sensation on the plantar aspect of the foot and in the first web space, and by assessing active contraction of the flexor and extensor hallucis longus.

Diagnosis and Initial Management

History and Physical Examination

There is pain, swelling, and a history of injury. There may be no discernible deformity, but there is a large knee effusion, which, when aspirated, has blood with fat in it, indicating an intraarticular fracture.

Radiographic Examination

Radiographs in the anteroposterior and lateral planes are of most use. Tilting the beam 10° caudally so that it profiles the articular surface gives more accurate information regarding the amount of depression. Tomograms and CAT scans are helpful.

Initial Management

A long leg splint with the knee in 20° of flexion is applied. The knee is iced.

Definitive Management

The goals of management of tibial plateau fractures are to decrease the risk of posttraumatic osteoarthritis and provide a stable knee with a normal axis of alignment. Indications for operative management are reducible intraarticular incongruity, intraarticular displacement (i.e., a gap without a step-off) of 3 mm or more, ligamentous instability, or a deviation in the alignment of the knee. Indications for nonoperative management are a fracture which cannot be satisfactorily reduced and stabilized, usually due to extensive comminution; blisters; and preexisting arthritis.

The **nonoperative management** of tibial plateau fractures which are minimally displaced or in which there is preexisting osteoarthritis consists of 4 to 8 weeks of immobilization in a long leg cast, followed by 4 to 8 weeks of nonweight-bearing and protected mobilization in an orthosis. Displaced fractures which are managed nonoperatively are placed in balanced skeletal suspension with the knee at 45°. A sling supports the calf, and 10 to 20 lb of traction is applied through a distal tibial pin. Alignment of the fracture is assessed radiographically every 2 to 3 days for the first 2 weeks, and traction is adjusted accordingly. At 2 to 3 weeks, passive motion in traction is initiated. At 4 to 6 weeks, there is usually enough healing clinically and radiographically that balanced suspension can be discontinued and a long leg cast can be applied. The cast is continued 8 to 10 weeks from injury. Nonweight-bearing is continued 12 weeks from injury.

The goal of **operative management** is anatomic alignment of the joint surface and stabilization adequate to allow early motion. The surgical exposure and method of stabilization is based on the type of fracture.

Split fractures are reduced closed under fluoroscopy and stabilized with percutaneous screws. To reduce the fracture, the knee is flexed to 30° and a varus stress is applied. At the same time, the lateral plateau is pushed medially toward the proximal tibia. If this maneuver does not result in reduction, the fracture is exposed through a lateral parapatellar approach. The block to reduction (frequently the lateral meniscus) is identified and removed. Postoperatively, the extremity is placed in a continuous passive motion machine and moved from 10 to 30°. When the patient can perform active range of motion, the continuous passive motion is discontinued. Nonweight-bearing is maintained for 6 to 8 weeks.

Depressed fractures are managed operatively through a straight anterior skin incision. The lateral plateau is elevated with a bone tamp inserted through a window in the lateral metaphysis. The tibial attachment of the meniscus is incised and the meniscus retracted superiorly to expose the plateau. The resulting defect is packed with autogenous bone graft. A plate is applied laterally with two large cancellous screws within 5 mm of subchondral bone. These screws function to support the articular surface.

Split-depressed fractures are exposed via a straight anterior incision. The anterior horn of the lateral meniscus is incised and the fracture is "booked open" through the split component, exposing the depressed segment. The depressed segment is elevated, bone grafted, and the split fragment is reduced and stabilized with a plate (Figs. 19–18 and 19–19).

Medial plateau fractures are managed operatively through a straight anterior incision. Depending on the location of the fracture, the anterior horn of the medial or lateral meniscus can be incised. There may be minimal compression with high-energy fractures in which case bone grafting is not necessary. A plate is used for stabilization.

Bicondylar fractures are exposed by incising one or both anterior horns of the menisci. The tibial tubercle can be osteotomized and the patellar tendon reflected. Fragments are reduced, bone graft is used to fill defects, and medial and lateral plates are applied.

Plateau fractures with an associated metaphyseal fracture are managed by first addressing the intraarticular fracture and then the metaphyseal fracture. Either flexible intramedullary nails or a plate are used to stabilize the metaphyseal fracture. Prolonged casting of the metaphyseal fracture is not an option because a stiff knee will result.

Early postoperative motion is encouraged. With the exception of split fractures, nonweight-bearing is maintained 12 weeks. Patients with split fractures are weight-bearing as tolerated at 6 weeks.

Complications

Complications of tibial plateau fractures are arthritis, nonunion, infection, and late subsidence of a reduced plateau. **Arthritis** results from articular incongruity or injury to the articular cartilage that occurred at the time of fracture. Patients under the age of 50 years are managed with nonsteroidal anti-inflammatories and local steroid injections. If the symptoms warrant, an arthrodesis or a varus or valgus high tibial osteotomy designed to "unload" the involved condyle is performed. Patients over the age of 50 with arthritis are managed with an arthroplasty.

Nonunion of tibial plateau fractures is rare; when it occurs it is often accompanied by infection. In evaluating the nonunion, it is important to determine if is infected, whether the knee joint is arthritic, and how much motion is occurring through the knee as opposed to through the nonunion. If there is no evidence of infection and there is severe arthritis, the nonunion is managed with an arthroplasty in patients over 50 years of age. In the same patient under 50 years of age, the nonunion is managed with an arthrodesis using an intramedullary nail. Management of aseptic nonunions without arthritis consists of rigid stabilization in the form of plates and screws and autogenous cancellous bone grafting. Restricted knee motion is associated with a high incidence of failure of fixation. The principles of management of **infected nonunions** of tibial plateau fractures are debridement of necrotic tissue and foreign bodies, stabilization of the nonunion with screws and plates, management of dead space with antibiotic impregnated beads or muscle flaps, soft tissue coverage with local or free tissue transfer, and antibiotic coverage based on the sensitivities of the pathogenic organisms. Septic nonunion of the tibial plateau is frequently associated with destruction of the joint. In these cases, knee arthrodesis is performed with an external fixater.

Late subsidence of a reduced tibial plateau occurs in osteopenic patients who have sustained a depressed fracture of the lateral plateau or a low-energy fracture of the medial plateau. At-risk patients are followed closely after weight-bearing has been initiated. If subsidence is suspected, weight-bearing is discontinued, and aggressive physical therapy, in particular strengthening and active range of motion, is instituted. After 2 to 4 weeks, partial weight-bearing in a varus (lateral plateau) or valgus (medial plateau) orthosis is reinstituted and gradually increased. Radiographs are obtained weekly until the patient is full weight-bearing. If subsidence has occurred and instability or alteration in the axis of the knee is symptomatic, management is osteotomy or arthroplasty.

INJURIES OF THE EXTENSOR MECHANISM

This section reviews fractures of the patella and injuries of the quadriceps tendon and patellar ligament.

FRACTURES OF THE PATELLA

Classification

Fractures of the patella are undisplaced or displaced, simple or comminuted, and transverse or vertical (Figs. 19–20 through 19–23). **Undisplaced** fractures are all fractures with less than 3 mm of displacement and no step-off. The patient has active knee extension. **Displaced** fractures are simple or comminuted and transverse or vertical. Fragments are displaced more than 3 mm or there is a step-off involving the articular surface. Frequently active knee extension is absent.

Associated Injuries

Fractures of the proximal femur and acetabulum are associated with patellar fractures sustained during high-energy trauma (i.e., the dashboard injury). Radiographs of the hip, femur, and tibia are obtained and examined. The knee is carefully stressed to detect any injury of the stabilizing ligaments. The hip is put through a range of motion to rule out associated fracture or dislocation.

Diagnosis and Initial Management

History and Physical Examination

There is pain and a history of direct trauma to the knee or forceful flexion of the knee (e.g., during a fall). There may be a gap at the fracture site. A large hemarthrosis with fat in it is present. Following aspiration, local anesthetic is injected. When some degree of anesthesia

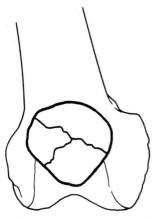

FIG. 19–20   Undisplaced comminuted patellar fracture.

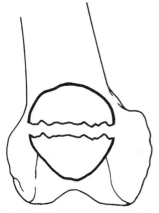

FIG. 19–21   Displaced simple transverse patellar fracture.

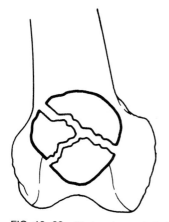

FIG. 19–22 Displaced comminuted patellar fracture.

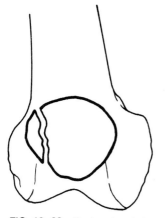

FIG. 19–23 Displaced vertical patellar fracture.

has been achieved, the patient's ability to actively extend the knee is determined. Loss of active extension is an indication for surgery.

Radiographic Examination

Anteroposterior and lateral radiographs are useful. A ''skyline'' view determines the presence of an intraarticular step-off. This view is obtained by flexing the knee 45°, placing the cassette at midcalf, and directing the beam from proximal to distal through the anterior aspect of the knee. Tomograms and CT scans are not helpful.

Initial Management

The knee is splinted in full extension and iced.

Definitive Management

Management is based on the type of fracture. Undisplaced transverse or comminuted fractures are managed by immobilizing the knee in extension, in a cylinder cast, or in a knee immobilizer. Partial weight-bearing is maintained for at least 3 weeks, during which time radiographs are obtained at weekly intervals. If displacement occurs, open reduction and internal fixation is necessary. At 6 weeks, immobilization is discontinued and active range of motion is initiated. Undisplaced vertical fractures are managed similarly, but the period of immobilization is only 4 weeks.

Displaced fractures are managed with open reduction and fixation. The fracture is approached through a straight anterior incision, extending from 4 cm proximal to the patella to 2 cm distal to the tibial tubercle. Fractures are reduced and stabilized with screws or Kirschner wires, or the comminuted segment is excised and the quadriceps tendon or patellar ligament is sutured to the remaining patella. The retinaculum is repaired. The repair is protected with a load-sharing cable extending from the tibial tubercle to the proximal patella (Figs. 19–24 and 19–25).

Complications

Complications of patellar fractures include posttraumatic arthritis and loss of fixation. **Posttraumatic arthritis** is managed conservatively with nonsteroidal anti-inflammatories and steroid injections. If this is not successful in managing the symptoms, a patellectomy is performed. **Loss of fixation** is managed with revision of the fixation.

INJURIES OF THE QUADRICEPS TENDON AND PATELLAR LIGAMENT

Classification

Disruption of the quadriceps tendon and patellar ligament is classified as either a bony avulsion or midsubstance tear.

Associated Injuries

There are no specific injuries associated with rupture of the quadriceps tendon and patellar ligament.

Diagnosis and Initial Management

History and Physical Examination

There is a history of the knee giving away, usually preceded by a forceful contraction of the quadriceps. There is pain and a palpable gap in the tendon or ligament. If active extension is present, the rupture is partial. Loss of active extension indicates a complete rupture and means that surgical repair is necessary.

Radiographic Examination

The radiographic signs are subtle and may consist only of an effusion. A bony avulsion from the patella or tibial tubercle and patella alta may be present.

Initial Management

The knee is splinted in full extension and iced.

Definitive Management

Partial rupture of the quadriceps tendon and patellar ligament is managed nonoperatively. The knee is immobilized in extension for 4 to 6 weeks, when gentle active and passive motion is initiated.

Complete ruptures are managed operatively. The surgical exposure is through a midline vertical incision centered over the site of injury. The type of repair depends on whether the injury is an avulsion or a midsubstance tear. Avulsions are reattached through drill holes in the patella or tibial tuberosity. Midsubstance tears are repaired by end-to-end repair with a Kessler suture technique. Associated tears in the retinaculum are repaired with figure of eight sutures. Patellar ligament repairs are protected with a load-bearing wire or cable loop extending from the proximal pole of the patella to the tibial tubercle.

Postoperatively, quadriceps tendon repairs are protected 4 to 6 weeks in a splint. Weight-bearing is as tolerated on crutches. At 4 to 6 weeks, the splint is removed daily for active range of motion exercises. At 8 weeks, the splint and crutches are discontinued. When the patellar tendon has been repaired, and a load-bearing cable or wire has been used, postoperative immobilization is not necessary. Active range of motion is initiated 2 weeks after surgery. Crutches are used for 4 weeks.

Complications

The complications of quadriceps tendon and patellar ligament rupture are primarily failure of the repair and infection. **Failure of the repair**

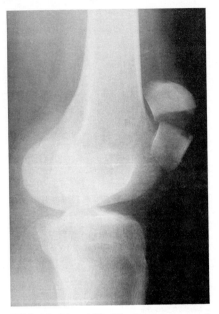

FIGS. 19–24 and 19–25   Simple transverse fracture before and after fixation.

is a serious complication. In the rare instance when it is caught early, the repair can be redone; however, the duration of immobilization must be extended. Usually failure of the repair is caught later, and a more extensive surgical procedure is required. V-Y advancement of the quadriceps, tendon grafts using the fascia lata, or transfer of semitendinous and gracilis muscles is performed to restore the continuity. **Infection** of the repair is relatively common because of its subcutaneous location. When infection occurs, it is treated aggressively with antibiotics. Surgical management of the infected repair is usually not necessary. The indications for surgery are a septic knee requiring drainage and loss of tissue over the patellar tendon requiring a soft tissue transfer (e.g., gastrocnemius flap).

LIGAMENTOUS INJURIES OF THE KNEE

This section describes the diagnosis and management of knee dislocations.

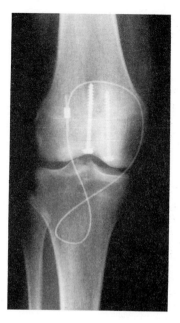

Classification

We classify knee dislocations according to which ligaments are disrupted.

There are four ligaments which may be disrupted: the anterior cruciate (ACL), posterior cruciate (PCL), lateral-collateral (LCL), and medial-collateral (MCL); in addition, the posterolateral corner (PLC) of the capsule is a major stabilizing structure which may be disrupted. The determination of which ligaments are disrupted is based on the physical examination either immediately following the injury or, later, under anesthesia.

For many years, the sine qua non of knee dislocations was complete disruption of both cruciate ligaments. Recently, it has become clear that the PCL is occasionally intact. This is a key point—a functioning PCL directs surgical management to the treatment of the torn ACL. In contrast, the dislocation in which both cruciate ligaments are torn is a much more complicated and unstable pattern.

One or both of the collateral ligaments may be disrupted during a knee dislocation. Disruption of a collateral ligament implies disruption of underlying capsular structures, and directs the surgical approach to ligamentous repair.

Using this system, there are five possible types of injury: type I—ACL/MCL/LCL torn, PCL intact; type II—ACL/PCL torn, MCL/LCL intact; type III—ACL/PCL/MCL torn, LCL/PLC intact; type IV—ACL/PCL/LCL/PLC torn, MCL intact; and type V—ACL/PCL/MCL/LCL/PLC torn.

Associated Injuries

Injuries associated with knee dislocations are vascular, neurologic, or skeletal.

Roughly one-third of all knee dislocations have an associated **popliteal artery** injury. The presence of pedal pulses does not rule out an arterial injury (e.g., an intimal tear). Therefore, arteriography, even in the presence of palpable postreduction pulses, is justifiable. Disruption of the popliteal artery is a surgical emergency. Circulation must be reestablished within 8 h or the chance of salvaging the leg is minimal. Stabilization of the knee protects the vascular repair. External fixation is the most effective method of accomplishing this. The external fixater can be left in place and used to manage the ligamentous injury.

The **peroneal and tibial nerves** are at risk. The peroneal nerve is injured more frequently than the tibial nerve with an incidence of about 20 percent. The peroneal nerve is most commonly injured in association with the lateral ligamentous complex (e.g., adduction injury to the knee ACL/PCL/LCL/PLC torn, MCL intact). It is usually a traction injury which cannot be repaired. The differential diagnosis of peroneal and tibial nerve injury is compartment syndrome.

Bony avulsions of ligamentous origins and insertions are distinct from fracture-dislocations of the knee in which ligamentous injury is associated with a fracture of the tibial or femoral condyles. Frequently, a bony avulsion facilitates ligamentous repair. The PCL is avulsed in approximately 80 percent of knee dislocations, and ACL in approximately 50 percent.

Diagnosis and Initial Management

History and Physical Examination

The mechanism of injury is important because the incidence of associated injuries, in particular popliteal artery disruption, is less with low-energy injuries (e.g., sports-related).

The diagnosis of a displaced knee dislocation is obvious because of the gross deformity. However, frequently the dislocation has been reduced at the site of the injury and massive swelling may be the only obvious physical finding. Lacerations are assumed to communicate with the joint unless proven otherwise. A medial skin furrow may indicate that the dislocation is irreducible with closed methods.

A focused vascular evaluation includes palpation of pedal pulses, examination of leg and foot compartments, and assessment of skin color and capillary refill. A focused neurologic evaluation includes examination of the peroneal nerve (i.e., sensation on the dorsum of the foot and ability to dorsiflex the ankle) and tibial nerve (i.e., sensation on the plantar aspect of the foot and ability to plantarflex the foot).

The initial ligamentous evaluation is performed in a standardized manner with reference made to the contralateral knee for comparison. The knee is stressed in full extension in varus and valgus; instability indicates a torn PCL along with a torn LCL and MCL, respectively. Instability in 30° of flexion indicates a torn MCL (valgus) or LCL (varus) (Fig. 19–26). Hyperextension indicates a torn PCL. A positive Lachman's test indicates a torn ACL. A Lachman's test is performed by flexing the knee to 25°. One hand stabilizes the thigh, the other stresses the tibia, attempting to displace it anteriorly and posteriorly (Fig. 19–27). If there is an abnormal amount of motion, the test is positive. Anterior and posterior drawer tests are performed by flexing the knee to 90° and applying anterior and posterior stresses. Instability indicates a torn ACL and capsule or PCL and capsule, respectively.

Radiographic Examination

The neurovascular and radiographic examinations are performed prior to reduction. Anteroposterior and lateral radiographs aid in classifying the injury according to the relative position of the tibia and femur, and determine whether there are associated fractures.

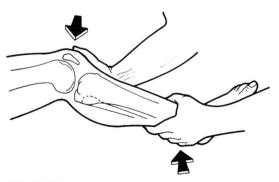

FIG. 19–26   Stressing the MCL.

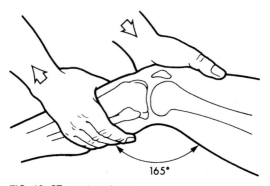

165°

FIG. 19–27 Lachman's test.

Following the initial closed reduction, the injury is further evaluated with MRI. MRI identifies which ligaments are disrupted and distinguishes midsubstance tears from avulsions. This is particularly useful in planning the management of a PCL disruption.

Finally, radiographs are obtained while the patient is anesthetized. The extended knee is stressed in varus and valgus. Joint line opening indicates complete disruption of both cruciate ligaments and of either the MCL or LCL.

Thus, with the initial evaluation, pre- and postreduction radiographs, MRI, examination under anesthesia, and stress radiographs, an accurate preincision prediction of the damaged structures is made.

Initial Management

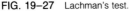

Reduction is usually straightforward and accomplished with longitudinal traction and manipulation. Once the joint is reduced, the vascular and neurologic examination is repeated. The knee is splinted and iced. Postsplinting radiographs are obtained to ensure maintenance of reduction. The patient is admitted for observation and arteriography.

Definitive Management

With the recent advances in ligament reconstruction and repair, it makes intuitive sense to perform acute ligamentous repairs. Furthermore, surgical repair allows early range of motion. Occasionally, closed management of knee dislocations is required because of associated injuries (soft tissue, multiple trauma, infection).

Closed management consists of immobilization of the knee in extension for 6 weeks, followed by range of motion exercises. This length of time allows satisfactory healing of the PCL. Frequently, manipulation under epidural anesthesia is required to regain full motion. Early range of motion as currently used to manage combined ACL/MCL injuries results in laxity.

Surgical Management

There are fundamental techniques and principles of surgical management. **Midline incisions** are utilized whenever possible to minimize the incidence of wound-healing problems if other surgical procedures are performed in the future. Repair of midsubstance ligament tears is accomplished with the **looping suture** technique as described by Marshall et al., or the **locking whip stitch** described by Krackow. Ligaments avulsed from their insertions or origins are **reattached with a screw and spiked washer.** Fixation of an autograft or allograft is accomplished by **fixing the graft in bony tunnels** in the femur and tibia. The key to reconstruction of the dislocated knee is **repair of the PCL.**

Simultaneous PCL/ACL surgery is not recommended, and ACL reconstruction is usually delayed. The exception to this rule is an ACL avulsion in which reattachment increases the stability of the knee without increasing the complexity or duration of surgery. Repair of collateral injuries adds to stability. **Arthroscopy** of the acute knee dislocation (within 14 days of injury) is contraindicated because of the risk of fluid extravasation due to the capsular disruption.

Specific Surgical Techniques

The following descriptions of surgical management of the dislocated knee are based on ligaments involved.

Type I ACL/MCL/LCL torn, PCL intact: PCL integrity directs the treatment of this type of dislocation to the anterior cruciate ligament. Repair of the ACL is performed either immediately or delayed until range of motion is restored and collateral healing has occurred.

Type II ACL/PCL torn, MCL/LCL intact: This injury pattern is rare, and the management is simplified by the intact collaterals. The key to successful management is repair of the PCL.

Type III ACL/PCL/MCL torn, LCL/PLC intact: The primary goal is repair of the PCL and MCL. Through a straight midline or paramedian incision, the knee joint is exposed and the menisci inspected. Gentle dissection medially exposes the MCL, which is repaired. The posterior cruciate ligament, if avulsed, can be reattached to the femur or tibia through this same incision. Midsubstance PCL tears are repaired using autograft obtained from the patellar ligament or an allograft. Final tensioning and fixation of the PCL and MCL repairs are performed with the knee flexed 20° and with the hip externally rotated, reducing the medial tibiofemoral compartment. The presence of a functioning posterolateral corner simplifies the treatment of this type of knee dislocation.

Type IV ACL/PCL/LCL/PLC torn, MCL intact: The torn LCL and PLC complicates treatment. It is important to reestablish the posterolateral corner and associated tendinous structures (i.e., biceps femoris and/or iliotibial band) in addition to the posterior cruciate ligament. The incision is posterolateral. The peroneal nerve is isolated and retracted, and the knee is inspected by subluxing the tibiofemoral joint. The locking-whip stitch is used to reattach or repair the lateral-collateral ligament and associated posterolateral structures if torn. Tibial avulsions of the PCL are reattached through the posterolateral incision. A medial incision is utilized to reattach the PCL when it has been avulsed from the femur or if a femoral tunnel is required for reconstruction.

Type V ACL/PCL/MCL/LCL/PLC torn: This pattern is most frequently a high-energy injury, characterized by gross instability and frequently accompanied by neurovascular compromise. Repair of the posterior cruciate ligament and posterolateral corner is the primary goal. Utilizing a posterolateral incision, these two structures are explored and repaired. A medial incision may be required to reattach the PCL to the femur or to reconstruct it with an autograft or allograft.

Complications

Complications unique to a dislocation of the knee are arthrofibrosis, residual laxity, and incompetent lateral structures.

Arthrofibrosis results in loss of motion. It is best avoided by following the surgical repair with rigorous physical therapy. If 90° of flexion has not been obtained by 6 weeks postsurgery, manipulation under epidural anesthesia and arthroscopic scar excision are performed. Epidural anesthesia is continued postoperatively 2 to 3 days to maintain motion.

Residual laxity is frequently due to reattachment of a stretched posterior cruciate ligament. Residual laxity is best avoided by reconstructing the stretched PCL with autograft or allograft at the initial repair.

Incompetent lateral structures result in **posterolateral rotary instability** (PLRI). Repair of the lateral structures can be difficult (midsubstance tears of the LCL are particularly difficult), but should be attempted. Unlike combined ACL/LCL injuries where the LCL is frequently treated nonoperatively, the LCL in a knee dislocation is repaired or reconstructed to promote lateral stability. Biceps tenodesis can be used to augment an LCL injury. The ACL reconstruction is frequently mandatory after initial LCL/PCL surgery (ACL functioning as an internal collateral) to provide stability in extension.

SELECTED READINGS

Supracondylar Fractures of the Femur

Giles JB, DeLee JC, Heckman JD, Keever JE: Supracondylar-intercondylar fractures of the femur treated with a supracondylar plate and lag screw. *J Bone Joint Surg* 66A:864–870, 1982.

Ker NB, Maempel FZ, Paton DF: Bone cement as an adjunct to medullary nailing in fractures of the distal third of the femur in elderly patients.

Mize RD, Bucholz RW, Grogan DP: Surgical treatment of displaced, comminuted fractures of the distal end of the femur. *J Bone Joint Surg* 64A:871–879, 1982.

Fractures of the Tibial Plateau

Fernandez D: Anterior approach to the knee with osteotomy of the tibial tubercle for bicondylar tibial fractures. *J Bone Joint Surg* 70A:208–219, 1988.

Perry CR, Evans LG, Rice S, Fogarty J, Burdge RE: A new surgical approach to fractures of the lateral tibial plateau. *J Bone Joint Surg* 66A:1236–1240, 1984.

Schatzker J, McBroom R, Bruce D: The tibial plateau fracture. The Toronto experience 1968–1975. *Clin Orthop* 138:94–104, 1979.

Injuries of the Extensor Mechanism

Levy M, Goldstein J, Rosner M: A method of repair for quadriceps tendon or patellar ligament (tendon) ruptures without cast immobilization. *Clin Orthop* 218:297–301, 1987.

Patellar Fractures

Levack B, Flannagan JP, Hobbs S: Results of surgical treatment of patellar fractures. *J Bone Joint Surg* 67B:416–419, 1985.

Perry CR, McCarthy JA, Kain CC, Pearson RL: Patellar fixation protected with a load-sharing cable: A mechanical and clinical study. *J Orthop Trauma* 2:234–240, 1988.

Dislocations of the Knee

Frassica FS, Franklin HS, Staeheli JW, Pairolero PC: Dislocation of the knee. *Clin Orthop* 263:200–205, 1992.

Green NE, Allen BL: Vascular injuries associated with dislocation of the knee. *J Bone Joint Surg* 59A:236–239, 1977.

Krackow KA, Thomas SC, Jones LC: Ligament-tendon fixation: Analysis of a new stitch and comparison with standard techniques. *Orthop* 11:909–917, 1988.

Marshall JL, Warren RF, Wickiewicz TL, Reider B: The anterior cruciate ligament: A technique of repair and reconstruction. *Clin Orthop* 143:97–106, 1979.

Schenck RC, Burke RL: The dislocated knee. *Perspect Orthop Surg* 2(2):119–34, 1991.

Schenck RC, Burke R, Walker D: The dislocated knee: A new classification system. *South Med* 85(9):3S–61, 1992.

Fractures of the Tibial Shaft

C.M. Court-Brown

This chapter reviews fractures of the tibial and fibular diaphysis.

ANATOMY

The proximal and distal 5 cm of the tibia are metaphyseal. The diaphysis of the tibia is triangular in cross-section, having medial, lateral, and posterior surfaces separated by anterior, medial, and lateral borders. The anterior border is sharp proximally, but distally it becomes blunt and runs into the medial malleolus. The medial border is blunt proximally, but sharpens distally as it runs into the posterior border of the medial malleolus. The lateral border of the tibia is also blunt proximally, but it sharpens as it runs distally into the lateral side of the inferior tibial metaphysis. The medial surface of the tibial diaphysis is subcutaneous, accounting for the high incidence of open tibial fractures. The lateral surface is hollowed proximally for the tibialis anterior muscle. The posterior surface is bounded by the medial and lateral borders and is crossed proximally by the soleal line. This ridge gives rise to the soleus muscle.

The shaft of the fibula is long and slender and has anterior, posterior, and lateral surfaces separated by anterior, posterior, and medial borders. This arrangement is modified by a slight spiral twist to the bone.

A major function of the tibia is to anchor the musculature that controls the movement of the ankle and foot. There are four myofascial compartments in the leg. These compartments are of considerable importance in tibial diaphyseal fractures.

The anterior compartment is bounded by the lateral border of the tibia, the interosseous membrane, the anterior fibula, and the deep fascia. It contains four muscles: tibialis anterior, extensor hallucis longus, extensor digitorum longus, and peroneus tertius. The muscles are supplied by the deep peroneal nerve and the anterior tibial artery that runs through the anterior compartment and continues below the ankle joint as the dorsalis pedis artery.

The lateral compartment is contained by the lateral border of the fibula, the deep fascia, and fascial connections between the fibula and deep fascia. It contains the peroneus longus and brevis muscles which are supplied by the superficial peroneal nerve.

There are two posterior compartments: deep and superficial. The deep posterior compartment, along with the anterior compartment, is most often involved in compartment syndrome. It is bounded by the posterior surface of the tibia, the medial and posterior borders of the fibula, the interosseous membrane, and the fascia which separates it from the superficial posterior compartment. It contains four muscles:

popliteus, flexor hallucis longus, tibialis posterior, and flexor digitorum longus. All these muscles are supplied by the posterior tibial nerve and the main neurovascular bundle containing the posterior tibial nerve and artery that runs through the compartment.

The superficial posterior compartment is bounded by fascia and contains gastrocnemius and soleus muscles in addition to the plantaris muscle. These are supplied by branches from the posterior tibial nerve.

The sural and saphenous nerves run between the skin and deep fascia.

Classification

Tibia fractures are classified according to the mechanism of injury, location, fracture configuration, and whether the fracture is open.

The three **mechanisms of injury** are excessive loading, pathologic fractures, and stress fractures. When considering the mechanism of injury, it is vital to distinguish between low- and high-energy injuries. The ultimate prognosis of tibial fractures is governed by the extent of associated soft-tissue injury, which is much greater in motor-vehicle accidents and gunshot injuries than it is in minor falls or sports-related injuries. The worst prognosis is seen in tibial fractures caused by prolonged crushing, as this destroys the soft tissue vasculature and frequently leads to muscle death. The most common mechanism of injury is **excessive loading of normal bone.** The force, or applied load, may be indirect (i.e., torsional), causing a spiral fracture in the weakest part of the diaphysis at the junction of the middle and distal thirds of the bone. Fracture may be due to a direct force such as a direct blow. These injuries usually involve a bending or shearing component and are usually higher energy than the torsional injuries.

Occasionally, the fracture is **pathologic** in that it occurs in abnormal bone as a result of a relatively minor force. The most common cause for a pathologic fracture is senile osteoporosis. The tibia may also be affected by metabolic bone diseases, such as Paget's disease or osteomalacia, or it may be the site of metastatic deposits from carcinomata or multiple myeloma.

Stress fractures of the tibial diaphysis are due to repeated submaximal loading of normal bone, usually in young people. In military recruits, the majority of stress fractures occur in the upper third. Whereas, with athletes the involvement is lower in the tibia, most frequently at the junction of the middle and lower third. In ballet dancers, most stress fractures are found in the middle third of the tibia. Stress fractures of the fibula are prone to occur just above the ankle in runners.

Location of the fracture is described as being in the proximal, middle, or distal thirds. Fracture **configuration** is described as transverse, oblique, or spiral. In addition, there may be a loose fragment that does not involve the complete cortex, which is commonly referred to as a "butterfly fragment." When the cortical fragmentation is circumferential, the fracture is referred to as comminuted. Segmental fractures have two separate fractures with an intervening intact cortical tube. Other factors used to determine the overall prognosis are the degree to initial displacement and the presence or absence of a segmental fibular fracture.

The classification of **open fractures** is presented in "Clinical Evaluation/Initial Management of Patients with Multiple Injuries" or Chapter 1. It has prognostic value in terms of the time to union and the patient's return to function. The type III subtypes are particularly important.

Diagnosis and Initial Management

History and Physical Examination

There is a history of trauma and the patient complains of pain. There may be obvious deformity. The skin is examined for open wounds, and distal pulses and sensation are documented.

Radiographic Examination

Anteroposterior and lateral radiographs are diagnostic of fractures due to excessive loading and pathologic fractures. Occasionally, oblique x-rays may be useful in visualizing the periosteal reaction associated with an occult stress fracture. Radiographs of the knee and ankle are examined to identify associated fractures. If a stress fracture is suspected, a technetium bone scan may be diagnostic.

Initial Management

Initial management is reduction of displaced fractures, application of a toe-to-groin splint, elevation, and application of ice. Reduction is accomplished by traction and manipulation while intravenous analgesia is administered (hematoma blocks are not used for tibial fractures).

Associated Injuries

Associated injuries include compartment syndrome and injuries of the knee and ankle. The term **compartment syndrome** is used to describe the collection of signs that occur when intracompartmental pressure rises beyond a critical point. The cardinal signs of compartment syndrome are pain, pain with passive stretch of muscles, tense compartments, and elevated pressures. The pathophysiology and diagnosis of compartment syndrome are described in detail in Chapter 1. Failure to diagnose a compartment syndrome has catastrophic consequences. Muscle necrosis and muscle death leads to significant soft tissue resection or even amputation. Undetected deep posterior compartment syndromes lead to clawing of the foot and toes. A delay in undertaking a fasciotomy for compartment syndromes in adults following tibial fracture results in a high incidence of nonunion. Once a diagnosis of compartment syndrome is made, the treatment is fasciotomy. This is a straightforward procedure and is best carried out through two incisions—one medial and one lateral. The medial incision allows for decompression of the superficial and deep posterior compartments, while the lateral incision permits decompression of the anterior and lateral compartments.

Injuries of the knee and ankle are ruled out by physical examination and radiographs.

Definitive Management

There are five methods used to manage tibial fractures: casts or braces, plating, intramedullary nailing, external fixation, and amputation.

The advantage of **cast management** is the low incidence of infection; however, there is a high incidence of joint stiffness, malunion, nonunion, and muscle wasting. The method is very labor intensive and relies on frequent outpatient visits for radiographic monitoring of fracture position and cast or brace adjustment.

The incidence of malunion and joint stiffness is much less with **plating** than with casts or braces. The infection rate associated with plating of closed fractures is about 4 percent, but it rises when plating is used for more severe open fractures. Failure of fixation is more commonly seen with plating than with other fixation techniques.

The advantages of closed **intramedullary nailing** are that the fracture site remains closed (Fig. 20–1). The absence of a cast allows for early joint movement and increases patient mobility. Muscle tone is also preserved. The union rate is high, and nonunion can often be treated by repeating the nailing procedure, a process known as exchange nailing. The disadvantage of intramedullary nailing is knee pain secondary to the infrapatellar incision and prominence of the underlying nail. This occurs in up to 40 percent of patients. Infection rate in closed fractures is higher than that following cast management or external fixation, but it is lower than plating. The major breakthrough in intramedullary nailing was the introduction of locking with proximal and distal screws which traverse both nail and bone cortices. This simple modification of the original intramedullary nail controls bone length, rotation, and angulation of even severely comminuted fractures.

The primary indication for **external fixation** is severe soft tissue injury. The disadvantages of external fixation are the high incidence of nonunion and pin tract infections, and restriction of soft tissue access (Fig. 20–2). The types of external fixation devices are described in Chapter 2.

There is a high incidence of eventual **amputation** following IIIC open fractures, with a lower but significant incidence following IIIB open fractures. Other than the severity of the soft tissue injury, indications for amputation include damage of the posterior tibial nerve, multiple trauma, and elderly patients with preexisting diseases such as

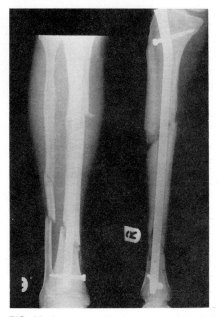

FIG. 20–1　Management with a statically locked nail.

arteriosclerosis or diabetes. When amputation is considered, the decision is made by two experienced orthopedic traumatologists and the amputation is carried out early in the patient's treatment to minimize medical, psychological, and social problems.

Choice of Method of Management

The choice of method of management is based on the type of patient and the type of fracture.

Casts or braces are used for **low-energy fractures** in young people that only require about 3 months immobilization. Under these conditions, joint stiffness is reduced to a minimum.

Other fractures are best managed with fixation. Intramedullary nailing provides the best results for fractures of the **middle and distal thirds** of the tibial diaphysis. Fractures of the **proximal third** of the diaphysis are technically difficult to nail. These usually are high-energy injuries and frequently are comminuted. Nailing does not adequately control this type of fracture and closed external fixation using a unilateral or multiplanar frame or plating provides better fixation. Similarly, some

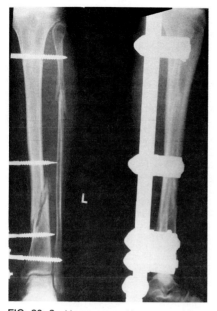

FIG. 20–2   Management with an external fixater.

distal metaphyseal fractures are difficult to nail, particularly if the fracture is oblique or spiral. These are to be managed with closed external fixation or plating. In the 5 percent of patients who present with a fracture of the tibia having a proximal or distal intraarticular fracture in addition to a diaphyseal fracture, fixation of both fractures is undertaken regardless of what the surgeon might choose to do for the equivalent isolated fractures. These are high-velocity injuries frequently associated with significant soft tissue damage, and fixation permits improved postoperative rehabilitation. The surgeon must select treatment methods appropriate for both fractures. The use of a proximal plate to stabilize a plateau fracture frequently renders nailing impossible, and closed external fixation is preferred for middle and distal third diaphyseal fractures. Plating is a good method of stabilizing a proximal diaphyseal fracture associated with a tibial plateau fracture. If there is an associated ankle fracture, it is managed in the conventional manner using plates and screws, with a nail used to stabilize the diaphysis.

The most important part of the management of **open fractures** is the surgery of the soft tissues. A thorough debridement is carried out as soon as possible. All devitalized and dubiously vital tissue is removed. This includes skin and muscle as well as bone fragments. The skin wound is never closed, primarily because closing inevitably causes tension and may lead to infection. Rather, the soft tissue defect is closed with a delayed primary closure, split thickness skin graft, or flap. Stabilization of open fractures is with either external fixation or intramedullary nailing using either a reamed or unreamed nail.

Stress fractures are managed with a cast or brace. There is rarely any indication for internal fixation, as these fractures are not associated with significant soft tissue damage and usually heal in a relatively short time.

Ideally, it is better to treat metastatic deposits in the tibia before the **pathologic fracture** occurs. The method of management depends on the overall prognosis of the patient. Unless the prognosis is very poor, the fracture should be stabilized. Because some of the bone will have been replaced by neoplastic tissue, these fractures are often unstable. Intramedullary nailing with filling of the bone defect with polymethylmethacrylate (PMMA) provides the best method of stabilization. The use of locked intramedullary nails has decreased the need for PMMA.

Complications

Complications of tibial diaphyseal fractures are infection, delayed union and nonunion, and malunion.

Infection following open tibial fractures is usually caused by severe soft tissue trauma and inadequate debridement. The most common pathogenic organism is *Staphylococcus aureus*. Posttraumatic osteomyelitis is difficult to treat if it has been present for a prolonged period. Management is relatively straightforward if the condition is detected early and treated adequately. Management involves stabilization of the fracture, drainage of abscess cavities, resection of devitalized and infected tissues, and antibiotic administration. Bone and soft tissue defects created by debridement are managed later with flap coverage and either corticocancellous bone grafting, vascularized bone transfer, or bone transport techniques.

Delayed union is overdiagnosed. In the past, surgeons have failed to adequately classify tibial fractures, grouping all tibial fractures together and expecting them to heal in a similar time. In contrast, **nonunion** is a definite entity indicating failure to heal. There are two forms of nonunion: hypertrophic and atrophic. In hypertrophic nonunion, there are clear radiologic signs of an attempt to heal the fracture and it is likely that the nonunion has occurred for mechanical reasons. Atrophic nonunions, however, show no evidence of fracture union radiographically and occur because of impaired vascularity at the fracture site. These are common following severe open fractures.

The management of hypertrophic nonunion is to alter the biomechanical environment of the fracture. If the nonunion has followed cast or brace treatment, then the application of a plate, external fixater, or an intramedullary nail will stimulate union. If the hypertrophic nonunion has followed the use of a plate or external fixation device, then closed intramedullary nailing is the treatment of choice if the nonunion is well aligned.

Atrophic nonunions are managed with autogenous cancellous bone grafting. Should the nonunion persist, the surgeon will have to consider vascularized bone grafts or bone transport.

There is no definition of what constitutes **malunion;** however, 5° of angulation or rotational abnormality and 1 cm of shortening provides a reasonable working definition. If a patient presents with a malunion, care must be exercised in determining whether further surgery is worthwhile. Experience suggests that if the patient presents with ankle osteoarthritis in conjunction with a tibial malunion, correction of the malunion may not lessen the degree of discomfort in the ankle joint, although it may slow down the deterioration of the joint. Management is corrective osteotomy and stabilization with any of the previously described methods.

FRACTURES OF THE FIBULAR SHAFT

Isolated fractures of the fibular diaphysis are usually the result of a direct blow and frequently occur during sporting activities. The most important diagnostic point relating to fractures of the diaphysis of the fibula is that the surgeon should exclude an associated ankle fracture. In suprasyndesmotic ankle fractures, the fibular fracture occurs in the diaphysis and may even occur as high as the fibular neck in the Maisonneuve fracture. If a fracture of the fibular diaphysis is encountered, it is important to check for the presence of an ankle injury.

If the fibular fracture is unrelated to an ankle injury, management is symptomatic. Usually the patient will manage with a light wrap, but if there is significant discomfort, the application of below-knee walking plaster is helpful.

SELECTED READINGS

Batten RL, Donaldson LJ, Aldridge MJ: Experience with the AO method in the treatment of 142 cases of fresh fracture of the tibial shaft treated in the UK. *Injury* 10:108–114, 1978.

Bone LB, Johnson KD: Treatment of tibial fractures by reaming and intramedullary nailing. *J Bone Joint Surg* 68A:877–887, 1986.

Court-Brown CM, Christie J, McQueen MM: Closed intramedullary tibial nailing: Its use in closed and type I open fractures. *J Bone Joint Surg* 72B:605–611, 1990.

Hooper GJ, Keddell RG, Penny ID: Conservative management or closed nailing for tibial shaft fractures. *J Bone Joint Surg* 73B:83–85, 1991.

| Fractures and Dislocations of the Ankle

Arsen M. Pankovich

This chapter reviews injuries of the distal tibia, fibula, and talus, and their ligaments and joint capsule. These are indirect fractures, direct fractures, and sprains.

ANATOMY

The ankle is a uniaxial joint. Articular surfaces are covered with hyaline cartilage. Range of motion of the talus in relation to the tibia is 10° of dorsiflexion and 20° of plantar flexion. The fibula moves laterally several millimeters and rotates externally as the talus dorsiflexes.

The **talus** consists of a head, body, and neck. The head articulates with the navicular, the body with the tibia (the superior articular surface of the body is called the trochlea) and the calcaneus. The neck extends between the body and head. In fractures of the ankle we are primarily concerned with the relationship between the body of the talus and the ankle mortise, composed of the medial malleolus, tibial plafond, and lateral malleolus. The trochlea of the talus is concave when viewed from the front and convex when viewed from the side. It fits perfectly in the ankle mortise which is reciprocally shaped. In most cases, the body of the talus is wider anteriorly than posteriorly. This difference averages 2.4 mm, although it may be as much as 6 mm. Dorsiflexion of the talus results in the "close pack" position (i.e., there is maximal contact between joint surfaces and maximal ligamentous tension). The greater width between the malleoli required for this position is afforded by the slight external rotation and lateral movement of the fibula. To prevent loss of dorsiflexion, syndesmotic screws are inserted with the talus dorsiflexed.

The **distal tibia** consists of the plafond or weight-bearing surface, the medial malleolus, the anterior and posterior processes, and the lateral surface.

The **plafond** has a convex shape when viewed in the anteroposterior projection. This convexity corresponds to the concavity of the trochlea. A seemingly insignificant medial or lateral shift of the talus markedly decreases the area of contact between the bearing surfaces and increases the pressure per unit area resulting in destruction of articular cartilage.

The **medial malleolus** is the medial process of the distal tibia and is formed by the anterior and the posterior colliculi which are separated by the intercollicular grove. The superficial deltoid ligament is attached to the anterior colliculus, and the deep deltoid to the posterior colliculus. Tendons of the posterior tibialis and flexor digitorum longus lay in a sulcus on the posterior surface of the posterior colliculus preventing its displacement when fractured.

The **anterior process** is the anterior edge of the distal tibia which laterally forms the anterior tibial tubercle or tubercle of Chaput. The **posterior process** is the posterior edge of the distal tibia which laterally forms the posterior tibial tubercle, often referred to as the posterior malleolus or Volkman's tubercle.

The **lateral surface** of the tibia between the anterior and posterior tubercles is concave and articulates with the corresponding convex surface of the distal fibula. Hyalin cartilage extends 1 mm into the tibiofibular joint, the remainder is covered with fibrocartilage.

The medial surface of the **distal fibula** is covered with hyaline cartilage and articulates with the lateral side of the talar body. The anterior tubercle, or tubercle of LeFort, and the posterior tubercle are the insertion of the anterior and posterior tibiofibular ligaments. The posterior surface of distal fibula has a sulcus for the peroneal tendons.

The three ligament complexes which stabilize the ankle are the **deltoid, syndesmotic,** and **lateral-collateral** (Figs. 21–1 and 21–2). These may be disrupted in the substance of the ligament or avulsed with a fragment of bone from either insertion. A "sprain" is an injury of a ligamentous complex and is grade I—rupture of intraligamentous fibers without damage to surrounding tissues and without lengthening of the ligament; grade II—partial rupture of the ligament with enough intra-ligamentous fibers ruptured to result in lengthening of the ligament and

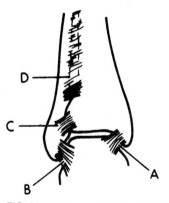

FIG. 21–1 Ligaments of the ankle: (a) the deep deltoid, (b) the anterior talofibular, (c) the anterior tibiofibular, and (d) the interosseous membrane and the interosseous ligament.

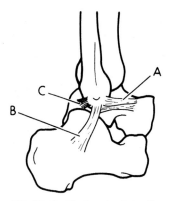

FIG. 21–2 The lateral-collateral ligaments of the ankle: (*a*) the anterior talofibular, (*b*) the calcanealfibular, and (*c*) the posterior talofibular.

damage of surrounding soft tissue; or grade III—rupture or avulsion of the ligament and significant damage of surrounding soft tissue.

The **deltoid ligament** consists of superficial (attaching to the anterior colliculus) and deep (attaching to the posterior colliculus) parts, and runs between the medial malleolus and the talus, os calcis, and navicular. It resists external rotation and lateral displacement of the talus.

The **syndesmosis complex** is the interosseous membrane, anterior tibiofibular ligament, posterior tibiofibular ligament, inferior transverse ligament, and interosseous ligament. Anterior and posterior ligaments are attached to the corresponding tubercles of the tibia and the fibula. The inferior transverse ligament reinforces the posterior tibiofibular ligament. The interosseous ligament is a strong and short band located at the distal extent of the interosseous membrane. In addition, the interosseous membrane extends from just above the interosseous ligament the entire length of the tibia and fibula.

Collateral ankle ligaments run from the fibula to the talus and calcaneus. They resist medial tilt (adduction) and anterior or posterior displacement of the talus. There are three ligaments: anterior talofibular, calcaneofibular, and posterior talofibular. The latter two ligaments lay under the peroneal tendons.

INDIRECT ANKLE FRACTURES

Indirect ankle fractures are caused by indirect torsional forces applied to the ankle. These forces result in motion of the talus in relation to the distal tibia and fibula. As these motions become pathologic, ligament complexes are disrupted and fractures occur resulting in predictable injury patterns on which the classification system is based. Prior to describing the classification system, the individual components of these injuries are reviewed.

In the majority of cases, the obliquity of the **fibular fracture** indicates the mechanism of injury, and the relationship of the fracture to the syndemosis (above, at, or below it) indicates the severity of the injury.

The **anterior tibiofibular ligament complex injury** is an avulsion of the tubercle of Chaput, rupture of the ligament itself, or avulsion of the anterior tubercle of the fibula.

Deltoid ligament complex injuries are fracture of the medial malleolus, rupture of the deep deltoid ligament complex, or fracture of the anterior and posterior colliculi. Superficial and deep deltoid ligaments remain attached to the fractured fragment. Only rupture of the deep deltoid results in loss of stability of the ankle. The deltoid normally allows only 2 mm of lateral shift of the talus. When the talus is grossly displaced, lateral rupture of the deep deltoid is obvious. When talar shift is more subtle, the precise amount of talar shift is determined by stress radiographs.

Classification

Indirect ankle fractures are classified according to the position of the foot at the time of the injury and the direction of the injuring force (Table 21–1). Thus, two words are used: The first word indicates the position of the foot (supination/pronation), and the second word indicates the direction of the force applied to the foot (adduction/abduction or external/internal rotation). Adduction and abduction occur around the long axis of the talus and result in medial and lateral tilt of the talus. Internal and external rotation occur around the long axis of the tibia. Occasionally, injuries which do not fit this "extended Lauge-Hanson" classification occur. These "atypical injuries" are the result of other factors (e.g., ligamentous laxity or osteopenia) overriding the primary determinants.

Two hints regarding this classification are supination injuries always start on the lateral side and pronation injuries on the medial side. The sequence in which structures are injured follows the direction of the force (e.g., adduction and abduction injuries proceed from lateral to medial or medial to lateral, respectively).

Supination-external rotation (SE) fractures of the ankle are the most common type of indirect ankle fracture (Figs. 21–3 through 21–5). They are characterized by the typical SE fibular fracture and, in complete injuries, a disrupted deltoid ligament complex. The fibula fracture is oblique and extends from anterior distal to posterior proximal. If the medial malleolus is fractured, it is oblique. The first stage of the injury is either disruption of the anterior tibiofibular ligament complex or fracture of the fibula below the anterior tibiofibular complex. If the

TABLE 21–1 Extended Lauge-Hanson Classification of Indirect
Ankle Fractures

1. Supination-external rotation
   a. Stage 1—anterior tibiofibular complex disruption
   b. Stage 2—fracture of fibula at or above the syndesmosis
   c. Stage 3—posterior tibiofibular complex disruption
   d. Stage 4—deltoid ligament complex disruption
2. Pronation-abduction at syndesmosis
   a. Stage 1—deltoid ligament complex disruption
   b. Stage 2—fracture of fibula at syndesmosis
3. Pronation-abduction above syndesmosis
   a. Stage 1—deltoid ligament complex disruption
   b. Stage 2—anterior and posterior tibiofibular ligament complex
      disruption
   c. Stage 3—fracture of the fibula above the syndesmosis
4. Pronation-external rotation
   a. Stage 1—deltoid ligament complex disruption
   b. Stage 2—anterior tibiofibular ligament complex disruption
   c. Stage 3—fracture of the fibula above the syndesmosis
   d. Stage 4—posterior tibiofibular ligament disruption
5. Supination-adduction
   a. Stage 1—lateral-collateral ligament complex disruption
   b. Stage 2—vertical fracture of the medial malleolus

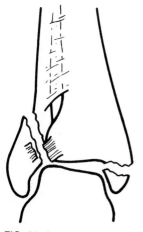

FIG. 21–3 Supination-external rotation injury.

anterior tibiofibular ligament is disrupted, the second stage is fracture of the fibula at or above the syndesmosis. Subsequent stages are the same regardless of where the fibula is fractured. These stages are injury of posterior tibiofibular complex and injury of the deltoid ligament complex. When there is an SE fibular fracture, an intact medial malleolus, and no widening of the medial clear space, an external rotation stress radiograph is mandatory to determine whether the deep deltoid ligament is ruptured.

Pronation-abduction (PA) fractures occur at two levels—at and above the syndesmosis—and are frequently complicated by compression of the lateral surface of the tibial plafond. The first stage of injury is rupture of the deltoid complex. The second stage is simultaneous rupture of the anterior and posterior tibiofibular complexes. If the interosseous ligament and membrane are not injured, diastasis does not occur, and the third stage of injury is the characteristic PA fracture of the fibula at the level of the syndesmosis. This fracture is comminuted laterally (Fig. 21–6). Occasionally, the interosseous ligament ruptures, the interosseous membrane also tears, and the fibula fractures 2 to 3 cm above the syndesmosis. The fracture characteristically has a lateral butterfly.

In atypical PA fractures, the anterior tibiofibular and interosseous complexes are disrupted with fractures below the syndesmosis.

Pronation-external rotation (PE) fractures are characterized by the typical PE fibular fracture, which is 2 to 4 cm above the syndesmosis and has a short oblique pattern which runs from the anterior edge of the fibula posteriorly and inferiorly (i.e., the opposite direction of an SE fibular fracture). The first stage is rupture of the deltoid ligament or transverse fracture of the medial malleolus. The second stage is rupture of the anterior tibiofibular and interosseous ligament. The final stage of injury is rupture of the posterior tibiofibular ligament (Fig. 21–7). Because the PE lesion starts with injury of the deltoid ligament, there is no need for stress radiographs even if the talus is reduced and a fracture of the medial malleolus is not present.

Supination-adduction (SA) fractures are characterized by a vertical fracture of the medial malleolus and disruption of the lateral-collateral ligaments (Fig. 21–8). The first stage is disruption of the lateral-collateral ligament complex, usually an avulsion fracture of the fibula distal to the syndesmosis. The second stage is a vertical fracture of the medial malleolus. The medial corner of the plafond is frequently compressed.

Atypical Indirect Injuries

In addition to the SE, PA, PE, and SA lesions described, there are several atypical lesions. Although the same forces are applied to the ankle, the usual patterns of injury do not occur. Why this is so is not

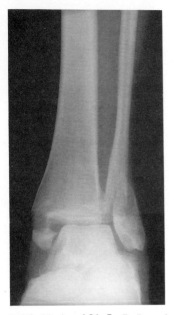

FIGS. 21–4 and 21–5 Radiographs of a supination-external rotation injury.

clear, although variability in the size and strength of ligament complexes plays a role.

The stages of a **Maisonneuve fracture** are: (1) injury of the anterior tibiofibular and interosseous ligament complexes, (2) injury of the posterior tibiofibular ligament complex of the syndesmosis, (3) rupture or avulsion of the anteromedial joint capsule, (4) PE- or SE-type fracture of the proximal fibula, and (5) injury of the deltoid ligament complex. The significance of this injury is that failure to recognize the diastasis and stabilize the syndesmosis results in loss of reduction, widening of the mortise, and eventual arthritis.

The mechanism of **Bosworth's fracture,** or posterior dislocation of the fibula behind the tibia, is external rotation on the supinated foot. There are seven stages of injury: (1) injury of the anterior tibiofibular complex, (2) rupture of the posterior tibiofibular complex, (3) rupture or stretching of the anteromedial capsule, (4) partial tear of the interosseous membrane, (5) dislocation of the fibula behind the tibia, (6) an oblique

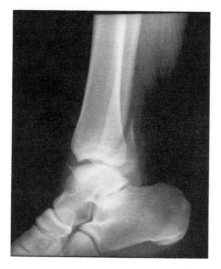

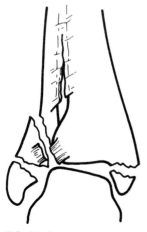

FIG. 21–6   Pronation-abduction injury at the level of the syndesmosis.

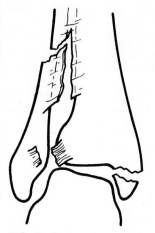

FIG. 21–7   Pronation-external rotation injury of the ankle.

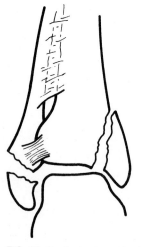

FIG. 21–8   Supination-adduction injury of the ankle.

fracture of the fibula (SE-type) at the level of the syndesmosis (if the fracture occurs above the syndesmosis, the proximal fragment of the fibula is too short to reach the tibia and be locked behind it), and (7) injury of the deltoid ligament complex.

Fracture dislocation of the ankle with translocation of the medial structures into the tibiofibular space is a distinct lesion. The talus, in a PA lesion, displaces the fibula sufficiently laterally to allow for translocation of the medial structures, which include tendons, vessels, and the nerve, into the interosseous space. These structures become trapped, thus resulting in an irreducible fracture-dislocation.

Diagnosis and Initial Management

History and Physical Examination

The history of injury is rarely helpful as the patient seldom can describe the direction of the injuring force. On physical examination, areas of ecchymosis, swelling, and tenderness are looked for over the anteromedial and posteromedial joint line and laterally over the entire length of the fibula. The condition of the skin is noted. Frequently, the skin will be badly contused or damaged. Gentle manipulation of the ankle may reveal gross instability.

Radiographic Examination

The standard radiographic examination consists of anteroposterior, lateral, and mortise views. The mortise view or true anteroposterior view of the ankle is obtained with the foot in 20° of internal rotation. The radiographs are examined with the following six points in mind: (1) Is there a fracture of the medial malleolus, and, if so, what type is it? This is important in order to plan a method of fixation. If there is compression of the medial plafond, bone grafting is anticipated. (2) The direction and location of the fibula fracture are noted. The direction is the mirror of the mechanism of injury. The location or level at which the fracture occurs is an approximate indicator of the extent of the injury. Thus, an SE fracture above the syndesmosis indicates, at the least, rupture of the anterior tibiofibular ligament. If there is a fracture of the medial malleolus, a complete lesion is present with all syndesmosis ligaments ruptured. (3) Is there a rupture of the deltoid ligament complex? This may be obvious if the injury is a pronation lesion. The initial stage of pronation injuries is rupture of the deltoid ligament complex. Therefore, if the medial malleolus is intact in association with a PA or PE fibular fracture, there is no need for stress films to demonstrate widening of the mortise. However, an SE lesion in which the medial malleolus is intact and the mortise appears normal will require a stress radiograph if there is any tenderness over the medial side. (4) When there is an injury of the medial ligament complex, without a fracture of the fibula at the ankle, the entire length of the fibula is radiographed to determine whether there is a high-fibular fracture. (5) Other associated fractures should be recognized, such as those involving the posterior tibial process (Volkmann), anterior tibial tubercle (Chaput), and fibular tubercle (Wagstaffe). (6) The dome of the talus is examined for osteochondral fractures.

External rotation stress radiographs are obtained when there is an indication that the deltoid ligament may be ruptured despite the fact that the mortise is reduced. The foot is gently externally rotated and a mortise view of the ankle is obtained. The width of the clear space between the lateral tibial plafond and the lateral talus is determined. Likewise, the width of the clear space at the corner where the tibial plafond joins the medial malleolus and the medial corner of the talus is determined. A difference greater than 3 mm between these two measurements indicates a ruptured deltoid ligament (Figs. 21–9 and 21–10).

Tomography, computed tomography, and arthrography are not necessary to evaluate indirect fractures of the ankle.

Initial Management

Subluxations or frank dislocations are reduced by pulling in line with the deformity. The ankle is splinted, elevated, and iced. Excessive swelling, ecchymosis, and blisters usually improve sufficiently with this regimen for surgery in 4 to 7 days.

Associated Injuries

Associated injuries of neurovascular structures are rare but they should be ruled out with a careful focused examination of the extremity. Compartment syndrome is occasionally associated with indirect fractures of the ankle, and if suspected on the basis of the clinical exam, compartment pressures are measured.

Definitive Management

Definitive management is by surgical or closed methods. The primary indications for surgery are unstable injuries and fractures of the medial malleolus. Surgery is rarely indicated for an isolated fibular fracture without ligamentous injuries.

All injuries involving the medial and lateral sides of the ankle (bimalleolar) are unstable. An undisplaced fracture may be maintained in a long leg cast, but the position of the fragments must be carefully monitored. A displaced bimalleolar fracture, even when anatomically reduced, tends to redisplace; therefore, it should be internally fixed.

Fractures of the medial malleolus are fixed if displaced because

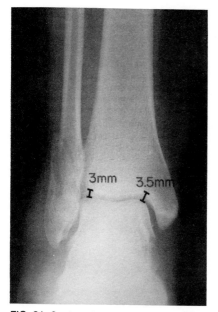

FIG. 21–9 A mortise view of an ankle indicating a fracture of the fibula slightly above the syndesmosis and a medial clear space measuring 3.5 mm. The width of the articular cartilage measures 3 mm laterally.

invariably the periosteum is interposed in the fracture site, resulting in a high incidence of delayed union or nonunion.

Closed Reduction

Closed reduction is performed by reversing the mechanism of injury and the position of the foot (e.g., SE fractures are reduced by internally rotating and pronating the foot). A short leg cast is applied while the reduction is maintained. It is then extended to a long leg cast with 30° of knee flexion. Cast immobilization is continued for 6 weeks. The position of the fragments is monitored with frequent radiographs.

Open Reduction

Under tourniquet control, an incision is made laterally over the fibula and extended distally and anteriorly directly over the distal syndesmosis. Exposure of the medial side is through a curved incision centered over the anterior medial corner of the mortise. The anterior skin bridge

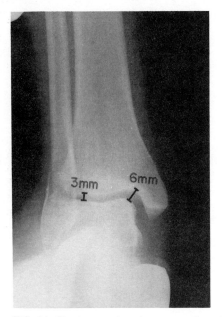

FIG. 21–10 A external rotation stress radiograph of the ankle shown in Fig. 21–9. The increase in the width of the medial clear space indicates that the deltoid ligament has been ruptured and that this is an unstable ankle injury.

formed by these two incisions must be a minimum of 6 cm wide. The skin is handled carefully to avoid injuring it further. The dome of the talus is examined, as are the anterior tibiofibular ligament complex and the anterior talofibular ligament. The fracture of the fibula and medial malleolus are reduced and stabilized. We use a one-third tubular plate posterolaterally on the fibula and two partially threaded cancellous screws in the medial malleolus. The presence of a diastasis is determined by distracting the fibula from the tibia after fixation. If a diastasis is present, a syndesmotic screw is inserted. If bone grafting of an impacted medial or lateral plafond is required, cancellous bone is obtained from the ipsilateral distal femur. If ruptured, the anterior tibiofibular ligament complex is repaired prior to closure. Postoperatively, a short leg cast is applied when the incisions are stable (usually at 2 days) and maintained for 2 weeks. At 2 weeks, the cast is taken off, the sutures are removed, and a removable cast is applied to facilitate skin care. At 6 weeks, range of motion of the ankle and partial weight-bearing are initiated.

Complications

Complications of indirect ankle fractures include arthritis, infection, and nonunion. These complications are more frequent following direct ankle fractures; therefore, their management is covered at the end of the ''Direct Ankle Fractures'' section.

DIRECT ANKLE FRACTURES

Direct ankle fractures are usually caused by the talus being driven into the distal tibia causing a pylon or burst fracture. Occasionally, they are caused by a direct impact (e.g., gunshots or crushing). These injuries are frequently open and associated with injuries of the foot, proximal tibia, and fibula. Fractures caused by direct impact will not be discussed further except to say that the rules to follow in their management are good wound care; reduction of the articular surfaces; maintenance of alignment; and early bone grafting, if necessary.

Classification

There are three types of pylon fractures: type I the articular surface is not involved or is undisplaced, type II a portion of the articular surface is displaced, but there is an undisplaced segment, type III and the entire plafond is involved (Figs. 21–11 and 21–12). The severity of injury parallels these fracture types.

Diagnosis and Initial Management

History and Physical Examination

The diagnosis of pylon fractures is usually obvious. There is typically a history of a fall and severe pain localized to the ankle. There may be deformity of the ankle. A careful neurovascular examination is performed, with particular attention to the anterior and posterior tibial pulses and capillary refill. The skin is examined for lacerations or blisters.

Radiographic Examination

The standard anteroposterior, lateral, and mortise views are of most value. Tomograms and CT scans help in determining the extent of articular damage and the degree of comminution.

Initial Management

Initial management consists of aligning the ankle by traction. These injuries are usually unstable and, therefore, easily aligned. The ankle is splinted, elevated, and iced.

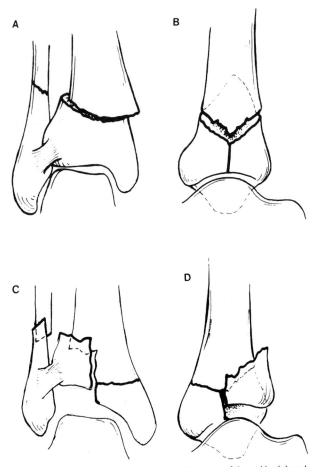

FIG. 21–11 The classification of direct fractures of the ankle: (*a*) and (*b*) type I fracture, (*c*) and (*d*) type II fracture, and (*e*) and (*f*) type III fracture.

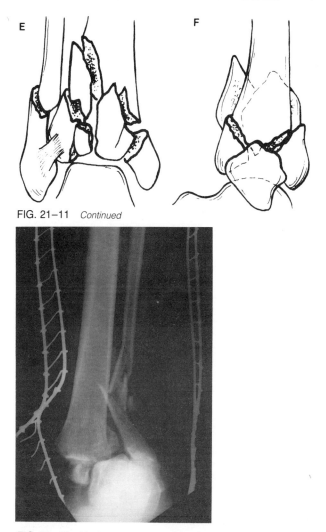

FIG. 21-11   *Continued*

FIG. 21-12   Mortise radiograph of a type II direct fracture of the ankle. Although there is intraarticular involvement, a portion of the articular surface is undisplaced.

Associated Injuries

Lumbar spine fractures are the injuries most frequently associated with pylon fractures due to a fall. They are ruled out with physical examination and radiographs. Neurovascular injuries are ruled out with a careful physical examination.

Definitive Management

Management of pylon fractures must be individualized. Ultimately, the severity of injury and the adequacy of reduction of the articular surfaces will determine the outcome. The extended surgical procedures necessary to reduce and stabilize displaced fractures are fraught with complications; therefore, attenuated soft tissue is a relative contraindication to an extended surgical procedure. Likewise, vascularity and sensation must be assessed. The presence of lymphedema, venous stasis, or peripheral neuropathy are relative contraindications to open reduction. Most importantly, the surgeon must decide if he is capable of reducing and stabilizing the fracture. Some fractures are so comminuted, with such extensive destruction of the articular surface, that open reduction and internal fixation is not an option. In these cases, closed management, early fusion, or external fixation must be relied on to give a stable painless ankle.

Closed initial management with early fusion is used when the tibial plafond or dome of the talus are irrevocably injured. Initially, the fracture is managed with external immobilization, often with a period in calcaneal traction. When swelling and blisters have subsided, a cast or external fixater with pins in the calcaneus and talus is applied. Tibiotalar fusion with autogenous cancellous bone graft is performed when the condition of the skin permits.

The goal of **open reduction and internal fixation** is anatomic, stable reduction of the joint. Usually medial and lateral incisions are made. Their exact location and length is based on the fracture pattern and tailored to each case. Once the fragments have been identified, the fibula, if fractured, is plated, thus aligning the anterior tubercle of the tibia around which other fragments are reduced and held in place with screws and plates. Bone graft is packed beneath depressed segments. An extended period of elevation following surgery is required to decrease the incidence of postoperative wound problems. The duration of nonweight-bearing depends on the severity of the fracture.

Complications

Complications are arthritis, infection, and nonunion.

Arthritis is due to an inadequate reduction of intraarticular fragments, varus or valgus malalignment of the entire articular surface, or damage to the articular cartilage that occurred at the time of the injury. If radiographically there is a joint space and clinically there is only minimal pain with motion, an osteotomy to realign the joint may help. If arthritic changes are advanced, or the articular surface is aligned, the only option other than steroid injections and nonsteroidal anti-inflammatories is arthrodesis. The techniques that we use are excision of the distal fibula, removal of the remaining articular cartilage from the joint surfaces, autogenous cancellous bone graft to fill gaps, and stabilization with an external fixater. The pins of the external fixater are placed in the tibia proximally and in the talus and calcaneus distally.

Infection, especially of a pylon fracture, is a severe complication and often the precursor of amputation. If the infection is controlled (i.e., the patient is not systemically ill), the hardware is left in place, as long as it is providing stability, until the fracture has healed. Systemic antibiotics are used to control flare-ups of the infection. Once the fracture is healed, the hardware is removed and all necrotic bone is debrided. Frequently, a free flap is required for coverage. Six weeks of systemic antibiotics are administered.

Nonunion of the fibula or medial malleolus, if symptomatic, is treated with autogenous bone grafting and stabilization.

INJURIES OF THE LATERAL-COLLATERAL LIGAMENT COMPLEX

There are several facts concerning ankle sprains: (1) Rupture of the anterior talofibular ligament is usually an isolated injury. (2) Simultaneous rupture of all three collateral ligaments is very rare, the posterior talofibular ligament being the least vulnerable. (3) Rupture of the anterior talofibular ligament is usually a complete or grade III injury. This is not the case with the calcaneofibular ligament injury which is frequently grade II. (4) Frequently, there are associated injuries of the anterior tibiofibular ligament.

Classification

Injuries of the lateral-collateral ligament complex of the ankle are classified into three groups. First degree—complete rupture of the anterior talofibular ligament only; the mechanism of injury is internal rotation of the pronated ankle. Second degree—complete rupture of the anterior talofibular and calcaneofibular ligaments, but an intact posterior talofibular ligament; the mechanism of injury is internal rotation of the supinated foot. Third degree—all three lateral-collateral ligaments of the ankle are ruptured; the mechanism of injury is adduction of the supinated ankle.

Two patterns of medial malleolar fracture are associated with lateral-collateral ligament injuries: a vertical supination-adduction (SA) pattern and a supination-internal (SI) rotation fracture. This is a transverse or slightly oblique fracture of the medial malleolus and indicates a second degree sprain.

Diagnosis and Initial Management

History and Physical Examination

The clinical evaluation is most important as radiographs frequently are of little help. Specifically, tenderness directly over the anterior tibiofibular ligament complex or over any of the three lateral-collateral ligaments is noted. In addition, stability of the talus in the coronal plane (adduction) and sagittal plane (anterior drawer) is assessed.

Radiographic Examination

Plain films are usually of little value and indicate only soft tissue swelling. An SA or SI medial malleolar fracture may be present on the mortise view.

Stress films are valuable. Stability in the coronal plane is assessed by adducting the midfoot while a mortise view is obtained. This is compared to a stress film of the uninjured side. Varus tilt of the talus, which is 10° greater than the uninjured side, indicates a third degree sprain. Stability in the sagittal plane is assessed with a lateral film of the ankle being taken while an anterior drawer test is performed. To perform the anterior drawer test, the heel is held in one hand while the other hand pushes the tibia posteriorly. Displacement anteriorly of greater than 3 mm when compared with the normal side indicates at least a first degree sprain.

Initial Management

There is no dislocation or deformity to reduce; therefore, ice and elevation are all that is required.

Definitive Management

A short leg walking cast is applied with the ankle in neutral position. The cast is maintained 4 weeks. A removable ankle splint is worn an additional 2 weeks.

If primary repair of the ligaments is indicated, the operative exposure is via an incision which parallels the peroneal tendons. The peroneal sheath is opened and the tendons retracted proximally to reach the posterior talofibular and calcaneofibular ligaments. The anterior talofibular ligament is the easiest to expose and repair. Postoperatively, the ankle is protected with a short leg cast for 4 weeks and a removable cast for 2 weeks.

Complications

The complication unique to this injury is laxity of the lateral-collateral ligament complex resulting in "giving out" when a varus force is applied to the foot (e.g., when the patient walks on uneven ground). Management is conservative with a lateral shoe wedge and peroneal strengthening exercises or operative. Numerous operative techniques have been described. Most use the tendon of the peroneus brevis to replace the injured ligaments.

SELECTED READINGS

Indirect Ankle Fractures

Ashhurst AP, Bromer RS: Classification and mechanism of fractures of the leg bones involving the ankle. *Arch Surg* 4:51–129, 1922.
Lauge-Hansen N: Fractures of the ankle. Combined experimental-surgical and experimental-roentgenologic investigations. *Arch Surg* 60:957–985, 1950.
Pankovich AM: Fracture of the fibula proximal to the distal tibiofibular syndesmosis. *J Bone Joint Surg* 60A:221–229, 1978.
Pankovich AM: Fractures of the fibula at the distal tibiofibular syndesmosis. *Clin Orthop* 143:138–147, 1979.
Phillips WA, Schwartz HS, Keller CS, Woodward HR, Rudd WS, Spiegel PG, Laros GS: A prospective, randomized study of the management of severe ankle fracture. *J Bone Joint Surg* 67A:67–78, 1985.

Direct Ankle Fractures

Ovadia DN, Beals RK: Fractures of the tibial plafond. *J Bone Joint Surg* 68A:543–551, 1986.
Ruedi TP, Allgower M: The operative treatment of intraarticular fractures of the lower end of the tibia. *Clin Orthop* 138:105–110, 1979.
Scheck M: Treatment of comminuted distal tibial fractures by combined dual-pin fixation and limited open reduction. *J Bone Joint Surg* 47A:1537–1553, 1965.

Injuries of the Lateral-Collateral Ligament Complex

Staples OS: Ruptures of the fibular collateral ligaments of the ankle. Result study of immediate surgical treatment. *J Bone Joint Surg* 57A:101–107, 1975.

Enes Kanlic   Clayton R. Perry

This chapter reviews injuries of the foot (i.e., distal to the ankle joint).

ANATOMY AND BIOMECHANICS

The foot is divided into the hindfoot, consisting of the Achilles tendon, talus, and calcaneus; the midfoot, consisting of the tarsal navicular, three cuneiforms, and cuboid; and the forefoot, consisting of the five metatarsals and corresponding phalanges.

The **talus** is unique in that no muscles insert on it, 60 percent of its surface is covered with cartilage, and its vascular supply is tenuous. Deltoid branches from the posterior tibial artery supply the medial talar body. The artery of the sinus tarsi is located in the sinus tarsi, plantar to the neck of the talus, and it gives off branches which enter the inferior neck. The dorsalis pedis gives off arterial branches which enter the superior neck. Most of the blood supply of the talus is via the talar neck; therefore, the body is susceptible to avascular necrosis following fracture.

The posterior portion of the **calcaneus** is the tuberosity and serves as the **Achilles tendon** insertion. The plantar fascia and the small muscles of the foot originate from the plantar surface. The anterior process is the origin of the bifurcate ligament which runs to the cuboid and navicular, stabilizing the midfoot. The superior aspect of the calcaneus has three facets which articulate with the talus. The posterior facet is more important than the middle and anterior. The talocalcaneal ligament runs from the superior surface of the calcaneus to the inferior surface of the talus. It lies in the sinus tarsi and is the primary stabilizer of the talocalcaneal articulation. The sustentaculum tali is on the medial side of the calcaneus. On its superior aspect is the middle facet, and on its inferior surface is the groove for the tendon of the flexor hallucis longus. The distal calcaneus articulates with the cuboid.

The **navicular** articulates with the head of the talus and the first and second cuneiforms. The posterior tibial tendon inserts on the tubercle of the navicular, supporting the medial longitudinal arch.

The bones of the foot form **longitudinal and transverse arches.** The longitudinal arch is higher medially than laterally. The medial segment (talus; navicular; cuneiform; and first, second, and third rays) is the dynamic portion of the foot and flattens during weight-bearing. The lateral segment (calcaneus, cuboid, and fourth and fifth rays) is flatter, more rigid, and contacts the ground first during weight-bearing. The transverse arch is due to the shape of the tarsals and base of the metatarsals which are broader on the dorsal aspect than the plantar, forming a ''Roman arch.''

The bones of the foot are connected by fibrous structures (e.g., the plantar fascia), intrinsic muscles, and extrinsic muscles. The muscles and the tensioned plantar fascia act as a "tie" at the base of the longitudinal arch which prevents it from flattening during weight-bearing.

The **subtalar joint** has four articulations. Three between the anterior middle and posterior facets of the calcaneus and talus, and one between the head of the talus and navicular. These articulations function as one multiaxial joint. Forty degrees of supination and pronation occur through the subtalar joint. The ankle and subtalar joints function together as a universal joint with 45° of dorsal and plantar flexion.

Chopart's joint, or transverse tarsal joint, consists of talonavicular and calcaneocuboid articulations (Fig. 22–1). The amount of motion occurring through Chopart's joint is greater when the calcaneus is pronated. Thus, subtalar fusion is performed with the calcaneus in slight pronation.

Lisfranc's joint, or tarsometatarsal joint, is a series of plane joints. The greatest degree of motion occurs through the first metatarsal medial cuneiform articulation. Motion through the remainder of the joint is restricted by dorsal and volar ligaments and the bony architecture (i.e., the second metatarsal is inset between the first and third cuneiforms).

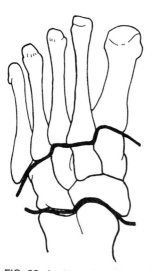

FIG. 22–1 Chopart's, or the transverse tarsal, joint, and Lisfranc's, or the tarsometatarsal, joint.

The five metatarsal heads are connected with strong interosseous ligaments, but only the lateral four metatarsal bases have strong interosseous ligaments. In place of the interosseous ligament between the first and second metatarsal bases is "Lisfranc's ligament" connecting the medial cuneiform and base of the second metatarsal (Fig. 22–2). Because of this structural anomaly, dislocations of the Lisfranc joint are frequently limited to the lateral side (i.e., second through fifth metatarsals) or medial side (i.e., first metatarsal).

The **metatarsophalangeal joints** function as hinge joints to tension the plantar aponeurosis.

The **interphalangeal joints** are hinge joints. They actively flex, but extend actively only to neutral.

Classification

Injuries of the foot are classified according to the mechanism of injury: indirect, direct, or due to repetitive stress. They are further classified according to which structures are involved. These structures are the hindfoot (i.e., the Achilles tendon, the talus, the subtalar joint, and the calcaneus); the midfoot (i.e., navicular, cuneiforms, and the cuboid); and the forefoot (i.e., the tarsometatarsal joint, the metatarsals, and the phalanges).

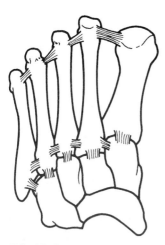

FIG. 22–2   The interosseous ligaments between the second through fifth metatarsals. In place of the ligament between the first and second metatarsal is the Lisfranc's ligament between the second metatarsal and the medial cuneiform.

DISRUPTION OF THE ACHILLES TENDON

Classification

Disruption of the Achilles tendon is due to direct injury (e.g., a laceration) or indirect injury (e.g., forced dorsiflexion of the ankle). Direct injuries disrupt any part of the tendon and are open. Indirect injuries, or ruptures, occur at the musculotendinous junction or the insertion on the calcaneus. The younger the patient, the greater the chance that the injury is at the musculotendinous junction.

Diagnosis and Initial Management

History and Physical Examination

Pain is localized to the posterior ankle. Direct injuries have a laceration. Indirect injuries have a palpable defect at the site of injury. Active ankle plantar flexion is absent or weak. The Thompson test determines if a complete rupture is present. The patient is prone with his feet extending off the examining table. The calf musculature is compressed by the examiner; if the ankle plantarflexes, the tendon is partially intact. If not, there is complete disruption.

Radiographic Examination

Decrease in soft tissue density indicates the location of the rupture; however, this is a subtle finding. MRI is useful in equivocal cases.

Initial Management

Initial management of a direct injury is debridement. If the tendon cannot be repaired within 12 h, the skin is closed. Indirect injuries are elevated and iced.

Associated Injuries

There are no injuries associated with an indirect injury of the Achilles tendon. Direct injuries are associated with injuries of surrounding tendons and neurovascular structures. Tendons frequently injured are the posterior tibialis, flexor hallucis longus, and flexor digitorum longus. The presence of tenodesis (i.e., flexion of the metatarsophalangeal and interphalangeal joints) with dorsiflexion of the ankle indicates that the long flexors are intact. The neurovascular structures at risk are the posterior tibial nerve and artery. Intact sensation on the plantar surface of the foot indicates that the posterior tibial nerve is intact. A palpable or doplerable posterior tibial pulse behind the medial malleolus indicates the artery is intact.

Definitive Management

Definitive management is dependent on the type of disruption and the patient's age.

Direct injuries are managed with primary repair. Indirect injuries are managed with operative repair in young, healthy patients, and with casting in older, less healthy patients. In comparison with a direct injury, the repair following an indirect injury is not as secure, and the incidence of complications is greater. The patient is positioned prone. The incision is over and parallel to the tendon. The peritenon is exposed and incised so that it can be repaired later. A Kessler-type suture approximates the ends. In indirect injuries, the ends are longitudinal strips, described as a "mop end," and it is key to place the Kessler suture in healthy tendon. If the disruption is extremely distal, the tendon is secured to the calcaneus via pull-through wires. Other lacerated tendons are repaired (direct injury). A short leg cast is applied with the ankle plantar flexed 20°. At 3 weeks, the cast is changed, the sutures removed, and another cast applied with the ankle in neutral. At 6 weeks, the cast is removed. If the repair is tenuous, immobilization is longer. A splint is prescribed which is removed for active range of motion exercises and while sleeping. At 8 to 10 weeks, external immobilization is discontinued.

Nonoperative management of indirect injuries starts with application of a long leg cast. The knee is flexed 30° (to relax the gastrocnemius) and ankle plantarflexed 30°. At 4 weeks, a short leg cast is applied with the ankle plantarflexed 30°. At 8 to 10 weeks, the ankle is positioned in neutral, and at 12 to 14 weeks, a removable splint is prescribed and active range of motion is initiated. Immobilization is discontinued at 16 to 20 weeks.

Complications

Complications of Achilles tendon disruption are failure of the repair and infection. Failure is managed with surgical revision. The plantaris tendon or strips of fascia lata are used to reinforce the repair. Infection is managed with administration of systemic antibiotics and debridement. Free tissue transfer or a split thickness skin graft may be required for coverage.

FRACTURES OF THE TALUS

The four types of talar fractures are fractures of the neck, body, head, and lateral process.

Fractures of the **neck of the talus** are the most common talar fracture and are classified into four groups (Fig. 22–3). Type I is undisplaced. Type II is displaced with subluxation or dislocation of the talocalcaneal articulation. Type III is displaced with a talocalcaneal and a talotibial dislocation. Type IV is a type III fracture with a dislocation of the head of the talus from the talonavicular joint. The incidence of avascular necrosis, delayed union, and nonunion is directly related to fracture displacement, length of time between injury and reduction, and quality of reduction. With early accurate reduction and stable fixation, the incidence of avascular necrosis and nonunion increases from approximately 10 percent in type I fractures to nearly 100 percent in type IV fractures.

Fifteen to twenty percent of talar fractures involve only the **talar body** (Fig. 22–4). Without an associated subtalar dislocation, the incidence of avascular necrosis is 25 percent. With an associated subtalar dislocation, the incidence of avascular necrosis is about 50 percent.

Fractures of the **head of the talus** comprise 5 to 10 percent of all talus fractures and frequently represent an injury of Chopart's joint (Fig. 22–5).

Fractures of the **lateral process** are the second most common type of talar fracture (Fig. 22–6). They are caused by hyperextension of the supinated foot and are nondisplaced.

Osteochondral fractures involving the lateral side of the talar dome are usually traumatic in origin; those of the medial side are usually degenerative (Fig. 22–7).

Diagnosis and Initial Management

History and Physical Examination

There is pain distal to the ankle in the midfoot. There is obvious deformity in cases of talocalcaneal dislocation. Open wounds and skin tented over bone, putting the patient at risk for pressure necrosis, is noted. The neurovascular status distal to the injury is assessed.

Radiographic Examination

Anteroposterior, oblique, and lateral radiographs are adequate to evaluate talar neck and body fractures and talocalcaneal dislocation. Lateral process fractures are best seen on the lateral projection. The presence of osteochondral fragments in the talocalcaneal articulation is determined with coronal CT scan.

The earliest signs of avascular necrosis are radiographic. Hawkin's sign is the appearance of a radiolucent line below the subchondral bone of the talar dome. This sign is best seen on a mortise view and appears between 6 to 8 weeks after injury. Hawkin's sign indicates resorption of subchondral bone and indicates that the talus is not avascular. MRI and radionuclide scans are useful in assessing vascularity.

Initial Management

Fractures without significant displacement or an associated dislocation are splinted and iced. If there is displacement or a dislocation, time is crucial. The greater the delay to reduction, the higher the incidence of

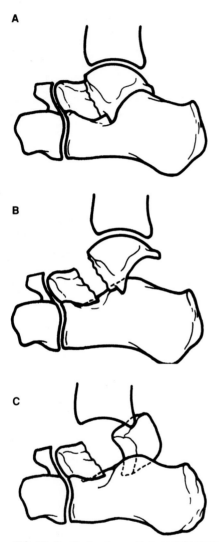

FIG. 22–3   The four types of talar neck fractures: (a) type I, (b) type II, (c) type III, and (d) type IV.

D

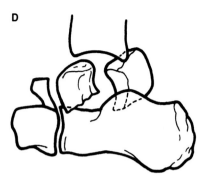

complications, such as skin necrosis, nonunion, and avascular necrosis. Closed reduction is attempted in the emergency room. If unsuccessful, open reduction is indicated. Closed reduction of talar neck fractures with subtalar subluxation (type II) is accomplished by gentle plantar flexion of the foot and traction to the heel. Talar neck fractures with dislocation of the talocalcaneal, talocrural, or talonavicular joints are more difficult. Reduction is attempted by flexing the knee and applying traction through the heel. Supination or pronation of the heel to increase the deformity as traction is applied frequently results in reduction. When reduction has been accomplished it is usually stable. The foot and ankle are splinted with the ankle in neutral and iced.

Associated Injuries

Fractures of the head of the talus indicate injury to Chopart's joint; therefore, the calcaneocuboid joint is examined. Neurovascular injuries are rare and are ruled out with a careful examination. There are no other injuries specifically associated with fractures of the talus.

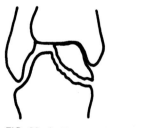

FIG. 22–4   Fracture of the talar body.

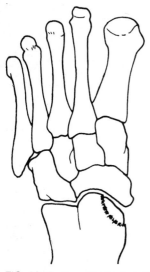

FIG. 22–5   Impaction fracture of the head of the talus.

Definitive Management

Type I fractures are managed nonoperatively with a nonweight-bearing short leg cast until the fracture heals, usually 6 to 10 weeks. Radiographs obtained weekly for the first 3 weeks determine whether displacement of the fragments has occurred. **Fracture types II, III, and IV** are managed with open reduction and internal fixation (Figs. 22–8 and 22–9). Reduction of the talar neck fracture is not possible unless the subtalar joint is reduced. If closed manipulation does not result in

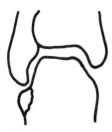

FIG. 22–6   Fracture of the lateral process of the talus.

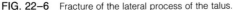

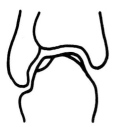

FIG. 22–7   Medial and lateral osteochondral fractures of the dome of the talus.

reduction, the subtalar joint is exposed through a lateral incision over the sinus tarsi. Loose bodies and soft tissue that are blocking reduction of the talocalcaneal joint are removed, and the joint is reduced. The talar neck fracture is exposed via an incision medial to the extensor hallucis longus. Stabilization of the talar neck fracture is with screws inserted through the talar head and directed proximally. The screws are countersunk to minimize impingement on the navicular. Postoperatively, nonweight-bearing is maintained until the fracture is healed, at least 10 weeks.

Displaced fractures of the talar body are managed with open reduction and fixation. Exposure is via osteotomy of the medial malleolus.

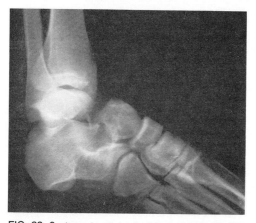

FIG. 22–8   Lateral radiograph of the foot and ankle following a type II talar neck fracture. There is an associated supination-adduction type fracture of the medial malleolus which is not evident on this projection.

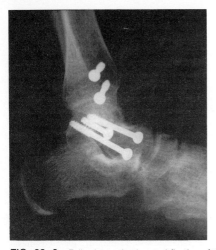

FIG. 22–9 Following reduction and fixation of the talar neck fracture with three screws. The fracture of the medial malleolus has been stabilized with two screws.

The fracture is reduced and stabilized with Kirschner wires, Herbert screws, or conventional screws. The fixation device cannot project above subchondral bone into the ankle joint or arthritis will result. If fixation is tenuous, an external fixater with pins in the tibia and the calcaneus neutralizes stresses across the fracture. Postoperatively, nonweight-bearing is maintained until healing occurs, at least 10 weeks. In most cases, immobilization is not necessary because fixation is stable.

Undisplaced **talar head fractures** are managed in a nonweight-bearing short leg cast for 6 weeks and with an arch support for an additional 3 to 6 months. Displaced fractures are managed with open reduction and fixation with screws or Kirschner wires. Small fragments are excised. An external fixater with pins in the calcaneus and first metatarsal neutralizes stresses across the fracture when fixation is tenuous.

Fractures of the **lateral process** of the talus are almost always undisplaced. They are managed symptomatically with immobilization in a cast for 4 to 6 weeks. If the fracture fails to heal, the fragment is excised.

Undisplaced **osteochondral fractures** of the talar dome are managed with nonweight-bearing in a short leg cast for 3 months. When conservative management fails, or the fragments are displaced, surgery is indicated. Lateral osteochondral fractures are located anteriorly on the talar dome and are exposed through an anterolateral approach. Osteotomy of the medial malleolus is required to expose medial osteochondral fractures. Small fragments are excised. Large fragments are pinned after curettage and drilling of their bed. Postoperatively, nonweight-bearing is maintained until healing is demonstrated radiographically.

Complications

Complications of fractures of the talus are avascular necrosis, nonunion, and posttraumatic arthritis.

Avascular necrosis of the body of the talus is the complication unique to fractures and dislocations of the talus. It is most likely to occur following a displaced fracture of the talar neck or body. The diagnosis is based on the absence of Hawkin's sign. Once avascular necrosis has occurred, the goal is to prevent collapse of the talus by an extended period of nonweight-bearing in a patellar tendon bearing orthosis. Revascularization takes up to 36 months, and the orthosis is worn until there is radiographic evidence of revascularization.

The diagnostic sign of **posttraumatic arthritis** of the subtalar joint is pain with pronation and supination of the foot. The patient complains of pain induced by walking over uneven ground. Management is conservative with nonsteroidal anti-inflammatories and local injections of steroids. If this fails, the involved joints are arthrodesed. It is important to accurately identify the symptomatic joints to minimize the number of joints that are arthrodesed. The greater the number of joints that are arthrodesed, the more stress across remaining functional joints and the sooner they develop arthritis. Symptomatic joints are identified by injection with local anesthetic and observation of symptom-relief.

Nonunion is a complication of fractures of the talar neck and is associated with avascular necrosis of the body. Management is stabilization with screws and grafting with autogenous cancellous bone.

SUBTALAR DISLOCATION

The term "subtalar dislocation" denotes dislocation of both the talocalcaneal and talonavicular articulations.

Classification

Subtalar dislocations are classified according to the position of the forefoot in relation to the talus and whether there is an associated dislocation of the tibiotalar joint. The types of subtalar dislocations commonly encountered are medial, lateral, and pantalar. Medial dislocation is by far the most common type of dislocation and is caused by forefoot supination. Lateral subtalar dislocation is less common and is the result of forefoot pronation. Lateral dislocations are the result of greater force and have a worse prognosis than medial dislocation. Pantalar dislocations are most frequently a medial subtalar dislocation associated with a tibiotalar dislocation. They have a poor prognosis due to the high incidence of avascular necrosis and associated soft tissue injury. Plantar and rotary dislocation have also been reported but are uncommon.

Diagnosis and Initial Management

History and Physical Examination

The patient has pain localized to the foot. Deformity of the foot is obvious. The foot appears shortened and is in equinus. The head of the talus can be palpated anterior to the medial malleolus (lateral dislocation) or anterior to the lateral malleolus (medial dislocation). Fifteen percent of subtalar dislocations are open. In an even greater percentage of subtalar dislocations, the skin over the talus is injured and later sloughs.

Radiographic Examination

The diagnosis of subtalar dislocation is obvious radiographically. Anteroposterior, lateral, and oblique radiographs of the foot are obtained (Fig. 22–10). Other radiographic views and studies are not necessary to make the diagnosis. After closed reduction, coronal CT scans of the talocalcaneal joint determine the presence of osteochondral fragments in the joint and the congruity of reduction.

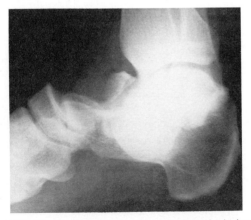

FIG. 22–10   Lateral of a foot following a lateral subtalar dislocation.

Initial Management

Once subtalar dislocation has been diagnosed, reduction is performed as quickly as possible to minimize the incidence of skin necrosis and avascular necrosis of the talus. The reduction maneuver is axial traction and pronation and supination of the heel. In addition, the head of the talus is relocated with digital pressure. Many subtalar dislocations cannot be reduced by closed means, and repeated forceful attempts at closed reduction are not indicated and jeopardize the viability of the skin over the head of the talus. If reduction is accomplished, a well-padded splint is applied with the ankle in neutral.

Associated Injuries

Fracture of the neck of the talus and intraarticular osteochondral fractures of the talus and calcaneus are frequently associated with subtalar dislocation. Talar neck fractures are ruled out by careful assessment of the lateral radiograph of the foot. The presence of intraarticular osteochondral fragments is determined with coronal CT scans through the talocalcaneal articulation. There are no other injuries specifically associated with subtalar dislocation.

Definitive Management

The goal of management is a congruous reduction. If this is obtained with closed reduction and the skin is viable, a short leg cast is applied. Nonweight-bearing is maintained for 4 weeks. Skin necrosis precludes casting.

In cases in which a closed reduction cannot be accomplished, open reduction is performed. The most common obstacle to reduction of medial dislocations is ''buttonholing'' of the talar head through soft tissue laterally (i.e., the extensor retinaculum, extensor digitorum brevis, and bifurcate ligament). The most common cause of irreducible lateral dislocation is displacement of the posterior tibial tendon inferior to the neck of the talus. Occasionally, fractures of the head of the talus or interposed osteochondral fragments may block reduction. The surgical exposure for open reduction is through a longitudinal skin incision over the head of the talus. Interposed soft tissue is identified and incised or retracted, and osteochondral fragments are removed. If the posterior tibial tendon is disrupted, it is repaired after reduction. A pin is driven across the talonavicular joint. The foot is immobilized in a short leg cast and nonweight-bearing is maintained for 6 weeks. Pantalar dislocations frequently must be reduced open. In addition to pinning of the talonavicular joint, the talocrural joint is also pinned. If the injury is open, an external fixater is used in place of a cast.

Complications

The complications of subtalar dislocation are avascular necrosis, subtalar arthritis, and infection secondary to an open injury or skin necrosis. Avascular necrosis and subtalar arthritis are managed as described in the "Complicating Section of Fractures of the Talus."

Infection is a devastating complication, particularly when it is coupled with avascular necrosis of the talus. The basic principles of debridement of necrotic tissue, early soft tissue coverage, stabilization of the foot and ankle, and appropriate antibiotic coverage must be followed. Debridement of necrotic tissue may result in a talectomy if the body of the talus is avascular. Stabilization is with an external fixater with pins in the tibia, metatarsals, and, if possible, calcaneus.

CALCANEUS

Classification

Fractures of the calcaneus are broadly classified as intraarticular or extraarticular. Intraarticular fractures involve the posterior facet. Extraarticular fractures involve the tuberosity, sustentaculum tali, and anterior process. In addition to being fractured, the calcaneus is occasionally dislocated.

Intraarticular fractures of the calcaneus are caused by axial loading of the talus which is driven into the calcaneus. The talus acts as a wedge, producing the primary fracture. This fracture is in the sagittal plane, starting at the calcaneocuboid articulation and continuing posteriorly and medially through the posterior facet to the medial wall of the calcaneus. The primary fracture divides the calcaneus into an anterior medial half and a posterior lateral half (Fig. 22–11a). If the force of the axial load is not dissipated, the impact of the talus produces a compression fracture of the lateral portion of the posterior facet. There are variations of this basic fracture pattern due to the position of the foot (e.g., supination of the foot medializes the primary fracture; pronation lateralizes it; dorsiflexion results in a joint depression fracture [Fig. 22–11b]; and plantar flexion results in a tongue-type fracture [Fig. 22–11c]).

Extraarticular fractures of the calcaneus are caused by axial loading or by the avulsion of bony insertions or origins of ligaments or tendons. Isolated fractures of the tuberosity of the calcaneus are caused by direct impact or avulsion of the tendo Achilles insertion. Fractures due to direct impact are minimally displaced; the plane of the fracture is sagittal (Fig. 22–12a). Avulsion fractures of the tendo Achilles are displaced, the plane of the fracture is horizontal (Fig. 22–12b). Fractures of the sustentaculum tali are caused by the medial side of the talus impacting the sustentaculum during axial loading of a supinated foot. Anterior process fractures are an avulsion of the origin of the bifurcate ligament

A

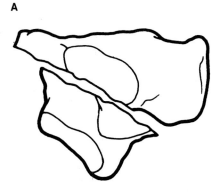

B

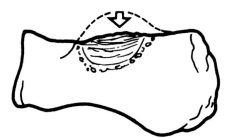

C

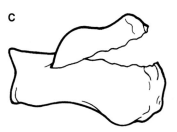

FIG. 22–11   Intraarticular fractures of the calcaneus: (*a*) the primary fracture viewed from above, (*b*) joint depression fracture, and (*c*) tongue-type fracture.

A

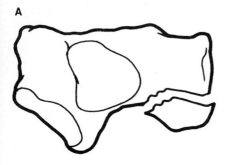

B

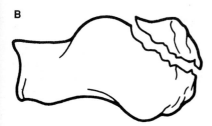

C

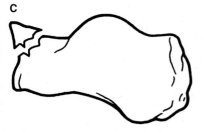

FIG. 22–12   Extraarticular fractures of the calcaneus. (*a*) Isolated fracture of the tuberosity caused by direct impact; the calcaneus is viewed from above. (*b*) Isolated fracture of the tuberosity caused by an avulsion of the tendo Achilles. (*c*) Fracture of the anterior process of the calcaneus.

caused by forefoot adduction and inversion (Fig. 22–12*c*). Dislocations of the calcaneus are extremely rare. There is usually a fracture of the calcaneus or cuboid at the calcaneocuboid articulation.

Diagnosis and Initial Management

History and Physical Examination

There is a history of a fall or a twisting injury and pain localized to the hindfoot. When seen shortly after injury, prior to diffuse swelling, the exact location of the fracture can be determined by gentle palpation. Fracture of the sustentaculum tali is indicated by painful passive motion of the great toe (the flexor hallucis longus runs beneath the sustentaculum). An avulsion fracture of the tendo Achilles is indicated by weakness of plantar flexion of the ankle. Loss of plantar flexion is not complete as the peroneal and posterior tibial muscles are intact.

Radiographic Examination

The four radiographic projections helpful in the evaluation of calcaneal fractures are the lateral, oblique, axial, and Broden's view. The **lateral projection** is the most helpful and is diagnostic of posterior facet depression and tuberosity avulsion. Bohler's angle, or the tuber angle, and the crucial angle of Gissane, which indicate the extent of displacement and angulation, are determined from the lateral projection (Fig. 22–13). The loss of parallelism of the articular surface of the posterior facet of the calcaneus and talus is determined from the lateral projection.

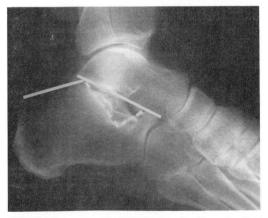

FIG. 22–13 A lateral radiograph of the foot illustrating Bohler's (solid line) and Gissane's (dotted line) angles.

The **oblique projection** is useful to assess the presence of a fracture of the anterior process of the calcaneus and to determine whether there is involvement of the calcaneal cuboid articulation.

The **axial projection,** or Harris or jumper's view, is obtained by placing the foot on the cassette with the ankle dorsiflexed and the beam angled 30° distally. The axial projection is useful in evaluating the tuberosity and sustentaculum tali and axial shortening.

Broden's view is used to assess the posterior and middle facets. To obtain this view, a lateral radiograph is obtained with the foot passively dorsiflexed, supinated, and internally rotated. The beam is centered on the sinus tarsi.

Initial Management

Initial management is with a splint, ice, and elevation.

Associated Injuries

Forty percent of calcaneus fractures incurred in a fall are associated with a fracture of the lumbar spine, usually a stable compression fracture. Injury of the medial and lateral plantar nerves results in decreased sensation on the plantar aspect of the foot. Compartment syndrome is suspected if there is massive swelling and severe pain not relieved by ice, elevation, and customary amounts of analgesics. The diagnosis and management of compartment syndrome is covered under the ''Injuries of the Forefoot'' section.

Definitive Management

Definitive management depends on the type of calcaneus fracture, the amount of displacement or angulation, and the presence of articular incongruity.

Intraarticular fractures of the calcaneus which are not signifi- cantly displaced are managed conservatively with nonweight-bearing for 4 weeks. Casting is counterproductive as it leads to stiffness of the subtalar joint.

Management of **displaced intraarticular fractures** is operative. Dis- placement is defined as loss of articular congruity of the posterior facet or at the calcaneal cuboid joint, loss of parallelism between the posterior facets of the calcaneus and talus, more than 4 mm of shortening of the tuberosity as seen on the axial projection, and Bohler's angle of 10° or less.

The surgical approach is via an extensile lateral incision or separate medial and lateral incisions. Because of flap necrosis, we reserve the extensile lateral approach for severely comminuted displaced fractures in young patients without a history of smoking or diabetes. Surgery is delayed until swelling has decreased to the point that the skin on the dorsum of the foot wrinkles with ankle dorsiflexion (usually 10 to 14 days). The incision starts over the tendo Achilles. It extends distally to the plantar skin, where it turns 90° and runs parallel with the plantar aspect of the foot. The incision is carried down to the calcaneus. A flap which includes the periosteum of the calcaneus is raised. The peroneal tendons along with their sheath are elevated with the rest of the flap and reflected anteriorly, exposing the entire lateral calcaneus, including the calcaneocuboid articulation and the posterior facet. Fragments are reduced and held in place with plates and screws.

In most cases, we prefer separate medial and lateral approaches. The goals of these surgical approaches are specific. The medial approach exposes the medial side of the calcaneus so that it can be brought out to length and its normal concavity can be restored. The lateral approach is designed to expose the posterior facet so that it can be reduced. These approaches have a low incidence of associated wound problems. The medial approach is via a skin incision which is parallel with the posterior medial border of the tibia. The incision starts proximal to the ankle joint and extends distally to the abductor hallucis brevis. The plantar branch of the posterior tibial nerve must be protected during the exposure. The medial wall of the calcaneus is reduced by disimpacting it with an elevator. The tuberosity fragment is stabilized with a staple or two-hole plate. The lateral approach is via a skin incision centered over the sinus tarsi. It starts at the lateral border of the extensor tendons and runs in a plantar direction posteriorly to the peroneal tendons. The fat in the sinus tarsi is excised exposing the posterior facet. This incision can be located slightly more anteriorly to expose fractures involving the calcaneocuboid articulation and fractures of the anterior process of the calcaneus. The posterior facet is reduced by elevating and rotating it posteriorly. If only the lateral part of the posterior facet is depressed, it is reduced and held in place with interfragmentary screws (i.e., the screws are inserted from the lateral fragment into the medial half of the facet). If the entire facet is depressed, it is held in its reduced position with Kirschner wires inserted through the fragment into the talus. Postoperatively, if the subtalar joint is not crossed by an implant, early motion is encouraged. Nonweight-bearing is maintained a minimum of 6 weeks. If the subtalar joint has been crossed with Kirschner wires, the extremity is immobilized in a short leg cast until the wires are removed at 6 weeks. At 8 weeks, partial weight-bearing is started and advanced.

Occasionally, tongue fractures can be reduced and stabilized with the Essex-Lopresti method of driving a large pin into the tongue fragment from posterior to anterior. The tongue fragment is then reduced under fluoroscopy by manipulating the pin, and the pin is advanced into the talus, stabilizing the fracture. This technique seldom results in anatomic reduction, but is of use when the patient has risk factors such as peripheral vascular disease or fracture blisters.

Isolated fractures of the **tuberosity caused by direct impact** are almost always minimally displaced and are managed with nonweight-bearing for 3 to 6 weeks. In the rare case of a displaced tuberosity fracture, the displaced fragment is on the medial side. The fracture is reduced and held in place with screws.

Isolated fractures of the **tuberosity caused by avulsion** of the tendo Achilles are usually displaced. They are exposed through a medial approach, reduced, and stabilized with a large cancellous screw and washer. Postoperatively, if the fixation is adequate, immobilization is not required; however, nonweight-bearing is maintained for 4 to 6 weeks. In the rare case in which there is minimal displacement, an acceptable alternative form of management is a long leg cast with the ankle plantar flexed 30° and the knee flexed 30°. At 3 to 4 weeks, the cast is changed to a short leg cast with the ankle in neutral. Immobilization is continued a total of 6 weeks. Throughout this period, the fracture is followed radiographically. Displacement is an indication for open reduction and stabilization.

Fractures of the **sustentaculum tali** are managed in a short leg weight-bearing cast for 4 to 6 weeks.

Undisplaced fractures of the **anterior process** are managed in a short leg weight-bearing cast for 4 to 6 weeks. Displaced fractures are managed with open reduction and fixation. Excision of the fragment is not indicated as it is the origin of the bifurcate ligament. The fragment is small and fixation is not stable; therefore, the foot is maintained in neutral for 3 to 4 weeks with a short leg cast.

Dislocations of the calcaneus are managed in the same fashion as subtalar dislocations. An emergent closed reduction is performed. If closed reduction cannot be achieved, an open reduction is performed. Following closed reduction, it is important to asses the talocalcaneal articulation for loose bodies; if present, these are removed. The reduction is usually stable and fixation not necessary. A short leg cast is maintained for 6 to 8 weeks.

Complications

Complications of fractures of the calcaneus are malunion resulting in a widened heel and plantar fasciitis, subtalar arthritis, calcaneocuboid arthritis, and peroneal tendonitis.

A **widened heel and plantar fasciitis** are managed conservatively. Footwear is altered, and a heel cup may be necessary. Injections of local anesthetic and steroids may relieve symptoms for extended periods. Rarely, excision of a spike of bone is indicated.

Subtalar and calcaneocuboid arthritis are managed conservatively with nonsteroidal anti-inflammatories and local injections. Arthrodesis is a last resort.

Peroneal tendonitis is caused by impingement of the peroneal sheath. Local injections of anesthetic and steroids may help. The sheath must be explored and decompressed frequently.

INJURIES OF THE MIDFOOT

Injuries of the midfoot include fractures and dislocations of the navicular, cuneiform, and cuboid bones; and dislocations of Chopart's joint.

Classification

There are three types of fractures of the tarsal **navicular:** dorsal chip fractures, fractures of the tuberosity, and fractures of the body of the navicular. Dorsal chip fractures, the most common type of navicular fracture, are a capsular avulsion and are caused by plantar flexion and pronation of the foot. Fractures of the tuberosity are an avulsion of the posterior tibial tendon and occur during eversion of the foot. Fractures of the body of the navicular are the least common type of fracture of the navicular and are caused by forceful hyperextension and inversion.

Fractures of the **cuneiforms** are rare and are usually caused by direct trauma. Subluxation of the first cuneiform from its articulations with the navicular and the second cuneiform frequently occurs as part of a Lisfranc dislocation.

Fracture of the **cuboid** is due to direct trauma, capsular avulsion during inversion or eversion of the forefoot, or compression during abduction of the forefoot.

Chopart's dislocation is a rare injury. There are three types: medial, lateral, and plantar. The mechanism of injury is, respectively, inversion, eversion, and plantar flexion of the forefoot. The bifurcate ligament ruptures while the talocalcaneal ligament remains intact; therefore, the talocalcaneal joint does not dislocate.

Diagnosis and Initial Management

History and Physical Examination

There is a history of either twisting or direct trauma to the midfoot and pain localized to the midfoot.

Radiographic Examination

The radiographic examination starts with anteroposterior, lateral, and oblique views of the foot. Stress views, obtained while inverting, everting, abducting, or adducting the forefoot, demonstrate instability of Chopart's joint. Other studies are seldom indicated.

Fracture of the navicular tuberosity can be confused with the os tibiale externum, an accessory ossicle. Distinguishing features are that the os tibiale externum is frequently bilateral, and its edges are rounded.

Initial Management

Initial management consists of splinting, ice, and elevation. Dislocations of Chopart's joint are usually reduced by axial traction and manipulation of the forefoot under hematoma block. If closed reduction is not accomplished, immediate open reduction is indicated. Subluxations of the first cuneiform are usually not significantly displaced. In cases in which the soft tissue is not at risk, these injuries are splinted in situ.

Associated Injuries

There are no specific injuries associated with injuries of the mid-foot.

Definitive Management

Dorsal chip fractures of the **navicular** are managed symptomatically with a short leg cast and weight-bearing as tolerated for approximately 4 weeks. Minimally displaced (2 mm or less) fractures of the tuberosity of the navicular are managed with a short leg cast with the forefoot inverted. At 4 weeks, the cast is changed and the foot is positioned in neutral; a short leg cast is applied and maintained an additional 2 weeks. Displaced fractures of the navicular are managed with open reduction and internal fixation. The surgical exposure is through an incision centered over the navicular, parallel to the anterior tibial tendon. The talonavicular joint is exposed and the navicular is reduced under direct vision when the joint is distracted with longitudinal traction. Interfragmentary screws or pins are used for fixation. Postoperatively, a short leg cast is applied. In cases in which the fixation is tenuous, an external fixater with pins in the calcaneus and first metatarsal is used to maintain length.

Fractures of the **cuneiforms** are usually managed with a short leg cast and weight-bearing as tolerated for 6 weeks. Indications for surgery include displacement which threatens overlying soft tissue or intraarticular displacement that can be improved.

Subluxation of the first cuneiform is managed operatively. The articulations between the first cuneiform and the navicular and second cuneiform are involved. If there are associated fractures, the procedure is performed open, through a dorsal incision. Because the fragments are small, pins are used for fixation. If there are no associated fractures, the joints are reduced closed under fluoroscopy and pinned. It is important to stabilize both articulations. Postoperatively, a short leg cast is applied and nonweight-bearing is maintained for 6 weeks. At 6 weeks, the pins are removed and the patient is allowed to bear weight in a shoe with a stiff sole and an arch support.

Dislocations of Chopart's joint are managed operatively because reduction is unstable. Dislocations without associated fractures are stabilized with a minimum of two pins inserted under fluoroscopy. The first pin crosses the calcaneocuboid joint. The second pin crosses the talonavicular joint. A short leg cast is applied and nonweight-bearing is maintained for 6 weeks. At 6 weeks, the pins are removed and a stiff soled shoe and arch support are worn.

Complications

The complication of midfoot injuries is arthritis. Management is nonsteroidal anti-inflammatories and alterations in footwear. If necessary, local injections of anesthetic agents and steroids are performed. Arthrodesis of an arthritic joint is a last resort.

INJURIES OF THE FOREFOOT

Injuries of the forefoot are Lisfranc's dislocation, fractures of the metatarsals and phalanges, and dislocations of the metatarsophalangeal joints and interphalangeal joints.

Classification

The mechanism of injury of **Lisfranc's dislocation** is hyperextension (Fig. 22–14). Lisfranc's dislocations are classified into one of three groups: total incongruity, partial incongruity, and divergent (Fig.

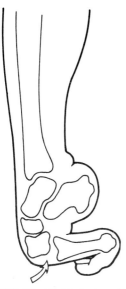

FIG. 22–14 Mechanism of injury of Lisfranc's dislocation. The tarso-metatarsal articulation is hyperextended causing the weaker dorsal ligaments to rupture.

22–15). **Total incongruity** is characterized by involvement of the entire joint and displacement in one direction (usually laterally). **Partial incongruity** is characterized by involvement of only part of the joint, usually either the first metatarsal or the second through fifth metatarsals. This break between the first and second metatarsal occurs because there is no stabilizing ligament between their bases, as there is between the bases of the other metatarsals. **Divergent** dislocations are characterized by involvement of the entire joint. Displacement is in two directions (usually the first metatarsal is displaced medially, the second through fifth metatarsals laterally).

   Metatarsal fractures are classified as stress fractures or traumatic fractures. Two types of traumatic fractures bear special mention: the Jones fracture and avulsion fractures of the base of the fifth metatarsal. The **Jones fracture** is a transverse fracture of the fifth metatarsal at the junction of the proximal metaphysis and diaphysis (Fig. 22–16), and has characteristics of a stress fracture in that it may initially be incomplete, involving only the lateral cortex of the metatarsal. Jones fractures frequently fail to heal when managed nonoperatively. **Avulsion fractures of the base of the fifth metatarsal** occur when the insertion of the peroneus brevis is avulsed during forced inversion of the forefoot. This fracture is distinguished from the Jones fracture by its metaphyseal location and its tendency to heal when managed with immobilization (Fig. 22–17).

   Fractures of the **phalanges** are classified as intraarticular, extraarticular, or tuft fractures.

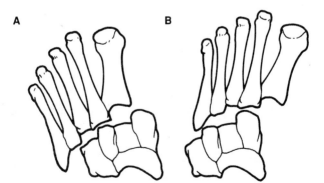

FIG. 22–15   Types of Lisfranc's dislocations: (*a*) and (*b*) total incongruity of Lisfranc's joint, (*c*) and (*d*) partial incongruity of Lisfranc's joint, and (*e*) divergent dislocation of Lisfranc's joint.

C

D

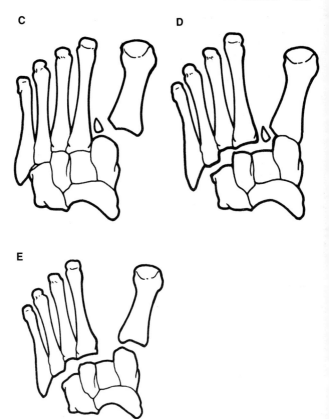

E

Dislocations of the metatarsal phalangeal and interphalangeal joints are classified according to the direction of displacement—dorsal or volar.

Diagnosis and Initial Management

History and Physical Examination

The patient complains of pain localized to the structure injured. The dorsum of the forefoot quickly becomes swollen and ecchymotic. Short-ening of the forefoot indicates an unreduced Lisfranc's dislocation or

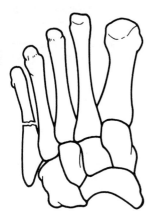

FIG. 22–16   Jones fracture.

displaced fractures of all five metatarsals. Apparent hyperflexion or hyperextension of a metatarsophalangeal or interphalangeal joint indicates dislocation.

Radiographic Examination

Anteroposterior, oblique, and lateral radiographs are obtained. A fracture of the base of the second metatarsal indicates that Lisfranc's joint

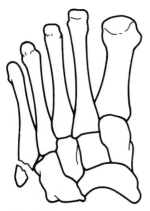

FIG. 22–17   Fracture of the base of the fifth metatarsal.

is disrupted. Loss of congruity between articular surfaces and double densities (i.e., one articular surface superimposed on another) indicates subluxation.

Stress radiographs assess the stability of Lisfranc's joint. Bone scans help diagnose stress fractures of the metatarsals prior to their radiographic appearance.

Initial Management

Initial management consists of alignment of severely displaced fractures, reduction of dislocations, immobilization, elevation, and ice.

Dislocations of Lisfranc's joint with an absent dorsalis pedis or posterior tibial pulse or compromised overlying skin are reduced closed emergently. A hematoma block is administered and axial traction is applied to the involved rays by suspending the foot by the toes with finger traps. Inability to obtain a closed reduction is an indication for immediate open reduction.

Displaced fractures of the metatarsals are rare; when they occur they are reduced with axial traction. If adequate reduction is achieved, the foot is immobilized in a short leg cast with a toe plate (i.e., the plantar surface of the cast extends distal to the toes). The cast is maintained 4 to 6 weeks. The Jones fracture and fracture of the base of the fifth metatarsal are seldom displaced and are casted. The Jones fracture may eventually require internal fixation. Stress fractures are managed with immobilization and nonweight-bearing.

Fractures of the phalanges are usually caused by direct trauma. Displaced fractures of proximal and middle phalanges are aligned with the aid of a digital block, and the toe is buddy taped to the neighboring toe. Nonweight-bearing is maintained until there is clinical and radiographic healing. Fractures of the distal phalanx are protected with a splint, and associated subungual hematomas are drained to relieve pain. Crushed open distal phalanges are managed with amputation in the operating room. Displaced intraarticular fractures of proximal and distal phalanges of the great toe are splinted and managed with open reduction and stabilization later.

Dislocations of metatarsophalangeal and interphalangeal joints are managed with closed reduction under hematoma block. Simple axial traction and gently increasing of the deformity reduce the dislocation. Occasionally, an interphalangeal dislocation of the great toe is irreducible because of interposition of the long flexor tendon and requires open reduction. Isolated cases of irreducible metatarsophalangeal dislocations have been reported, but are extremely rare. When reduction of a metatarsophalangeal or interphalangeal dislocation has been achieved, the toe is immobilized with a dorsal alumafoam splint and buddy taping. Immobilization is continued 4 to 6 weeks.

Associated Injuries

Compartment syndrome of the foot is associated with forefoot injuries. Increased pain made worse by passive motion is the cardinal sign of compartment syndrome. The diagnosis is confirmed by measuring the compartment pressures and finding a value greater than 30 mmHg. Management is surgical release of the four osteofascial spaces of the foot. All four compartments are surgically released via two dorsal longitudinal incisions. The first centered over the second interspace and the second centered over the fourth metatarsal. The dissection is carried around each metatarsal and the central compartment is opened between the first and second metatarsals.

Definitive Management

The definitive management of **Lisfranc's dislocation** is reduction and stabilization with pins or screws. We prefer open reduction, as we have been impressed with the amount of displacement and comminution which is routinely present (Figs. 22–18 and 22–19). The surgical exposure is via two longitudinal incisions, the first centered over the first interspace and the second over the third interspace. Only one incision is required for partial incongruity type dislocations. The dorsalis pedis is at risk in the first interspace. The joint is debrided of free fragments of bone and cartilage, and intraarticular fragments are reduced and held in place with small diameter Kirschner wires. The joint is reduced and stabilized with large diameter Kirschner wires. The number and location of the Kirschner wires required to stabilize the reduction is dependent on the type of dislocation. Total incongruity dislocations require a minimum of two Kirschner wires, one in the first ray and the second in the fourth or fifth ray. Divergent dislocations require a minimum of three Kirschner wires, one in the first ray and the second and third wires in the second and fifth ray. Partial incongruity dislocations require a minimum of two Kirschner wires. The location of the wires is dictated by the rays involved. Postoperatively, the foot must be immobilized in a short leg cast and the patient is not allowed to bear weight until the wires are removed at 6 to 8 weeks. After the wires are removed, a short leg cast is reapplied and the patient is allowed to bear weight as tolerated. The cast is maintained for 2 to 4 weeks. After the cast is removed, the patient wears a stiff-soled shoe with an arch support for 6 months.

The definitive management of **metatarsal** fractures depends on the amount and direction of angulation and displacement. Dorsal or plantar angulation and displacement result in abnormal pressure on the plantar aspect of the foot and must be reduced and stabilized. Lateral displacement is usually not significant unless the first metatarsal is fractured. The closed management of metatarsal fractures is covered in the "Initial Management" section. Open management consists of surgical exposure

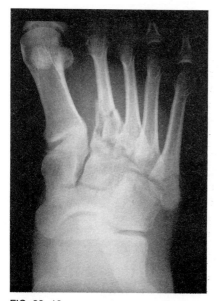

FIG. 22–18   An anteroposterior radiograph of a foot following a partial incongruity Lisfranc's dislocation involving the bases of the second through fifth metatarsals. There are fractures of the second, third, and fifth metatarsal bases.

of the fracture through dorsal longitudinal incisions, reduction, and stabilization with Kirschner wires. Small plates and screws are used to stabilize fractures of the first metatarsal. An intramedullary screw inserted from proximal to distal is used to stabilize the Jones fracture. Postoperative management is based on stability of fixation, quality of reduction, and is tailored to the individual case.

Intraarticular fractures of the proximal and distal phalanges of the great toe are reduced and stabilized if displaced. The goal of surgery is to restore stability (frequently these fractures are the result of a ligamentous, capsular, or tendinous avulsion) and to minimize the incidence of posttraumatic arthritis. Fractures of the metatarsophalangeal joint are approached via a straight dorsal incision. Fractures of the interphalangeal joint are approached via a midlateral incision. Fragments are reduced and held in place with small screws or small diameter Kirschner wires. Postoperatively, the toe is splinted and nonweight-bearing is maintained for 4 to 6 weeks.

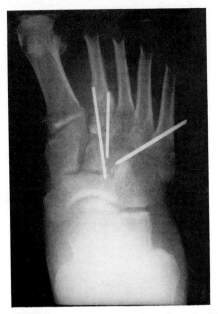

FIG. 22–19   An anteroposterior radiograph of the foot in Fig. 22–18 following open reduction of Lisfranc's joint and fixation with three Kirschner wires.

Complications

Complications of forefoot injuries include posttraumatic arthritis of Lisfranc's joint and malunion of the metatarsals. **Posttraumatic arthritis of Lisfranc's joint** is managed with arch supports, nonsteroidal anti-inflammatory medication, and local injections of steroids. If these measures fail, the joint is fused. **Malunion of a metatarsal fracture** results in a localized area of increased pressure on the plantar aspect of the foot. A metatarsal bar or custom-molded shoe insert may compensate for the malunion and resolve the pain. If conservative measures are not acceptable, an osteotomy of the proximal metatarsal is performed. Fixation is not required, and the patient is encouraged to bear weight postoperatively so that the involved metatarsal head will heal in the proper location.

SELECTED READINGS

Injuries of the Hindfoot

Canale ST, Kelly FB Jr: Fractures of the neck of the talus. Long-term evaluation of seventy-one cases. *J Bone Joint Surg* 60A:143–156, 1978.

Comfort TH, Behrens F, Gaither DW, Denis F, Sigmond M: Long-term results of displaced talar neck fractures. *Clin Orthop* 199:81–87, 1985.

DeLee JC, Curtis R: Subtalar dislocation of the foot. *J Bone Joint Surg* 64A:433–437, 1982.

Hawkins LG: Fractures of the neck of the talus. *J Bone Joint Surg* 52A:991–1002, 1970.

Leung KS, Chan WS, Pak PPL, So WS, Leung PC: Operative treatment of intraarticular fractures of the os calcis—The role of rigid fixation and primary bone grafting: Preliminary results. *J Orthop Trauma* 3:232–240, 1989.

Sclamberg EL, Davenport K: Operative treatment of displaced intra-articular fractures of the calcaneus. *J Trauma* 28:510–516, 1988.

Injuries of the Midfoot

Main BJ, Jowett RL: Injuries of the midtarsal joint. *J Bone Joint Surg* 57B:89–97, 1975.

Tountas AA: Occult fracture subluxation of the midtarsal joint. *Clin Orthop* 243:195–199, 1989.

Injuries of the Forefoot

Arntz CT, Veith RG, Hansen ST Jr: Fractures and fracture-dislocations of the tarsometatarsal joint. *J Bone Joint Surg* 70A:173–181, 1988.

Hardcastle PH, Reschauer R, Kutscha-Lissberg E, Schoffmann W: Injuries to the tarsometatarsal joint. Incidence, classification and treatment. *J Bone Joint Surg* 64B:349–356, 1982.

Kavanaugh JH, Brower TD, Mann RV : The Jones fracture revisited. *J Bone Joint Surg.* 60A:776–782, 1978.

General

Hansen ST Jr: Foot injuries, in Browner B (ed): *Skeletal Trauma*, 2d ed. Philadelphia, WB Saunders, pp 1959–1991.

Heckman JD: Fractures and dislocations of the foot, in *Rockwood and Green's Fractures in Adults*. New York-Hagerstown, JB Lippincott, 1991, pp. 2041–2182.

Myerson M: Diagnosis and treatment of compartment syndrome of the foot. *Orthop* 13:711–717, 1990.

Glossary

Abduction   Motion in the coronal plane. The extremity is moved away from the midline; the opposite of adduction.

Adduction   Motion in the coronal plane. The extremity is moved toward the midline (e.g., adduction of the right hip crosses the right leg over the left).

Allograft   Donor bone graft.

Ankylosis   Fusion of a joint; it may be fibrous or bony.

Arthrodesis   Surgical fusion of a joint.

Autograft   Bone graft from the patient who is being grafted.

Buddy taping   Splinting a finger or toe by taping it to a neighboring finger or toe.

Caudad   Toward the foot (e.g., the x-ray beam is angled caudad).

Cephalad   Toward the head (e.g., the x-ray beam is angled cephalad).

Comminuted   Term applied to fractures indicating that there are several fragments of bone and that the fracture is not simple (i.e., fractured into only two pieces).

Compound   Term applied to fractures indicating that the fracture is open.

Contralateral   Opposite side (e.g., a femur fracture and contralateral knee dislocation indicates that the fracture and knee dislocation are not in the same leg).

Coronal plane   A two-dimensional surface in the frontal plane (e.g., medial and lateral angulation is in the coronal plane).

Coxa   The hip and proximal femur (e.g., "coxa magna"—large femoral head).

Cubitus   The elbow; cubital pertains to the elbow.

Diastasis   Separation of bones attached by fibrous tissue, which is distinct from a dislocation in which the articular surfaces of a diarthrodial joint are separated (e.g., symphysis pubic diastasis or tibiofibular diastasis in a Maisonneuve fracture).

Dislocation   Disruption of the joint with complete loss of continuity between the articular surfaces, as opposed to subluxation.

Dorsiflexion   Describes motion away from the palmar, plantar, or volar surfaces of the hand or foot (e.g., dorsiflexion of the ankle lifts the forefoot superiorly off the ground).

Eversion   Forefoot position in which the sole of the foot faces laterally; opposite of inversion.

Genu The knee (e.g., genu valgum—knock-kneed).

Inversion Forefoot position in which the sole of the foot faces medially; opposite of eversion.

Ipsilateral Same side (e.g., ipsilateral femur and tibia fractures indicate that the fractures both involve the right or left leg).

Kessler suture Suture technique used to repair tendons (Fig. G–1).

Lateral Away from the midline (e.g., apex lateral angulation).

Medial Toward the midline (e.g., apex medial angulation).

Palmar Toward or on the palm (e.g., palmar flexion of the wrist or a palmar incision).

Plantar Toward or on the sole of the foot (e.g., plantarflexion of the ankle or a plantar incision).

Pronation Forearm rotation resulting in the palm facing down. Rotation of the foot and ankle around the axis of the neck of the talus, resulting in the sole facing laterally.

Prone Describes face-down position of patient.

Sagittal plane Two-dimensional surface in the lateral plane (e.g., anterior and posterior angulation is in the sagittal plane).

Subluxation Disruption of a joint with partial loss of continuity between the articular surfaces.

Supination Forearm rotation resulting in the palm of the hand facing up. Rotation of the foot and ankle around the axis of the neck of the talus resulting in the sole of the foot facing medially.

Supine Describes face-up (lying on the back) position of the patient.

Valgus Used to describe angulation in the coronal plane. Varus and valgus are always used in conjunction with a joint. They indicate that the extremity distal to the named joint goes toward the midline (varus) or away from the midline (valgus) (e.g., ''genu varum''—

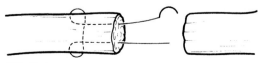

FIG. G–1 Kessler suture.

the calf [i.e., the extremity distal to the knee] goes toward the midline, resulting in bowing).

Varus   Used to describe angulation in the coronal plane. (*See* "*Valgus*")

Volar   Refers to the palmar surface of the hand and flexor or anterior surface of the wrist and forearm (e.g., volar flexion of the wrist is opposite of wrist dorsiflexion).

Index

345

303.
886